MASSACHUSETTS

GENERAL

HOSPITAL

MANUAL
OF ORAL AND
MAXILLOFACIAL
SURGERY

MASSACHUSETTS
GENERAL
HOSPITAL

MANUAL
OF ORAL AND
MAXILLOFACIAL
SURGERY

R. Bruce Donoff, D.M.D., M.D.

Dean and Professor
Department of Oral and Maxillofacial Surgery
Harvard School of Dental Medicine
Visiting Oral and Maxillofacial Surgeon
Massachusetts General Hospital
Boston, Massachusetts

Third Edition

with 32 illustrations

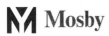 Mosby

St. Louis   Baltimore   Boston   Carlsbad   Chicago   Naples   New York   Philadelphia   Portland
London   Madrid   Mexico City   Singapore   Sydney   Tokyo   Toronto   Wiesbaden

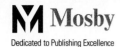

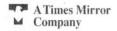

A Times Mirror
Company

Vice President and Publisher: Don Ladig
Executive Editor: Linda L. Duncan
Managing Editor: Penny Rudolph
Project Manager: Deborah L. Vogel
Production Editor: Mamata Reddy
Designer: Pati Pye
Manufacturing Manager: Linda Ierardi

NOTICE

Every effort has been made to ensure that the drug dosage schedules and current therapy contained herein are accurate and in accord with the standards accepted at the time of publication. However, as new research and experience broaden our knowledge, changes in treatment and drug therapy occur. Therefore, the reader is advised to check the product information sheet included in the package of each drug he/she plans to administer to be certain that changes have not been made in the recommended dose or in the contraindications. This is of particular importance in regard to new or infrequently used drugs.

THIRD EDITION

Printed in the United States of America
Composition by Compset, Inc.
Printing/binding by R. R. Donnelley and Sons Company

Mosby–Year Book, Inc.
11830 Westline Industrial Drive
St. Louis, Missouri 63146

Library of Congress Cataloging-in-Publication Data
Massachusetts General Hospital manual of oral and maxillofacial
    surgery / [edited by] R. Bruce Donnoff. — 3rd ed.
        p.   cm.
    Prepared by current and former members of the Oral and
Maxillofacial Surgery Service of the Massachusetts General Hospital.
    Includes index.
    ISBN 0-8151-2755-3
    1. Mouth—Surgery—Handbooks, manual, etc.   2. Maxilla—Surgery—
Handbooks, manuals, etc.   3. Face—Surgery—Handbooks, manuals,
etc.   I. Donoff, R. Bruce.   II. Massachusetts General Hospital.
Oral and Maxillofacial Surgery Service.
    [DNLM: 1. Surgery, Oral—handbooks.   2. Dentistry, Operative—
handbooks.   3. Stomatognathic Diseases—surgery—handbooks.   WU 49
M414 1997]
RK529.M37   1997
617.5'2059—dc20
DNLM/DLC
for Library of Congress   96-43578
                                                                        CIP

96 97 98 99 00 / 9 8 7 6 5 4 3 2 1

CONTRIBUTORS

MEREDITH AUGUST, D.M.D., M.D.
Instructor, Department of Oral and Maxillofacial Surgery
Harvard School of Dental Medicine
Assistant Oral and Maxillofacial Surgeon
Massachusetts General Hospital
Boston, Massachusetts

ROBERT CHUONG, D.M.D., M.D.
Private Practice, Oral and Maxillofacial Surgery
St. Petersburg, Florida
former Instructor, Department of Oral and Maxillofacial Surgery
Harvard School of Dental Medicine
former Clinical Associate, Oral and Maxillofacial Surgery Service
Massachusetts General Hospital
Boston, Massachusetts

R. BRUCE DONOFF, D.M.D., M.D.
Dean and Professor
Department of Oral and Maxillofacial Surgery
Harvard School of Dental Medicine
Visiting Oral and Maxillofacial Surgeon
Massachusetts General Hospital
Boston, Massachusetts

RAY ENGLISH, JR., D.M.D.
Private Practice, Oral and Maxillofacial Surgery
Warwick, Rhode Island
former Clinical Fellow, Department of Oral and Maxillofacial Surgery
Harvard School of Dental Medicine
former Senior Resident, Oral and Maxillofacial Surgery Service
Massachusetts General Hospital
Boston, Massachusetts

EARL G. FREYMILLER, D.M.D., M.D.
Acting Chair and Associate Professor
Section of Oral and Maxillofacial Surgery
University of California
Los Angeles School of Dentistry
Los Angeles, California
former Resident, Oral and Maxillofacial Surgery Service
Massachusetts General Hospital
Boston, Massachusetts

DAVID A. KEITH, B.D.S., F.D.S.R.C.S., D.M.D.
Associate Professor, Department of Oral and Maxillofacial Surgery
Harvard School of Dental Medicine
Visiting Oral and Maxillofacial Surgeon
Massachusetts General Hospital
Chief, Oral Surgery
Harvard Community Health Plan
Boston, Massachusetts

DAVID H. PERROTT, D.D.S., M.D.
Associate Professor, Department of Oral and Maxillofacial Surgery
Harvard School of Dental Medicine
Visiting Oral and Maxillofacial Surgeon
Massachusetts General Hospital
Boston, Massachusetts

EDWARD B. SELDIN, D.M.D., M.D.
Associate Professor, Department of Oral and Maxillofacial Surgery
Harvard School of Dental Medicine
Visiting Oral and Maxillofacial Surgeon
Massachusetts General Hospital
Boston, Massachusetts

WILLIE L. STEPHENS, D.D.S.
Oral and Maxillofacial Surgeon
Department of Surgery
Brigham and Women's Hospital
Instructor, Department of Oral and Maxillofacial Surgery
Harvard School of Dental Medicine
Assistant Oral and Maxillofacial Surgeon
Massachusetts General Hospital
Boston, Massachusetts

JOSEPH W. WILKES, III, D.M.D., M.D.
Instructor, Department of Oral and Maxillofacial Surgery
Harvard School of Dental Medicine
Assistant Oral and Maxillofacial Surgeon
Massachusetts General Hospital
Boston, Massachusetts

To

Dr. Walter C. Guralnick

Professor Emeritus of Oral and Maxillofacial Surgery,
Harvard University, Chief of Service Massachusetts General Hospital,
1970–1982.

The epitome of a teacher, mentor, and caring, compassionate doctor.
You represent the most important ingredient in clinical education
without which books like this manual never truly reach
their intended level of usefulness.

PREFACE

This is the third edition of the *Massachusetts General Hospital Manual of Oral and Maxillofacial Surgery.* It reflects the broadened scope of the specialty with the addition of chapters in pertinent areas. In the ten years since the preface for the first edition was written, we have witnessed the explosion of the era of the information highway and electronic means of information transfer. Yet, the functionality of a manual such as this one has not decreased. The paper-based book still has many advantages over its digital counterparts. It is small, lightweight, high resolution, and inexpensive. This manual is meant to be carried and always available. It still fulfills its primary goal of providing the essentials for diagnosis, treatment, and management of the oral and maxillofacial surgery patient. Over the years it has been most gratifying to hear feedback both in America and around the world from colleagues on how useful it has been to students, house staff, and practitioners in dentistry, dental specialties, and medicine. Our goal is to maintain that level of usefulness in this third edition.

The manual was prepared by current and former members of the Oral and Maxillofacial Surgery Service of the Massachusetts General Hospital and reflects their knowledge, skills, and clinical judgment. It is not meant to be all-inclusive. The preface of the second edition states it best: "There are no substitutes for textbooks, journals, and clinical experience. The development of good doctors and surgeons should be a continuous preoccupation of educator-clinicians. Without thought, there is little learning. Without reading, there is little to think about. Without discussion, it is difficult to distinguish beween good and bad thinking."

My thanks to Ms. Penny Rudolph and Ms. Mamata Reddy and to the editorial staff of Mosby-Year Book, Inc., for their assistance, guidance, and coaxing to complete this new edition. Special thanks to all my colleagues who contributed to this work and its success.

R. Bruce Donoff

CONTENTS

SECTION I
Algorithms

KNOWN DIABETIC PATIENT UNDERGOING ELECTIVE SURGERY

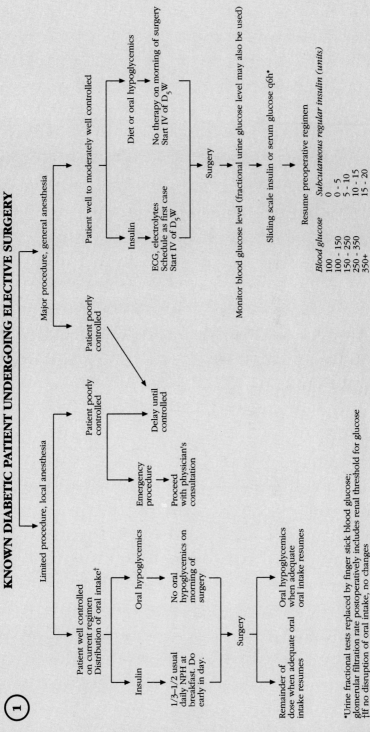

(1)

Major procedure, general anesthesia

Patient well to moderately well controlled

Diet or oral hypoglycemics — No therapy on morning of surgery Start IV of D₅W

Insulin — ECG, electrolytes Schedule as first case Start IV of D₅W

Surgery

Monitor blood glucose level (fractional urine glucose level may also be used)

Sliding scale insulin or serum glucose q6h*

Resume preoperative regimen

Blood glucose	Subcutaneous regular insulin (units)
100	0 - 5
100 - 150	0 - 5
150 - 250	5 - 10
250 - 350	10 - 15
350+	15 - 20

Patient poorly controlled

Limited procedure, local anesthesia

Patient poorly controlled

Emergency procedure → Proceed with physician's consultation

Delay until controlled

Patient well controlled on current regimen Distribution of oral intake†

Oral hypoglycemics — No oral hypoglycemics on morning of surgery

Insulin — 1/3–1/2 usual daily NPH at breakfast. Do early in day.

Surgery

Oral hypoglycemics when adequate oral intake resumes

Remainder of dose when adequate oral intake resumes

*Urine fractional tests replaced by finger stick blood glucose; glomerular filtration rate postoperatively includes renal threshold for glucose
†If no disruption of oral intake, no changes

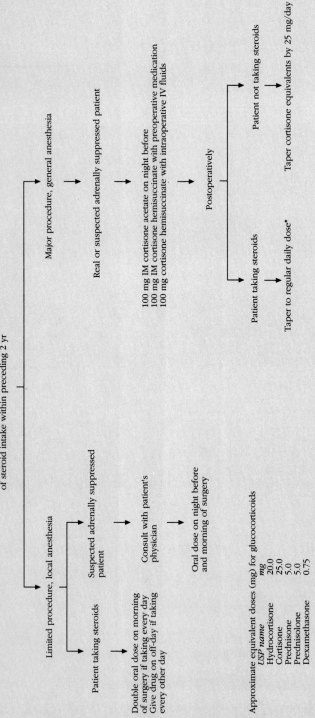

STEROID COVERAGE

Patient taking glucocorticoids or with 2-wk history of steroid intake within preceding 2 yr

Limited procedure, local anesthesia

- Patient taking steroids

  Double oral dose on morning of surgery if taking every day
  Give drug on off-day if taking every other day

- Suspected adrenally suppressed patient

  → Consult with patient's physician

  → Oral dose on night before and morning of surgery

Major procedure, general anesthesia

→ Real or suspected adrenally suppressed patient

→ 100 mg IM cortisone acetate on night before
100 mg IM cortisone hemisuccinate with preoperative medication
100 mg cortisone hemisuccinate with intraoperative IV fluids

→ Postoperatively

- Patient taking steroids

  Taper to regular daily dose*

- Patient not taking steroids

  Taper cortisone equivalents by 25 mg/day

Approximate equivalent doses (mg) for glucocorticoids

USP name	mg
Hydrocortisone	20.0
Cortisone	25.0
Prednisone	5.0
Prednisolone	5.0
Dexamethasone	0.75

(2)

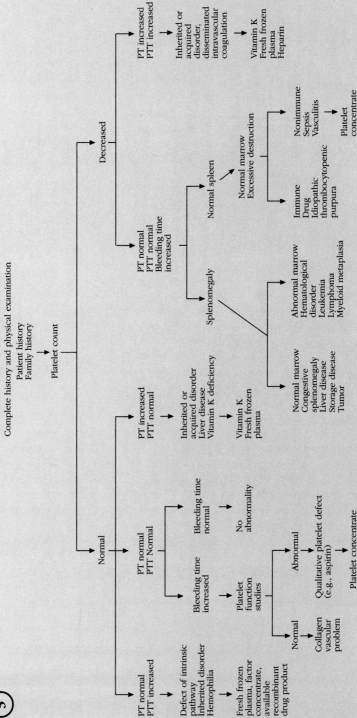

BLEEDING DISORDERS

Complete history and physical examination
Patient history
Family history

Platelet count

Normal

- PT normal
  PTT increased
  → Defect of intrinsic pathway
    Inherited disorder
    Hemophilia
    → Fresh frozen plasma, factor concentrate, available recombinant drug product

- PT normal
  PTT Normal
  - Bleeding time increased → Platelet function studies
    - Normal → Collagen vascular problem
    - Abnormal → Qualitative platelet defect (e.g., aspirin) → Platelet concentrate
  - Bleeding time normal → No abnormality

- PT increased
  PTT normal
  → Inherited or acquired disorder
    Liver disease
    Vitamin K deficiency
    → Vitamin K
    Fresh frozen plasma

Decreased

- PT normal
  PTT normal
  Bleeding time increased
  - Splenomegaly
    - Normal marrow
      Congestive splenomegaly
      Liver disease
      Storage disease
      Tumor
    - Abnormal marrow
      Hematological disorder
      Leukemia
      Lymphoma
      Myeloid metaplasia
  - Normal spleen
    → Normal marrow
    Excessive destruction
    - Immune
      Drug
      Idiopathic thrombocytopenic purpura
    - Nonimmune
      Sepsis
      Vasculitis
      → Platelet concentrate

- PT increased
  PTT increased
  → Inherited or acquired disorder, disseminated intravascular coagulation
  → Vitamin K
  Fresh frozen plasma
  Heparin

(3)

PAROTID ENLARGEMENT

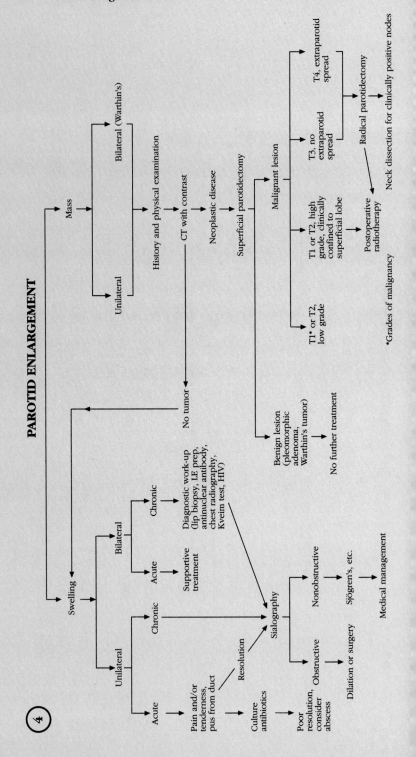

Mass

Unilateral — Bilateral (Warthin's)

History and physical examination

CT with contrast

Neoplastic disease

Superficial parotidectomy

Malignant lesion

Benign lesion (pleomorphic adenoma, Warthin's tumor) → No further treatment

T1* or T2, low grade

T1 or T2, high grade, clinically confined to superficial lobe → Postoperative radiotherapy

T3, no extraparotid spread

T4, extraparotid spread

Radical parotidectomy → Neck dissection for clinically positive nodes

*Grades of malignancy

No tumor

Swelling

Unilateral — Bilateral

Bilateral:
Acute → Supportive treatment
Chronic → Diagnostic work-up (lip biopsy, LE prep, antinuclear antibody, chest radiography, Kveim test, HIV)

Unilateral:
Acute → Pain and/or tenderness, pus from duct → Culture antibiotics → Resolution / Poor resolution, consider abscess
Chronic

Sialography

Obstructive → Dilation or surgery
Nonobstructive → Sjögren's, etc. → Medical management

④

ZYGOMATIC COMPLEX FRACTURES

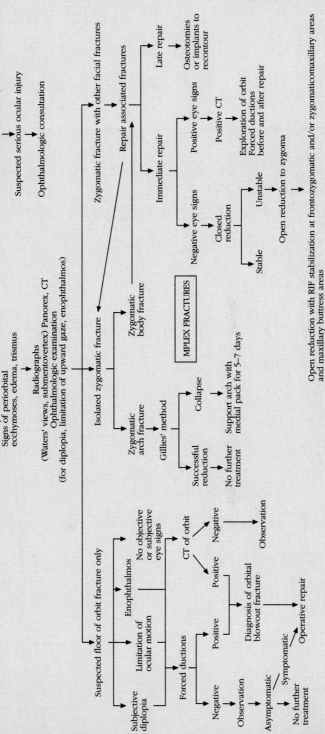

Complete history and physical examination
History of trauma
Signs of periorbital echymoses, edema, trismus

→ Radiographs (Waters' views, submentovertex) Panorex, CT
Ophthalmologic examination
(for diplopia, limitation of upward gaze, enophthalmos)

Signs of decreased visual acuity
Blood in anterior chamber, etc. → Suspected serious ocular injury → Ophthalmologic consultation

MPLEX FRACTURES

Suspected floor of orbit fracture only

Subjective diplopia — Limitation of ocular motion — Enophthalmos — No objective or subjective eye signs

Forced ductions
- Negative → Observation — Asymptomatic → No further treatment / Symptomatic → Operative repair
- Positive → Diagnosis of orbital blowout fracture → Operative repair

CT of orbit
- Positive → Diagnosis of orbital blowout fracture
- Negative → Observation

Isolated zygomatic fracture

Zygomatic arch fracture
Gillies' method
- Successful reduction → No further treatment
- Collapse → Support arch with medial pack for 5–7 days

Zygomatic body fracture

Zygomatic fracture with other facial fractures

Repair associated fractures
- Late repair → Osteotomies or implants to recontour
- Immediate repair
  - Negative eye signs → Closed reduction
    - Stable
    - Unstable → Open reduction to zygoma
  - Positive eye signs → Positive CT → Exploration of orbit
    Forced ductions before and after repair

Open reduction with RIF stabilization at frontozygomatic and/or zygomaticomaxillary areas and maxillary buttress areas

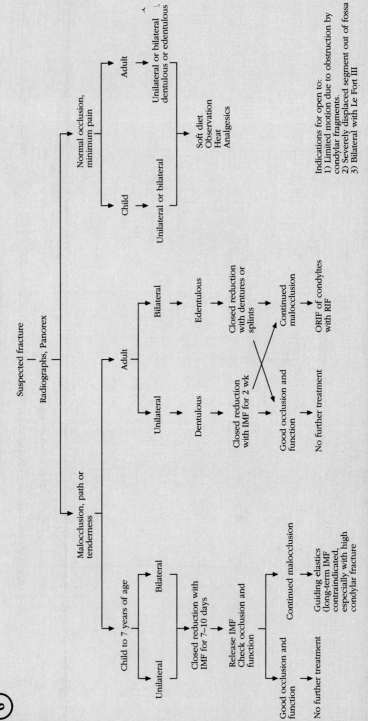

ISOLATED CONDYLAR FRACTURES

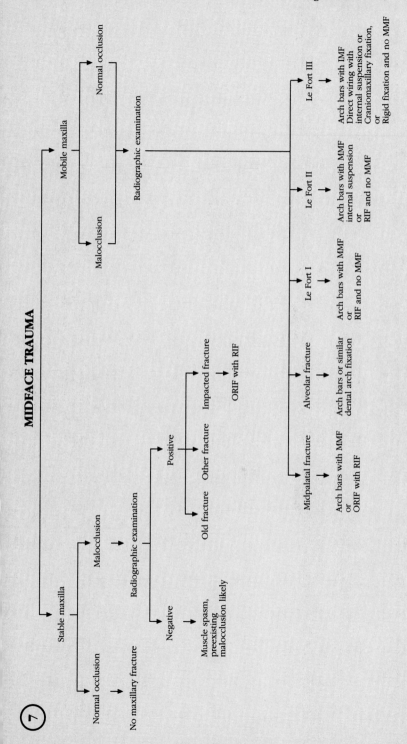

MIDFACE TRAUMA

TREATMENT PLANNING PROTOCOL

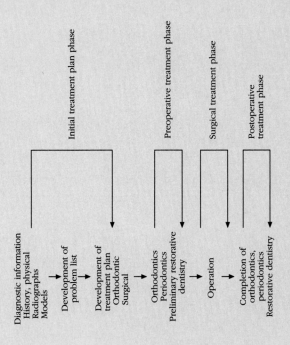

Diagnostic information
History, physical
Radiographs
Models

→ Development of
problem list

→ Development of
treatment plan
Orthodontic
Surgical

⎫
⎬ Initial treatment plan phase
⎭

Orthodontics
Periodontics
Preliminary restorative
dentistry

⎫
⎬ Preoperative treatment phase
⎭

→ Operation

⎫
⎬ Surgical treatment phase
⎭

→ Completion of
orthodontics,
periodontics
Restorative dentistry

⎫
⎬ Postoperative
treatment phase
⎭

⑧

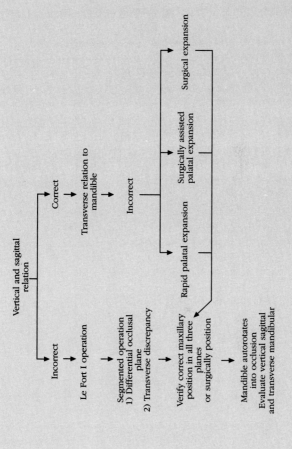

MAXILLARY CORRECTION

⑨

Vertical and sagittal relation

Correct — Transverse relation to mandible → Incorrect

Rapid palatal expansion | Surgically assisted palatal expansion | Surgical expansion

Incorrect → Le Fort I operation → Segmented operation
1) Differential occlusal plane
2) Transverse discrepancy
→ Verify correct maxillary position in all three planes or surgically position →
Mandible autorotates into occlusion
Evaluate vertical sagittal and transverse mandibular

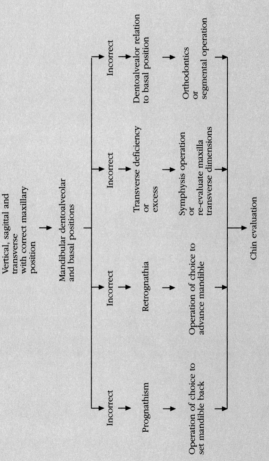

MANDIBULAR CORRECTION

Vertical, sagittal and transverse with correct maxillary position

→

Mandibular dentoalveolar and basal positions

Incorrect → Prognathism → Operation of choice to set mandible back →

Incorrect → Retrognathia → Operation of choice to advance mandible →

Incorrect → Transverse deficiency or excess → Symphysis operation or re-evaluate maxilla transverse dimensions →

Incorrect → Dentoalvealor relation to basal position → Orthodontics or segmental operation →

Chin evaluation

10

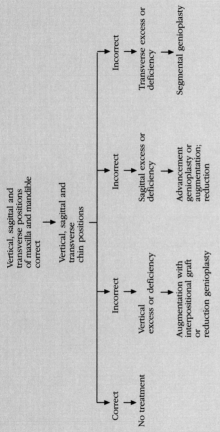

CHIN CORRECTION

Vertical, sagittal and transverse positions of maxilla and mandible correct

→ Vertical, sagittal and transverse chin positions

Correct → No treatment

Incorrect → Vertical excess or deficiency → Augmentation with interpositional graft or reduction genioplasty

Incorrect → Sagittal excess or deficiency → Advancement genioplasty or augmentation; reduction

Incorrect → Transverse excess or deficiency → Segmental genioplasty

⑪

MANDIBULAR RECONSTRUCTION

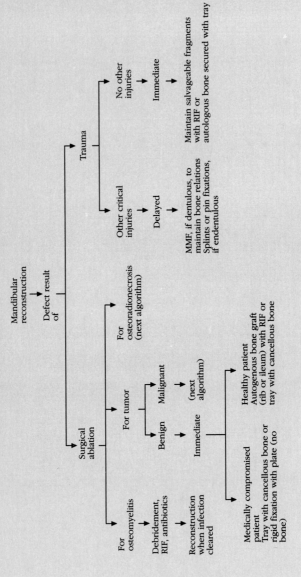

Mandibular reconstruction

Defect result of

Surgical ablation

For osteomyelitis → Debridement, RIF, antibiotics → Reconstruction when infection cleared

For tumor
- Benign → Immediate
- Malignant → (next algorithm)

For osteoradionecrosis (next algorithm)

Medically compromised patient
Tray with cancellous bone or rigid fixation with plate (no bone)

Healthy patient
Autogenous bone graft (rib or ileum) with RIF or tray with cancellous bone

Trauma

Other critical injuries → Delayed
MMF, if dentulous, to maintain bone relations
Splints or pin fixations, if endentulous

No other injuries → Immediate
Maintain salvageable fragments with RIF or autologous bone secured with tray

12

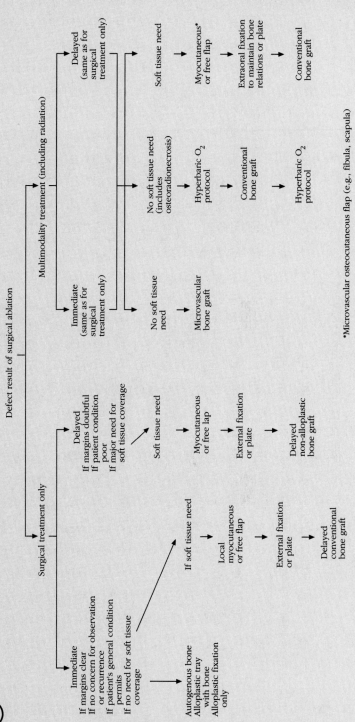

(13)

MANDIBULAR RECONSTRUCTION FOR MALIGNANCIES

Defect result of surgical ablation

Surgical treatment only

Immediate
If margins clear
If no concern for observation
or recurrence
If patient's general condition
permits
If no need for soft tissue
coverage

→ Autogenous bone
Alloplastic tray
with bone
Alloplastic fixation
only

If soft tissue need → Local
myocutaneous
or free flap → External fixation
or plate → Delayed
conventional
bone graft

Delayed
If margins doubtful
If patient condition
poor
If major need for
soft tissue coverage

→ Soft tissue need → Myocutaneous
or free lap → External fixation
or plate → Delayed
non-alloplastic
bone graft

Multimodality treatment (including radiation)

Immediate
(same as for
surgical
treatment only)

No soft tissue
need → Microvascular
bone graft

No soft tissue need
(includes
osteoradionecrosis) → Hyperbaric O$_2$
protocol → Conventional
bone graft → Hyperbaric O$_2$
protocol

Delayed
(same as for
surgical
treatment only)

Soft tissue need → Myocutaneous*
or free flap → Extraoral fixation
to maintain bone
relations or plate → Conventional
bone graft

*Microvascular osteocutaneous flap (e.g., fibula, scapula)

THE "ATROPHIC MANDIBLE"

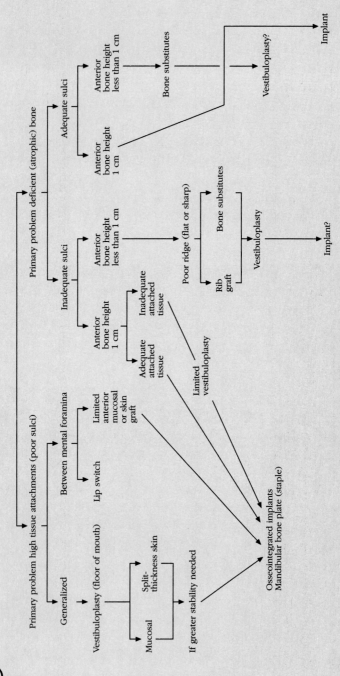

(14)

OROFACIAL PAIN

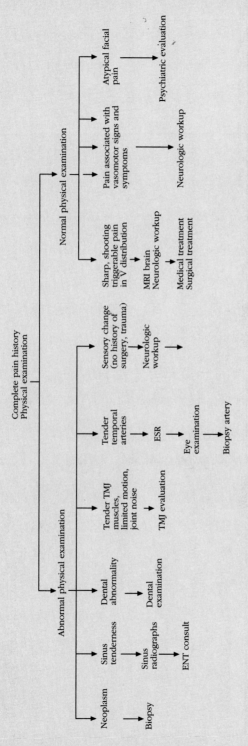

(15)

Complete pain history
Physical examination

Abnormal physical examination

- Neoplasm
  - Biopsy
- Sinus tenderness
  - Sinus radiographs
    - ENT consult
- Dental abnormality
  - Dental examination
- Tender TMJ muscles, limited motion, joint noise
  - TMJ evaluation
- Tender temporal arteries
  - ESR
    - Eye examination
    - Biopsy artery
- Sensory change (no history of surgery, trauma)
  - Neurologic workup

Normal physical examination

- Sharp, shooting triggerable pain in V distribution
  - MRI brain
  - Neurologic workup
    - Medical treatment
    - Surgical treatment
- Pain associated with vasomotor signs and symptoms
  - Neurologic workup
- Atypical facial pain
  - Psychiatric evaluation

NERVE INJURY

Clinical neurosensory examination

Noninvasive

A. Pin pressure nociception—mediated by small-diameter nerve fibers with and without myelin (A-delta and C)

B. Two-point detection—primarily tests for quantity of larger myelinated axons innervating pacinian corpuscles

C. Directional stroke determination mediated by specific receptors innervated by larger myelinated nerve fibers (A-delta and B)—tests for rapidly adapting mechanoreceptors

D. Weinstein-Semmes static light pressure—same as C but tests slowly adapting mechanoreceptors

E. Examination for Tinel's sign—shooting sensation distally or pain directly when palpating over surgical site or lingual alveolus

Invasive

A. Diagnostic nerve blocks—failure of peripheral block to alleviate pain suggests psychological, sympathetic, or central origin to dysesthesia despite original cause (deafferentation)

B. Somatosensory evoked potentials—noninvasive technique, experimental

Indications for microsurgery

1. Peripheral dysesthesia confirmed by diagnostic nerve blocks

2. Known or highly suspicious nerve injury with acute anesthesia and/or pain

3. No improvement at monthly sensory examinations over 6 mo

4. Continued deterioration at monthly sensory examination

5. Sudden halt in improvement at monthly sensory examination

6. Immediate microsurgical reconstruction of nerve resected during ablative surgery

Injury noted at surgery

1. Lingual nerve or inferior alveolar nerve torn

2. IAN torn at sagittal split osteotomy

3. IAN avulsed with malformed root structure

Intraoperatively

A. Repair immediately with tendon transfer technique using smallest absorbable suture available

or

B. Repair under magnification with 9-0 or 10-0 suture if possible

Postoperatively

A. Document and map sensory loss and recovery

B. Follow monthly

C. If pain a problem with sensory return, use analgesics and/or Dilantin 300mg/day

---

SUSPICION OF NERVE INJURY AT SURGERY

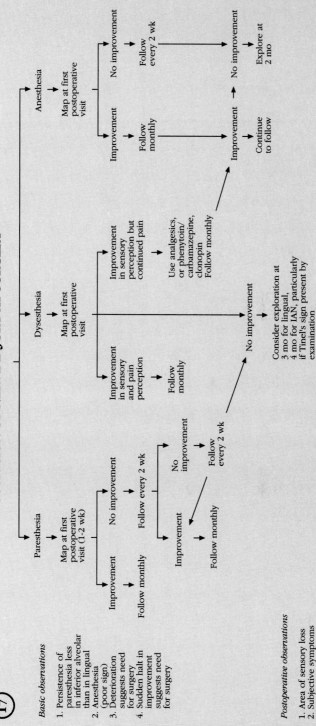

(17)

Basic observations

1. Persistence of paresthesia less in inferior alveolar than in lingual
2. Anesthesia (poor sign)
3. Deterioration suggests need for surgery
4. Sudden halt in improvement suggests need for surgery

Postoperative observations

1. Area of sensory loss
2. Subjective symptoms

NO SUSPICION OF NERVE INJURY AT SURGERY

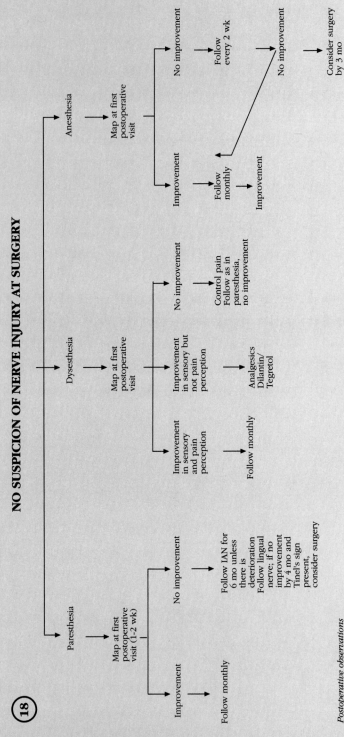

Paresthesia

Map at first postoperative visit (1-2 wk)

Improvement → Follow monthly

No improvement → Follow IAN for 6 mo unless there is deterioration Follow lingual nerve; if no improvement by 4 mo and Tinel's sign present, consider surgery

Dysesthesia

Map at first postoperative visit

Improvement in sensory and pain perception → Follow monthly

Improvement in sensory but not pain perception → Analgesics Dilantin/ Tegretol

No improvement → Control pain Follow as in paresthesia, no improvement

Anesthesia

Map at first postoperative visit

Improvement → Follow monthly → Improvement

No improvement → Follow every 2 wk → No improvement → Consider surgery by 3 mo

Postoperative observations

1. Area of sensory loss
2. Subjective symptoms

(18)

SECTION II
Basic Care of the Surgical Patient

Hospital Procedures

R. BRUCE DONOFF

RULES AND REGULATIONS

I. Medical records
  A. The chief of the service or department should be responsible for ensuring that an adequate medical record is established for every patient rendered care by that service or department.
  B. All clinical entries must be dated and authenticated.
  C. Notes sufficient to document the progress of the patient must be entered in the medical record.
  D. The medical record should contain evidence of the patient's informed consent for any procedure or treatment that is appropriate.
  E. Reports of ancillary services requiring interpretation by the doctor must be authenticated by the interpreting doctor and filed in the medical record.
  F. Reports of clinical laboratory examinations must be filed in the medical record.
  G. The entire contents of the medical record should be legible.
  H. The use of abbreviations should be limited to those approved by the medical staff.
  I. All consultation requests should be written in the medical record, and the name of the doctor requesting the consultation and the reason for consultation should be indicated.
  J. All medical records are the property of the hospital. The records must not be removed, except by a court order or subpoena.
  K. All diagnoses and procedures should be recorded on the face sheet or discharge summary, or both, without the use of abbreviations or symbols.
II. Admission records
  A. The inpatient record should include the following:
    1. Identification data
    2. Chief complaint
    3. Personal and family histories
    4. History of present illness
    5. Physical examination

6. Report of special examinations (e.g., clinical and radiologic examinations)
7. Consultant's notes
8. Provisional or working diagnosis
9. Medical and surgical treatments
10. Gross and microscopic findings
11. Progress notes
12. Final diagnosis
13. Condition on discharge
14. Discharge summary
15. A final autopsy report of the gross and microscopic diagnosis, if necessary. The complete autopsy protocol should remain on file in the pathology department.

B. Within 24 hr of admission, the patient's history, physical examination, summary of findings, provisional diagnosis, and diagnostic or treatment plan must be recorded.

C. The doctor responsible must review and authenticate the admission history, physical examination, therapeutic treatment plan, and summary, or must enter his or her own appropriate admission note.

III. Operative records

A. Immediately after surgery, a brief operative note is dictated, authenticated, and entered in the medical record. It contains a description of the findings, the technical procedures used, the

---

Name of patient: Date: Hospital number:

Service and floor: Surgeon: Assistants:

Preoperative diagnosis:

Postoperative diagnosis:

Name of operation:

Procedures
1. Description of surgical approach:
2. Findings:
3. Technical procedures used:
4. Specimens removed:
5. Type of closure and sutures used:
6. Drains placed if any:
7. Estimated blood loss and replacement:

Fig. 1-1 Operative report.

specimens removed, the postoperative diagnosis, and the name of the primary surgeon and any assistants (Fig. 1–1).
   B. The use of all anesthetic agents must be fully recorded and authenticated. A postanesthesia note in the medical record describing the presence or absence of anesthesia-related complications must be authenticated by the anesthesiologist.
   C. Reports of pathologic examinations should be authenticated promptly and filed in the medical record.
IV. Discharge records
   A. In all cases a concise discharge summary, either written or dictated, must be prepared within 15 days after discharge.
   B. The clinical resumé should recapitulate the reason for hospitalization, the significant finding(s), the procedures performed and treatment rendered, the condition of the patient on discharge, and special instructions given to the patient and/or family.

DOCTOR'S ORDERS
I. General requirements
   A. Clear, concise, and complete orders are essential for safe patient care. They ensure optimal communication and expeditious implementation of the patient care plan.
   B. The following guidelines are designed to assist the house officer in the preparation of a written plan of care. A complete set of orders must include:
      1. Medication orders only
         a. Medications
            (1) Complete name of drug
            (2) Metric dose
            (3) Dose frequency
            (4) Route of administration
            (5) Variables (when appropriate)
         b. Intravenous drugs
      2. All other orders
         a. Diagnosis (upon admission)
         b. Condition (upon admission)
         c. Allergies (upon admission)
         d. Activity
         e. Diet
         f. Diagnostic studies, including radiographs
         g. Vital sign frequency
         h. Wound care
         i. Respiratory orders, including O_2
         j. Special equipment
            (1) Cardiac monitor
            (2) Wire cutter at bedside
   C. Additional requirements
      1. Written orders must be dated and signed.
      2. All verbal orders must be signed by the doctor within 24 hr.

3. There should be automatic termination of all narcotic orders at noon of the third day following the order.
4. There should be automatic termination of all antibiotic orders at noon of the tenth day following the order.
5. IV orders must be rewritten daily.
6. IV orders and narcotic orders must be specific. "Same IV" or "renew pain med" is not acceptable.
7. Orders must be written in indelible blue or black ink.
8. The most current page must be used for new orders.
9. Abbreviations must be limited to those in the accepted list.
10. Deletion of errors is legally prohibited. If an error occurs, a line must be drawn through the incorrect entry and must be initialed and dated.
11. All orders must be flagged on the front of the order book.
12. Stat orders must be brought to the attention of the nurse.
13. When diagnostic studies are ordered, the clinical indication should be included to assist in the preparation of a requisition.
14. Medication doses must be specified (a dosage range is not acceptable).
15. Verbal or telephone orders may be taken by a registered nurse from a doctor who is unable to write the order because of unusual circumstances; the order can be for a single dose of medication, with one repetition of the order. The nurse must read the order back to the doctor for verification and sign it with the doctor's name and the nurse's name and licensure status. The prescribing doctor must sign these orders within 24 hr, preferably sooner.

II. Intravenous orders
   A. IV orders must be completely rewritten daily.
   B. They must be specific.
   C. A written order is required for a heparin lock.

III. Discharge orders
   A. The discharge plan must be communicated to the nursing staff well in advance to allow time for teaching appropriate referrals and for coordination of patient care.
   B. Orders for discharge must be written.
   C. When at all possible, discharge plans should enable the patient to leave the hospital by 11 AM.

INFORMED CONSENT (Fig. 1-2)

I. Communication and consent
   A. A doctor performing a medical or surgical procedure must obtain the patient's written informed consent to the procedure. This is essential to good medical practice (and is also required by law).
   B. Informed consent involves effective communication in which the doctor must provide enough information for the patient to make a judgment on the proposed treatment. Specifically, the

DATE:

PATIENT:

UNIT NO:

PROCEDURE:

Patient Identification Stamp

I have explained to the patient the nature of his/her condition, the nature of the procedure, and the benefits to be reasonably expected compared with alternative approaches.

I have discussed the likelihood of major risks or complications of this procedure including (if applicable) but not limited to loss of limb function, brain damage, paralysis, hemorrhage; infection, drug reactions, blood clots and loss of life. I have also indicated that with any procedure there is always the possibility of an unexpected complication.

Additional comments (if any):

All questions were answered and the patient consents to the procedure.

_____ M.D.

Dr. _____
has explained the above to me
and I consent to the procedure.

_____
Signature

If signature cannot be obtained, indicate reason in comments section above.

Fig. 1-2 Surgical consent form.

doctor must disclose, in a reasonable manner, all significant medical information that he or she possesses or reasonably should possess as a practitioner in that specialty and that is pertinent to an intelligent decision by the patient. This information should include:

1. The nature of the patient's condition
2. The proposed treatment and possible alternatives (including no treatment)
3. The benefits of the proposed treatment and alternatives
4. The nature and probability of risks of the proposed treatment and alternatives
5. The inability of the doctor to predict results and the irreversibility of the procedure

C. The information that must be provided will vary according to the patient's intelligence, experience, and age, as well as to other factors. Information that the doctor reasonably believes is already known to the patient (e.g., the risk of infection associated with any surgical procedure) need not be disclosed.

II. Documentation
  A. Procedures requiring documentation of consent
    1. The doctor must document, on the approved hospital form, consent for all therapeutic and diagnostic procedures for which disclosure of significant medical information, including major risks involved, would assist the patient in making an intelligent decision as to whether to undergo the procedure. Such procedures will vary from institution to institution but should include, although not necessarily be limited to, the following:
      a. Any operation performed under general or local anesthesia, including paracentesis, thoracentesis, and arthrocentesis, as well as biopsies and excisions, but not simple extractions
      b. Cardiac catheterizations and angiography
      c. All endoscopies, excluding sigmoidoscopy and proctoscopy without biopsy
      d. Invasive diagnostic and therapeutic radiologic procedures
      e. Extracorporeal and peritoneal dialysis
      f. Radiation therapy
      g. Invasive cancer chemotherapy
      h. Electroconvulsive therapy
      i. Administration of general or regional anesthesia
      j. Insertion of centrally placed venous lines
    2. Except in an emergency, when the patient's well-being may be seriously endangered, these procedures require the doctor to obtain the patient's informed consent, documented on the proper form with the patient's signature.

  B. Securing the patient's consent
    1. Although the best practice is for the person performing the procedure to obtain and document the informed consent, another licensed doctor who is also a member of the group responsible for administering care to the patient may obtain the consent and complete and file the form, indicating on the form the name of the doctor for whom the

consent has been obtained. If a surrogate doctor obtains the informed consent, the doctor with the ultimate responsibility needs to countersign the form.

    2. The consent may be obtained and the form completed in a doctor's office, but the form must ultimately be placed in the hospital record.

C. Concessions for patients who are physically incapable of signing or who are mentally incompetent to sign a consent form

    1. If the patient is physically unable to sign the form, after full discussion with and consent by the patient, the doctor may sign the form, which must include a written note indicating the reason for the absence of the patient's signature.

    2. If the patient does not have the mental capacity to consent, the doctor should document that with an appropriate note on the form, and a family member or close friend may sign on the patient's behalf.

D. Selection of consent form

    1. The standard hospital form should be used for documenting consent.

    2. It is also desirable that a written note be placed on the chart indicating that consent has been obtained.

Commonly Used
Medications

JOSEPH W. WILKES III

MEDICATIONS FOR AFFECTIVE DISORDERS

I. Affective disorders include the following:
   A. Depression
      1. Reactive—usually a specific cause, and usually self-limited
      2. Endogenous—no precipitating cause; tricyclic antidepressant (TCA) therapy is often used
      3. Drug induced (e.g., alcohol, barbiturates, and some antihypertensives)—dosage is often reduced or the drug may be discontinued
   B. Manic depression
      1. Manic form—often responds to lithium
      2. Depressed form (endogenous)—may respond to electroshock and antidepressant therapy
      3. Circular (bipolar) form—usually responds to lithium with or without initial antidepressant therapy
   C. Phobias and anxiety/panic attacks—frequently accompanied by depression and often provoked by a specific situation. TCA therapy (especially imipramine) or a monoamine oxidase inhibitor (MAOI) can be used.
   D. Schizoaffective disorders—usually responsive to neuroleptic drugs. They may require simultaneous administration of a TCA or lithium.

II. Classes of medication used for affective disorders (along with psychotherapy) include:
   A. *TCA*s inhibit neurotransmitter reuptake at the presynaptic membrane.
   B. *MAOI*s block the intracellular metabolism of biogenic amine neurotransmitters.
   C. *Lithium* is used for manic illnesses.
   D. *Stimulants* (e.g., amphetamines) are sometimes used for short periods in depression refractory to other modalities, but there is considerable disagreement regarding their efficacy.

Tricyclic antidepressants (Table 2-1)

I. Action and uses
   A. TCAs include:
      1. Desipramine (Norpramin)
      2. Amitriptyline (Elavil)
      3. Imipramine (Tofranil)
      4. Doxepin (Sinequan)
   B. These agents will often increase physical activity as well as elevate mood. They may also improve alertness, sleep patterns, and appetite while reducing morbid preoccupations.
   C. TCAs are absorbed orally, extensively metabolized, highly bound by plasma proteins, and slowly eliminated (their half-lives range from 8–93 hr).
      1. Reduced doses are given to elderly and debilitated patients.
      2. The drug is initially given twice a day in increasing doses until symptoms are controlled, and then a lower maintenance dose is used daily. If insomnia is a side effect, the dose need not be given at bedtime.
   D. Imipramine is often used for enuresis in children and adolescents.
   E. Constant central pain syndromes frequently respond to amitriptyline, doxepin, or imipramine.

II. Adverse reactions
   A. Anticholinergic activities and alpha-adrenergic blockade may induce any of the following symptoms:
      1. Flushing
      2. Sweating
      3. Xerostomia
      4. Visual disturbances
      5. Constipation (in adolescents)
      6. Tachycardia
      7. Orthostatic hypotension
      8. Glaucoma
      9. Urinary retention
   B. Sedation, tremor, and paradoxical anxiety have been reported.
   C. Cardiac reactions include heart block and bundle branch block. A baseline electrocardiogram (ECG) should be obtained before therapy, and the width of the QRS complex should be monitored on subsequent ECGs.

III. Precautions
   A. Elderly patients and those with hepatic failure metabolize the drugs slowly, so reduced doses are given or the drugs are avoided.
   B. TCAs are administered with caution in any patient who has a history of the following:
      1. Urinary retention or glaucoma
      2. Cardiac disease (congestive heart failure, angina, recent myocardial infarction, ECG changes)
   C. The dose must be tapered to avoid a withdrawal syndrome.

Table 2-1   MEDICATIONS USED FOR AFFECTIVE DISORDERS

Drug	Usual dose (mg) Adult	Usual dose (mg) Elderly	Adverse effects Sedation	Adverse effects Anticholinergic
TCAs (oral route preferred)				
Desipramine (Norpramin)	50–100 noct., maintenance	25–50 q.d., divided	+	+
Amitryptyline (Elavil)	50–160 noct., maintenance	Up to 10 t.i.d.	+++	+++
Imipramine (Tofranil)	50–150 noct., maintenance	30–40 q.d.	++	++
Doxepin (Sinequan)	25–150 q.d.		+++	+++
MAOIs				
Phenelzine (Nardil)	15–25 t.i.d.			
Antimanics				
Lithium	200–700 t.i.d.	Use with caution		

+ Moderately effective

++ Effective

+++ Strongly effective

TCA = tricyclic antidepressant; MAOI = monoamine oxidase inhibitor; noct. = nocturnal.

IV. Drug interactions
  A. TCAs may interfere with antihypertensive agents that involve action on the biogenic amines (e.g., guanethidine or clonidine), and hypertension may return.
  B. The effects of epinephrine and vasoconstrictors in local anesthetic agents are potentiated by TCAs. Local anesthetic agents without vasoconstrictors must be used.
  C. The anticholinergic effects of TCAs are additive when antipsychotic drugs are given simultaneously; also, delirium and gastric hypomotility may occur. The TCA should be given 1–2 hr before or after the antipsychotic drug if the two must be used together.
  D. Concomitant use of MAOIs with TCAs may produce tremors, muscle rigidity, excitability, or death.
    1. Stop the TCA several days before giving an MAOI.
    2. Stop the MAOI 2 wk before giving a TCA.
  E. The effect of sedatives is potentiated when they are given with TCAs.
  F. Barbiturates increase the metabolism of TCAs (hepatic) but also potentiate the effects of toxic levels of TCAs in TCA overdose situations.
  G. Alcohol has an increased sedative effect when used with a TCA, but it also potentiates the effects of toxic levels of TCAs.

Monoamine oxidase inhibitors (see Table 2-1)

  I. Action and uses
  A. Phenelzine (Nardil) is most often prescribed.
  B. MAOIs are useful in the treatment of atypical depressions, anxiety reactions, and amphetamine-like psychomotor stimulation. They are possibly also useful in migraine syndromes.
  C. After initial therapy, maintenance may be by one daily dose. Because of psychomotor stimulation, an MAOI should not be given at bedtime. Unlike TCAs, the MAOIs may be terminated abruptly.
  II. Adverse reactions
  A. Sedation, xerostomia, visual disturbances, constipation, and orthostatic hypotension are most common.
  B. Insomnia, tremors, or hypomania may reflect overdosage.
  C. Tachycardia, palpitations, and hypertension may occur together, so these drugs should be used cautiously in any cardiac patient.
  D. Coma may occur in overdosage.
  III. Precautions
  A. Strict dietary control must be followed to avoid hypertension induced by interaction with tyramine.
  B. Foods high in tyramine include cheese, red wines, chocolate, beer, yeast, meat extracts, fava beans, yogurt, herring, and pickles.
  IV. Drug interactions
  A. Simultaneous ingestion of tyramine can cause hypertension with headaches, tachycardia, nausea, vomiting, pulmonary edema,

intracranial hemorrhage, unconsciousness, or syncope. Symptoms are treated with phentolamine and propranolol.

B. Indirect-acting adrenergic drugs (e.g., amphetamines or the sympathomimetic amines in proprietary cold medicines) are potentiated and should be avoided.

C. Direct-acting adrenergic drugs (e.g., catecholamines) appear to be safe since MAOIs do not strongly block the reuptake of catecholamines, as do TCAs.

D. Simultaneous use with levodopa, tryptophan, and 5-hydroxytryptamine is contraindicated. These drugs must be withdrawn at least 2–4 wk before starting an MAOI.

E. Concomitant use of meperidine with an MAOI can produce hyperpyrexia and excitement, so meperidine must be avoided. The alternative narcotic chosen should have its dose reduced by one half to one fourth.

F. General anesthetic agents may require lower doses since the CNS depressant effects are potentiated by MAOIs.

G. The action of insulin is increased by administration with an MAOI, so hypoglycemia may result. The insulin dosage may need to be reduced.

H. Convulsions and death have been noted experimentally when tranylcypromine was administered in the presence of disulfiram (Antabuse).

LITHIUM (see Table 2-1)

I. Action and uses
   A. Lithium counteracts mood changes without sedation.
   B. Administration of lithium for 3–5 da may be necessary to reach therapeutic tissue levels. Then any antipsychotic drugs can be withdrawn gradually.
   C. Lithium is indicated for
      1. Bipolar depression, when clearly diagnosed
      2. Cluster headaches

II. Precautions
   A. Serum lithium levels must be measured every 2–3 wk.
   B. Lithium may cause irreversible morphologic changes in the kidney.
      1. Renal function must be monitored with renal function tests (e.g., creatinine clearance, serum and urine osmolality).
      2. Lithium is contraindicated in known renal disease.
   C. Vomiting and diarrhea may occur, leading to dehydration and salt loss. Lithium is discontinued, and salt and fluids are given.
   D. Lithium is contraindicated if the patient has cardiac disease (e.g., sick sinus syndrome).
   E. In the elderly patient, lithium may reduce renal function.
   F. Lithium is generally contraindicated during the first trimester of pregnancy.

III. Drug interactions
   A. When used with diuretics, lithium may be selectively absorbed because of relative dehydration and sodium potassium depletion. Close monitoring of serum lithium and electrolyte levels is necessary; the lithium dose is reduced if needed.
   B. Lithium increases the serum insulin levels. Blood sugar levels need periodic monitoring in patients with diabetes.
   C. Iodine-containing medications (e.g., cough medicines, multivitamins) used with lithium are toxic to the thyroid gland and may produce hypothyroidism.

Stimulants

   I. Stimulants include
   A. Dextroamphetamine
   B. Methylphenidate (Ritalin)—sometimes used in children for extreme hyperkinetic syndrome
   II. They are not recommended for most patients with affective disorders because they have a high potential for abuse or tolerance.

NEUROLEPTICS (Table 2-2)

   I. Action and uses
   A. Neuroleptic (antipsychotic) drugs are indicated in the treatment of
      1. Schizophrenia (acute and chronic)—a thought process disorder
      2. Schizoaffective disorders
      3. Organic brain syndromes with psychosis
      4. Huntington's chorea
      5. Intractable hiccups (chlorpromazine)
      6. Ballismus
      7. Nausea and vomiting (prochlorperazine)
   B. Routes of administration include
      1. Oral—preferred for convenience
      2. Intramuscular—one fourth to one half the oral dose is used with reliable absorption and uptake; preferred in aggressive treatment of patients with acute psychoses
   C. Half-lives range from 10–30 hr.
   D. The maintenance dose after the acute symptoms have subsided should be the minimum necessary to obtain a therapeutic response and allow the patient to function (usually once or twice daily).
   E. Overdoses are rarely fatal in adults, and addiction does not occur.
   F. Neuroleptic agents (e.g., haloperidol) are sometimes used for their sedative effect but may be poorly tolerated (especially in elderly patients). Antianxiety drugs are often more effective.
   II. Adverse reactions
   A. Behavioral effects include

1. Sedation—the dose is reduced, or a single dose may be given at bedtime.
2. Toxic psychosis—the dose is reduced. Toxic psychosis must be differentiated from an exacerbation of the underlying psychosis.

B. Extrapyramidal effects include
   1. Acute torsion dystonia (bizarre posturing, spasms, tics, dysphasia)—this occurs early in the course of (especially) parenteral therapy, (e.g., prochlorperazine).
      a. Reduce the dose.
      b. Administer benztropine or an antihistamine parenterally.
   2. Akathisia (restlessness, agitation, inability to sit still)
      a. Reduce the dose.
      b. If dose reduction is not possible, then give diazepam temporarily.
   3. Parkinsonism (tremors, rigidity, masklike facies, shuffling gait)—these occur after longer term therapy.
      a. Reduce the dose.
      b. Alternatively, substitute a central-acting anticholinergic drug.
   4. Tardive dyskinesia (choreiform movements, ballismus)—this is seen in older patients especially. (Reduce the dose.)

C. Autonomic nervous system effects include both alpha-adrenergic and anticholinergic reactions.
   1. Orthostatic hypotension if symptoms are severe—IV fluids are given since vasopressors may paradoxically worsen the hypotension
   2. Xerostomia, tachycardia, visual disturbances, urinary retention, and constipation

D. Idiosyncratic and allergic reactions consist of
   1. Cholestatic jaundice (usually self-limited)—the drug is withdrawn
   2. Allergic reaction of the skin
   3. Photosensitivity

E. Neuroendocrine effects include delayed ovulation, amenorrhea, galactorrhea, gynecomastia, loss of libido, and weight gain.

F. Cardiac effects consist of ECG changes resembling those seen in hypokalemia (which can be ruled out by checking the serum K^+).

G. Hematologic effects are as follows:
   1. Agranulocytosis may occur.
   2. Fever, cellulitis, or other evidence of infection—these warrant discontinuation of the drug and a check of the white blood cell (WBC) count.
   3. The patient should recover after drug withdrawal.

III. Precautions
   A. These drugs can cause inhibition of growth hormone release in children.

Table 2-2 NEUROLEPTICS

Drug	Type	Usual dose (mg)			Effects			
		Adult	Elderly	Child	Autonomic	Sedation	Extrapyramidal
Fluphenazine (Prolixin)	Phenothiazine	IM (acute): 1.25–2.5 q.d., divided PO: 2.5–3.0 q.d., divided	0.9–1.25 q.d., divided	NA	+	++	+++
Haloperidol (Haldol)	Butyrophenone	IM (acute): 2–5 q4–8h PO: 1–4 q.d., divided	Poorly tolerated Poorly tolerated	Poorly tolerated Poorly tolerated	+	+	+++
Trifluoperazine (Stelazine)	Phenothiazine	IM (acute): 2–5 to start, then 1–2 q4–6h	0.6–2.5 to start, then 0.3–1.0 q6–8h	1 b.i.d. if >5 yr	+	++	+++

Prochlorperazine Available rectally Dose for nausea and vomiting: Adult: 5–10 mg, IM-PO-PR q6h Child: 0.1 mg/kg, IM-PO-PR q6h	Phenothiazine	IM (acute): 10–20 q1–4h PO:15–75, divided	0.13/kg, age >2 yr 0.4/kg, age >2 yr	+	++	+++
Chlorpromazine (Thorazine)	Phenothiazine	IM (acute): 25–100 q1–4h PO: 200– 800 q.d.	0.5/kg q6–8h 0.5/kg q4–6h	+++	+++	
Thioridazine (Mellaril)	Phenothiazine	PO: 150– 300 q.d., divided	1/kg q.d.	+++	+++	+

+ Moderately effective

++ Effective

+++ Strongly effective

NA = Not applicable; IM = intramuscular; PO = oral; PR = rectal.

B. Sleep disturbance and psychiatric syndromes may occur in the elderly and may require drug withdrawal.

ANALGESIC AGENTS
Opiates and opioids (Table 2-3)

I. Action and uses
   A. The opiates are
      1. Purified alkaloids of opium
         a. Morphine
         b. Codeine
      2. Semisynthetic modifications of morphine
         a. Hydromorphone (Dilaudid)
         b. Nalbuphine (Nubain)
         c. Oxymorphone (Numorphan)
         d. Oxycodone (Percocet and Percodan)
   B. The opioids, which are synthetic compounds that resemble morphine in action, include
      1. Meperidine (Demerol)
      2. Methadone
      3. Propoxyphene (hydrochloride and napsylate)
      4. Pentazocine (Talwin)
   C. Both categories interact with the several postulated opiate receptors to produce varying degrees of analgesia, behavioral effects, and dependence.
   D. These drugs are indicated for use in
      1. Acute pain—to obtain analgesia and to alter the psychological response to pain, reducing anxiety and apprehension.
         a. Morphine used for severe pain; small to moderate doses for dull, constant pain, and large doses for intermittent, sharp pain
         b. Other opiates or opioids used for mild to moderate pain
      2. Chronic pain management with opiates or opioids is questionable because dependence may occur.
         a. Opiates and opioids should be withdrawn and the patient reevaluated.
         b. Consideration should be given to the nonopiates (acetaminophen, aspirin, and nonsteroidal anti-inflammatory agents).
         c. Antidepressants, sedatives, or antianxiety agents may possibly be needed.
         d. Nerve blocks should be considered.
         e. Pain of neoplastic disease is a special consideration, especially in terminal phases.
            (1) A nonopiate is the first choice of treatment.
            (2) Opiates or opioids are used in increasing strength as required, on a fixed schedule rather than as needed, to keep the patient free of pain.

      (3) The oral route is preferred for convenience. Adjusting the oral dose may compensate for the usually poor oral effectiveness of meperidine and morphine.

  3. Myocardial infarction

    a. Morphine is used for analgesia.

    b. Peripheral pooling of blood may occur, decreasing venous return.

      (1) Cardiac work load is decreased.

      (2) Pulmonary edema is reduced. (Note: equipment for artificial ventilation should be available if needed.)

    c. Any resultant excessive bradycardia, hypotension, or respiratory depression can be counteracted with naloxone (Narcan).

  4. Obstetric analgesia

  5. Preanesthetic medication and general anesthesia

    a. Drugs cause sedation and reduce anxiety when given as a preanesthetic medication. (Note: also consider other antianxiety agents, such as diazepam.)

    b. They are used with nitrous oxide–oxygen in a "balanced" general anesthetic technique. Equipment for artificial ventilation must be at hand.

II. Adverse reactions

  A. Respiratory depression, especially in the elderly or debilitated patient or in one with pulmonary disease, is rare in the common dose ranges. It can be reversed with intravenous naloxone administered repeatedly (because naloxone's half-life is shorter than that of the opiates).

  B. Hypotension—the drugs should be withheld from any patient in shock.

  C. Increased intracranial pressure and cardiovascular dilation may result from hypoventilation and hypercapnia, so the drugs should be withheld from the patient with head injuries or delirium tremens.

  D. Miotic drugs may mask pupillary response, an important diagnostic sign in the patient with a head injury.

  E. Drowsiness and altered sensorium can follow administration of opiates or opioids, or both.

  F. Increased ventricular work may be noted, especially with pentazocine; therefore, this drug should be used cautiously in cardiac patients.

  G. Reduced urinary output by release of antidiuretic hormone (ADH) may be an important consideration in the patient with renal insufficiency.

  H. Increased sphincter tone can lead to biliary colic, urinary retention, and constipation.

III. Drug interactions and precautions

  A. Reduced doses should be used in the patient with hypothyroidism, myxedema, or hypoadrenalism.

Table 2-3 OPIATES AND OPIOIDS

| | Usual dose (mg) | | Effectiveness of route | | | Hours of analgesia | Remarks |
	Adult	Child	PO	IM	IV	(maximum/duration)	
Opiates							
Morphine	IM: 0.1–0.2/kg q3–4h IV: 2.5–15 slowly (1–3/kg for general anesthetics) PO: 10–30 q3–4h	0.1–0.2 q3–4h	+	++	+++	1/4	For severe pain
Codeine	IM/PO: 30–60 q4–6h	0.5/kg q4–6h	++	+++	NA	1/4–6	For mild to moderate pain
Hydromorphone (Dilaudid)	IM: 1–1.5 q4–6h IV: 1–1.5 slowly PO: 2 q4–6h	NA	+	+++	+++	1/4–6	Potency 8 times that of morphine
Nalbuphine (Nubain)	IM/IV: 10 q3–6h	NA	NA	+++	+++	0.5/3–6	For moderate to severe pain
Oxymorphone (Numorphan)	IM: 1–15 q4–6h IV: 0.5 q4–6h PR: 5	NA	NA	++	+++	0.5–1/4–6	Available rectally
Oxycodone (Percocet, Percodan)	PO: q4–6h	NA	+++	NA	NA	1/4–6	Usually in combination

Opioids

Drug	Dose (mg)						Comments
Meperidine (Demerol)	IM and PO: 50–150 q3–6h	1–1.5/kg, q3–6h	+	++	+++	0.5–1/3–6	Spasm of smooth muscle (e.g., GI tract)
Methadone	IM and PO: 2.5–10, repeated when pain recurs	NA	+	++	NA	1.5	Half-life 25 hr; strict FDA regulations to its use in severe pain; detoxification possible in mild to moderate pain
Propoxyphene hydrochloride napsylate	PO: 65 q6–8h	NA	+++	NA	NA	1–1.5/6–8	Half the potency of codeine; 65 mg usually less effective than 650 mg aspirin or acetaminophen; frequently abused, especially with ethyl alcohol
	PO: 100 q6–8h	NA	+++	NA	NA		
Pentazocine (Talwin)	PO: 50 q3–4h	NA	+++	NA	NA	0.5–1/2–3	Potency one-fourth to one-sixth that of morphine; for moderate pain; less dependence than with morphine; increased cardiac workload; injection sites rotated to avoid "sterile abscess"

+ Moderately effective

++ Effective

+++ Strongly effective

NA = not applicable; IM = intramuscular; IV = intravenous; PO = oral; GI = gastrointestinal; FDA = U.S. Food and Drug Administration.

   B. Reduced doses also should be used in any patient taking other central nervous system–depressing medications (e.g., barbiturates, antipsychotics, anxiolytics).
   C. Severe adverse reactions may occur when meperidine is administered to the patient taking an MAOI. These reactions are not observed with morphine.
IV. Tolerance and dependence
   A. These vary with the individual patient.
   B. The abuse potential with morphine is greater than that with pentazocine, propoxyphene, or codeine.
      1. Dependence is unlikely with short-term use of even large doses.
      2. One must be aware of undermedicating in a patient with acute pain.
      3. The smallest effective doses must be given.
      4. Physical dependence may develop without psychological dependence after prolonged use.
      5. Any patient with a history of dependency needs careful observation.

Nonopiates (analgesic-antipyretic) (Table 2-4)

I. Action and uses
   A. Nonopiates do not bind to opiate receptors.
   B. The postulated mechanisms of action are
      1. Analgesic blockade of pain impulse generation peripherally
      2. Antipyretic stimulation of the hypothalamic nuclei and thermal regulatory center
      3. Anti-inflammatory inhibition of prostaglandin synthesis
   C. Indications include
      1. Mild pain (e.g., headache, myalgia)
      2. Fever (the underlying cause needs to be sought)
      3. Inflammation

Aspirin

I. Action and uses
   A. Aspirin is given for headache, neuralgia, myalgia, arthralgia, and pain affecting integumental structures.
   B. Buffered formulations improve aspirin's absorption but have little effect on its onset of action or its analgesic or dyspeptic properties. Effervescent preparations have faster absorption and less gastric irritation than does regular aspirin but alkalize the urine, resulting in faster excretion.
II. Adverse effects
   A. Gastrointestinal distress is reduced if aspirin is taken with food or a glass of water.
      1. Dyspepsia and nausea
      2. Gastrointestinal hemorrhage—rarely life-threatening and rarely correlated with dyspepsia; caused by direct action of the gastric mucosa and platelet dysfunction; results from a

Table 2-4 NONOPIATES (ANALGESIC-ANTIPYRETIC)

Drug	Usual dose (mg) Adult	Child	Half-life (hr)	Absorption	Remarks
Aspirin	650 q4h	0.25/m² q4h	3–3.5	+++	
Sodium salicylate	650 q4h	NA	3–4	+++	Less effective; less GI bleeding than with aspirin
Acetaminophen	325–650 q4h	0.25/m² q4h	1–3	++++	Rare adverse reactions; rectal potency half that of oral potency
Ibuprofen (Motrin)	400 q4h	NA	4–6	++	Low incidence of adverse reactions
	600 q4h	NA			Some GI bleeding, especially in patients with ulcers
Naproxen (Naprosyn)	Doses for analgesia not well established			+++	Useful for moderate to severe postoperative pain

++ Moderately well

+++ Well

++++ Very well

NA = Not applicable.

synergistic effect with alcohol. Aspirin should be avoided in any patient with ulcers or a history of GI tract bleeding.

B. Hypoprothrombinemia may occur with large doses of aspirin taken over several days but is reversed with vitamin K. It is usually insignificant unless the patient is also taking anticoagulants. The degree of hypoprothrombinemia can be measured by a partial thromboplastin time (PTT) test.

C. Platelet inhibition, as measured by bleeding time, may be seen, even with the usual analgesic doses.

D. Reversible hepatotoxicity is caused by large doses in a patient with preexisting liver disease.

E. Anaphylaxis results from common cross-sensitization with other prostaglandin inhibitors (e.g., ibuprofen). It is uncommon to find sensitization with salicylic acid and acetaminophen.

F. Tinnitus can result from long-term aspirin overdosage. Children should be monitored closely.

G. Preexisting renal disease may be exacerbated by the decreased glomerular filtration rate.

III. Precautions

A. Aspirin is contraindicated in any patient with a coagulopathy or in one taking anticoagulants.

B. It should be discontinued at least 1 wk before surgery to reverse its anticoagulant effect. Bleeding time must be checked.

IV. Drug interactions

A. Aspirin enhances the effects of oral hypoglycemic drugs and decreases blood glucose levels. The dose of an oral hypoglycemic drug must be decreased if concomitant administration is necessary.

B. Aspirin antagonizes uricosuric agents, so it should be avoided in patients with gout.

C. Concurrent use with corticosteroids or indomethacin may increase the incidence of gastric ulceration.

D. Aspirin decreases serum protein binding of sulfonamides, increasing their toxicity.

Sodium salicylate

I. Action and uses

A. No platelet effect has been found, and there is less occult GI bleeding than is seen with aspirin.

B. It does produce hypoprothrombinemia, although rarely.

C. It may be tolerated by the patient who is hypersensitive to aspirin.

II. Precautions—avoid in the patient on a low-sodium diet.

Acetaminophen

I. Action and uses

A. Acetaminophen's analgesic and antipyretic properties are equivalent to those of aspirin. It has no anti-inflammatory or antiplatelet action.

B. It is preferred in the patient with ulcer disease, hemophilia, or allergy to aspirin.

C. It does not antagonize uricosuric agents.

D. The rectal form is about half as potent as the oral tablet.

II. Adverse reactions—large doses (15 g single) may cause hepatic damage and death. Overdose is treated with acetylcysteine.

III. Drug interactions—large doses can potentiate the action of oral anticoagulants.

Ibuprofen (Motrin)

I. Action and uses

A. Ibuprofen's analgesic, antipyretic, and anti-inflammatory properties are similar to those of aspirin.

B. It is often tolerated by the patient who cannot tolerate aspirin.

II. Adverse reactions include nausea, vomiting, diarrhea, constipation, heartburn, and epigastric pain (low incidence).

III. Precautions—ibuprofen has a lower incidence of gastrointestinal bleeding than aspirin, but it must be used with caution in any patient known to have ulcer disease.

Naproxen (Naprosyn)

I. Action and uses

A. It has analgesic, anti-inflammatory, and antipyretic actions.

B. Its principal uses are in rheumatoid arthritis, ankylosing spondylitis, osteoarthritis, and moderate to severe postoperative pain.

C. Approximate dose equivalents (in milligrams) are as follows:

220–330	600 (aspirin)
250	50 (indomethacin)
400	70–150 (oral meperidine)
400	>65 (propoxyphene) or 30 (codeine with aspirin)

II. Adverse reactions—GI effects occur, even though the gastric mucosa is less severely affected than with the other agents in this group. GI bleeding with naproxen is less than with aspirin.

III. Precautions—the rare ulcerative reaction can be severe, and thus caution is indicated in the patient with a history of ulcer disease.

Analgesic mixtures

I. Theoretically, these provide greater pain relief, a wider range of therapeutic uses, and less severe side effects than a single agent.

II. Commonly used mixtures include

A. Codeine with aspirin (for moderate pain):

1. Ascriptin with codeine—325 mg aspirin and 16.2 or 32.4 mg codeine phosphate

    2. Empirin with codeine—325 mg aspirin and 15 or 30 mg codeine phosphate

B. Codeine with acetaminophen (for moderate to severe pain):
1. Empracet with codeine—300 mg acetaminophen and 30 or 60 mg codeine phosphate
2. Tylenol with codeine—300 mg acetaminophen and 7.5 (no. 1), 15 (no. 2), 30 (no. 3), or 60 mg (no. 4) codeine phosphate
3. Tylenol with codeine elixir—120 mg acetaminophen and 12 mg codeine phosphate per 5 ml

C. Oxycodone's (available only in mixtures in the United States), potency and dependency potential are greater than those of codeine. It is used for moderate to severe pain:
1. Percodan—4.5 mg oxycodone hydrochloride, 0.38 mg oxycodone terephthalate, and 224 mg aspirin
2. Percocet-5—5 mg oxycodone hydrochloride and 325 mg acetaminophen
3. Tylox—4.5 mg oxycodone hydrochloride, 0.38 mg oxycodone terephthalate, and 500 mg acetaminophen

D. Pentazocine's effectiveness is comparable to that of combinations containing codeine and oxycodone (e.g., Talwin compound [pentazocine hydrochloride, equivalent to 12.5 mg base and 325 mg aspirin]).

ANTICONVULSANTS (Table 2-5)

I. Action and uses
  A. Seizures—barbiturates, hydantoins, other antiepileptics
    1. Seizures represent a focal or generalized brain disturbance caused by
      a. Infection, neoplasms, congenital defects, or head trauma
      b. Fever, metabolic disturbances, or drug withdrawal
      c. Epilepsy (recurrent pattern with sudden disturbances in consciousness accompanied by uncontrolled motor activity, unusual sensory phenomena, and inappropriate behavior)
    2. Types of seizure include
      a. Partial (locally benign, usually remain focal)
        (1) Elementary—consciousness unimpaired (e.g., jacksonian seizures)
        (2) Complex—consciousness impaired (e.g., temporal lobe epilepsy)
      b. Generalized
        (1) Absences—staring, subtle clonic movements (petit mal epilepsy)
        (2) Bilateral myoclonic without loss of consciousness
        (3) Tonic-clonic (grand mal epilepsy)
        (4) Atonic—loss of postural tone
        (5) Akinetic—relaxation of all musculature
      c. Unilateral

3. General principles of drug therapy for seizures include the following:
   a. There should be few or no adverse reactions from the medication.
   b. Therapy is individualized.
   c. Seizures may "escape" control if liver enzymes are induced over time to augment metabolism of the anticonvulsant (e.g., barbiturates). The dose may need to be increased, or another agent tried.
   d. Discontinuation of the anticonvulsant should be considered with time, because spontaneous resolution of seizure disorders may occur. The dose should be gradually reduced.

B. Trigeminal neuralgia (tic douloureux)—carbamazepine or phenytoin
C. Certain cardiac arrhythmias—phenytoin

II. Adverse reactions
A. Gastrointestinal disturbances may necessitate a dose reduction.
B. Sedation may (rarely) induce personality changes and psychoses.
C. Ataxia may be found, especially with phenytoin. Cerebellar damage is possible if the dose is not reduced.
D. Hypersensitivity reactions may make drug discontinuance necessary, and an anticonvulsant drug of another class can then be tried. Skin eruptions may precede Stevens-Johnson syndrome. Anaphylaxis is rare.
E. Acute, intermittent porphyria may be precipitated by barbiturates and phenytoin. Therefore, these agents are contraindicated in this disease.
F. Visual disturbances may occur but are reversible by decreasing the dose or discontinuing the drug.
G. Gingival hyperplasia is found, especially with phenytoin use in children. If hygiene becomes a problem, gingivectomy (especially with an electrocautery) may provide temporary improvement.
H. Lymphadenopathies (generally rare) may be caused by any of the hydantoins but are reversible with discontinuation of the drug. A few cases of lymphoma that seemed to be possibly related to hydantoin use have been reported.
I. Megaloblastic anemias have been found, especially with hydantoin and barbiturate use. They are treated with folic acid. Blood counts must be monitored, and the agent may need to be discontinued.
J. Severe blood dyscrasias are rare. If sore throat, fever, petechiae, epistaxis, or signs of infection develop, blood tests are in order.
K. Hepatitis also is rare. Hydantoins and valproic acid are the most common causes. Baseline liver function tests must be per-

Table 2-5 ANTICONVULSANTS

| | Usual dose (mg) | | Common adverse reactions |
| | Type | | |
	Adult	Child	
Barbiturates Phenobarbital	PO: 50–100 b.i.d. IM: 200–300 q6h IV (slow): 200–300 q6h	PO: 15–50 b.i.d. IM: 3–5/kg q6h IV (slow): 3–5/kg q6h	Sedation, ataxia, paradoxical hyperactivity
Hydantoins Phenytoin	PO: 100 b.i.d.–t.i.d. IV (slow): 10–15/kg (slow infusion for status epilepticus only)	PO: 1.5–2.5/kg to 1 g IV (slow): 750/m² body surface	Skin eruptions (rarely serious), gingival hyperplasia (children), hepatitis, blood dyscrasias, Stevens-Johnson (all rare); hypotension from too rapid IV administration (exceeding 50 mg/min); GI disturbances
Succinimides Ethosuximide (Zarontin)	PO: 500 q.d.	PO: 250 q.d.	Sedation, headache, depression (rare)
Benzodiazepines Diazepam (Valium)	PO: 2–10 b.i.d.–q.i.d. (2 in elderly) IV (slow): 5–10 injected at 5 mg/min	PO: 0.5–1 b.i.d.–q.i.d. IV (slow): 0.5–1 q2–5min (max. 5–10 mg)	CNS depression, GI disturbances, sensitivity reactions, dependence, respiratory depression (parenteral route)

Carbamazepine (Tegretol)	PO: 400–800 b.i.d., maintenance	PO: 200–400 b.i.d., maintenance	CNS depression, nausea, vomiting, visual disturbances, confusion, dysphasia, paresthesias, dermatological reactions, aplastic anemia and thrombocytopenia (rare but may be fatal): follow blood counts and cross-sensitivity with TCAs
Valproic acid (Depakene)	PO: 5/kg b.i.d.–t.i.d.		Enhances sedative effect of phenobarbital, increases plasma phenytoin levels, interferes with platelet aggregation; GI disturbances, sedation, rare hepatic dysfunction
Acetazolamide (Diamox)	PO: 2–10/kg b.i.d.–t.i.d.		Rapid development of tolerance

PO = oral; IM = intramuscular; IV = intravenous; GI = gastrointestinal; CNS = central nervous system; TCA = tricyclic antidepressant.

formed before therapy is begun and repeated if symptoms of liver dysfunction occur.

L. Nephropathies, likewise, are rare and necessitate discontinuation of the agent being used.

III. Precautions—abrupt withdrawal of anticonvulsants can precipitate seizures. The dose must be reduced gradually. Abrupt withdrawal can be achieved only if another anticonvulsant is substituted intravenously.

IV. Common drugs (by seizure type)

A. Generalized clonic-tonic (grand mal epilepsy) or elementary partial seizures—phenytoin (Dilantin), a hydantoin, or phenobarbital; acetazolamide (Diamox) or valproic acid (Depakene) may be used as adjuncts.

B. Complex partial seizures (temporal lobe epilepsy)—carbamazepine (Tegretol) or phenytoin

C. Absence seizures—ethosuximide (Zarontin) or valproic acid (Depakene)

D. Status epilepticus (tonic-clonic)—vigorous emergency treatment is required; IV diazepam is given initially and may need to be repeated for control; load and maintenance doses of phenytoin or phenobarbital follow; if status persists, a general anesthetic administered by an anesthesiologist, with resuscitative equipment at hand, may be necessary.

DIGITALIS GLYCOSIDES (Table 2-6)

I. Action and uses

A. The digitalis glycosides enhance myocardial contractility, lengthen atrioventricular node conduction time and refractory period, and shorten atrial and ventricular refractory periods.

B. These drugs are indicated for

1. Treatment of congestive heart failure from coronary artery disease or hypertension, if antihypertensive drugs do not adequately control the condition

2. Control of ventricular rate in the patient with atrial fibrillation

3. Control of supraventricular tachycardias unresponsive to other interventions

C. Commonly used digitalis glycosides include

1. Digoxin

a. Onset is 5–30 min, half-life is 30–40 hr, and therapeutic serum level is 0.5–2.5 mg/ml.

b. It is excreted largely unchanged in the urine; therefore, care is needed in any patient with renal disease. It may be necessary to reduce the dose or use liver-metabolized digitoxin.

c. The usual dose varies. Maintenance for adults is 0.125–0.5 mg daily. For rapid digitalization, 0.25 mg IV is given every 4–6 hr to a total of 1 mg. A pediatric text should be consulted for children's dosages.

2. Digitoxin
    a. Onset is 1–4 hr, and half-life is 5–9 da.
    b. It is metabolized in the liver to inactive substances, which are excreted in the urine. It is useful in impaired renal function but not in hepatic dysfunction.
    c. The usual dose (in a patient who has not received digitalis for 2 wk or longer) is 0.1 mg daily for maintenance. For rapid digitalization, 0.8 mg and then 0.2 mg are given q6–8 hr in 2–3 doses. A pediatric text should be consulted for children's dosages.

II. Adverse reactions (digitalis intoxication)
    A. Therapeutic and toxic dose ranges are very close. Serum digoxin levels can be determined for the therapeutic range.
    B. Predisposing factors include alkalosis, hypercalcemia, hypokalemia, and hypoxemia.
    C. Signs include
        1. Noncardiac
            a. Gastrointestinal—nausea, vomiting, anorexia, and rarely diarrhea
            b. Neurologic—fatigue, sedation, vertigo, personality changes, and confusion
            c. Ophthalmologic—visual disturbances and photophobia
            d. Hypersensitivity (urticaria)—rare
        2. Cardiac (may be the first evidence of intoxication)
            a. Multifocal premature ventricular contractions (PVC) and junctional tachycardia
            b. Sinus bradycardia and sinus arrest
            c. Paroxysmal ventricular tachycardia
    D. Treatment includes discontinuation of the glycoside and administration of potassium (if the serum K is low) and other antiarrhythmics as indicated.

III. Precautions
    A. Quinidine increases the serum digoxin level. GI disturbances and ventricular arrhythmias may result.
    B. Propranolol may need to be added if the ventricular rate in atrial fibrillation is not controlled by maximal therapeutic doses of a digitalis glycoside.
    C. Diuretics that cause hypokalemia predispose to digitalis toxicity. Potassium chloride supplements or a potassium-sparing diuretic (e.g., spironolactone) are used.

CALCIUM CHANNEL BLOCKERS

These drugs inhibit the influx of calcium ions during membrane depolarization of cardiac and smooth vascular muscle. Two mechanisms of action have been postulated: (1) Angina during exertion, which reduces heart rate and systemic blood pressure during work load, thus reducing myocardial oxygen demand. (2) Angina from spasm of coronary arteries—dilation of coronary arteries. In patients with good left ventrical function, no negative inotropic effect has been revealed. Ven-

Table 2-6 ANTIARRHYTHMICS

	Action	Common indications	Common adverse reactions	Remarks
Digitalis glycosides	Depress AV conduction time and refractory period; prolong atrial and ventricular refractory period	Control ventricular rate in atrial fibrillation; treat congestive heart failure	Intoxication	
Quinidine gluconate (Quinaglute) Procainamide (Pronestyl)	Depresses automaticity; prolongs refractory period	Controls supraventricular and ventricular tachyarrhythmias; prevents PVCs with digitalis in atrial fibrillation	GI disturbances, AV block	Increases serum digoxin levels and can be given IM with less severe local reactions
Disopyramide (Norpace)	Depresses automaticity; prolongs refractory period; depresses myocardial contractility	Controls ventricular and supraventricular tachyarrhythmias	Anticholinergic activity, GI disturbances, AV block, hypoglycemia	Avoid in poorly compensated congestive heart failure
Lidocaine	Depresses automaticity; decreases refractory period; does not decrease conduction velocity in therapeutic doses	Controls ventricular tachyarrhythmias; prophylaxis against ventricular tachycardia in acute myocardial infarction	CNS depression, convulsions	Avoid in hepatic insufficiency

Phenytoin	Depresses automaticity; decreases refractory period	Controls digitalis-induced arrhythmias	Fatigue, GI distress, hepatitis (rare), blood dyscrasias	Needs *slow* IV push
Bretylium	Prevents norepinephrine release at sympathetic nerve terminals	Controls refractory supraventricular tachyarrhythmias	Uncommon angina	
Beta blockers (propranolol)	Block cardiac beta receptors; reduce rate and contractility; prolong AV conduction; suppress automaticity	Control supraventricular and ventricular tachyarrhythmias, atrial flutter, and fibrillation	Congestive heart failure and bronchospasm	Avoid in patients with asthma; needs slow withdrawal
Calcium channel blockers	Interfere with calcium transport at cell membrane; delay AV conduction; suppress automaticity at sinus node	Control supraventricular tachyarrhythmias	Hypotension	
Atropine	Increases sinus rate; speeds AV conduction	Controls sinus bradycardia, sinoatrial arrest, and second-degree AV block (type I)	Xerostomia, glaucoma (rare), urinary retention	
Isoproterenol	Enhances automaticity; increases contractility and rate; stimulates cardiac beta receptors	Controls second- and third-degree block (propranolol-induced) and myocardial depression	Tachycardia, PVCs	

AV = atrioventricular; CNS = central nervous system; GI = gastrointestinal; IM = intramuscular; PVC = premature ventricular contraction.

tricular end-diastolic falling pressure, cardiac output, and ejection fraction are not affected.

Diltiazem (Cardizem)

I. Indications
   A. Angina pectoris due to coronary artery spasm
   B. Chronic stable angina in patients who cannot tolerate, or who are still symptomatic on, nitrates or beta-blockers, or both
II. Precautions
   A. Renal or hepatic dysfunction
   B. Beta-blockers—bioavailability increased by concomitant diltiazem
   C. Cimetidine increases peak diltiazem levels when given concomitantly
   D. Digitalis—Cardizem increases plasma digoxin levels
   E. Anesthetic agents may potentiate the decreased cardiac contractility, conductivity, automaticity, and vascular dilation caused by diltiazem: 0.6 mg to 1.0 g atropine for bradycardia and for high-degree atrioventricular block; dopamine or dobutamine for cardiac failure; dopamine or levarterenol for hypotension
III. Adverse reactions (rare)
   A. Angina and atrioventricular block
   B. Bradycardia
   C. Congestive heart failure
   D. Amnesia and depression
   E. Insomnia and nervousness
   F. Paresthesia and tremor
   G. Somnolence
   H. Constipation and diarrhea
   I. Dyspepsia and vomiting
IV. Administration
   A. 30 mg PO qid, before meals and at bedtime, adjusted up to 180–300 mg/da to achieve optimal response

Nifedipine (Procardia)

I. Indications
   A. Angina pectoris due to coronary artery spasm
   B. Chronic stable angina
II. Precautions
   A. Hypotension, rarely excessive
   B. May occur in fentanyl anesthesia if nifedipine was used with a beta-blocker
   C. Peripheral edema responds to diuretic
   D. If congestive heart failure is suspected, care is necessary to determine whether edema was caused by nifedipine or failure
   E. See also Diltiazem (Cardizem) under Calcium Channel Blockers
III. Adverse reactions
   A. Peripheral edema, transient hypotension, dizziness, nausea, diarrhea, constipation, and muscle cramps

IV. Administration
    A. 10 mg tid adjusted up to 10–20 mg PO tid

Verapamil (Calan, Isoptin)

  I. Indications
    A. Angina during coronary artery spasm
    B. Chronic stable angina
    C. Control of ventricular rate with digitalis in chronic atrial flutter and fibrillation
    D. Prophylaxis for repetitive paroxysmal atrial tachycardia
    E. Essential hypertension
  II. Precautions
    A. Heart failure (negative inotropic effect)
    B. Hypotension
    C. Elevated liver enzymes
    D. AV block
    E. Patients with hypertrophic cardiomyopathy
    F. Impaired hepatic function
    G. Decreased neuromuscular transmission in patients with muscular dystrophy
    H. Additive effect with oral vasodilating antihypertensive drugs
    I. Inhalational anesthetic agents may potentiate effects
 III. Adverse reactions
    A. Constipation and nausea
    B. Congestive heart failure and peripheral edema
    C. Headache, dizziness, and fatigue
 IV. Administration
    A. Angina: 80–120 mg PO tid
    B. Atrial fibrillation on digoxin: 240–320 mg/da divided doses
    C. Paroxysmal supraventricular tachycardia not on digoxin: 240–480 mg/da divided doses
    D. Essential hypertension: 240–300 mg/da divided doses

All dosages start at the lower end and are titrated upward to the desired effect, not exceeding the maximum.

GENERAL REFERENCE

Goodman LS, Gilman A: *Pharmacologic basis of therapeutics*, ed 8, New York, 1990, McGraw-Hill.

Smith CM, Reynard AM: *Essentials of pharmacology*, Philadelphia, 1995, WB Saunders.

Frequently Requested
Oral Surgical Consultations

3

JOSEPH W. WILKES III

GENERAL CONSIDERATIONS

  I. Health care providers will have occasion to request oral surgical consultation. An appropriate response depends on determining the referring doctor's purpose for seeking the consultation.

    A. The purpose might simply be to obtain assistance in establishing a diagnosis or suggestions for managing a problem. In this case the oral surgeon is being asked for opinions and should not automatically presume to take over the patient's care.

    B. Alternatively, the referring doctor might specifically request assistance in the care of a patient (or even transfer of the patient to the oral surgeon's care). The oral surgeon will then become actively involved in managing the case.

    C. If no clear reason for the consultation exists, the referring doctor should be called to establish the purpose and ascertain the questions to be answered. Often a note in the chart or a discussion with the patient will make the purpose clear.

  II. When practical, inpatient consultations should be done in the oral surgical clinic, where adequate light, instruments, and radiographic studies are readily available. If the patient is confined to the ward, a bedside consultation will require adequate lighting and assistance in holding the light for the bimanual portions of the examination. Anything less can lead to a suboptimal bedside consultation.

  III. Outpatient consultations are most efficient when the referring doctor sends in any radiographs and copies of records. These should be requested in advance of the appointment when possible.

CONSULTATIVE METHOD

  I. When a consultation is requested, the oral surgeon should see the patient promptly to expedite patient care.

  II. The following outline of procedural care may prove useful:

    A. Purpose for the consultation—the reason for the patient's referral must be identified.

B. Review of the record—this will ensure that recommendations for therapy are consistent with the general stability of the patient and the medicines currently being administered. One must carefully review the record to:
   1. Ascertain the patient's overall condition.
   2. Determine the relationship and importance of the problem to the patient's situation.
   3. Review orders for the patient's medical regimen.
C. Patient history—one must assess the acuteness and severity of the problem.
D. Patient examination.
E. Additional studies—any indicated radiographs and blood studies or other consultations should be available.
F. Response—a written note should be placed in the record, and if the problem is urgent, a call made to the referring doctor. A diagnostic opinion and recommendations for further evaluation or therapy may be included. If requested, the response should include therapeutic intervention.
G. Follow-up—one must determine whether further therapy will be needed and coordinate such care with the patient's other health care providers.

FREQUENT REASONS FOR SEEKING CONSULTATION
Patient assessment before cardiac surgery

I. Purpose
   A. The oral surgeon must identify and eliminate actual and potential sources of orofacial infection that could, through bacteremia, infect prosthetic materials implanted in the heart or great vessels. Included are valve replacements, septal repairs, and replacement of aortic or pulmonic roots. Intervention to eliminate these sources of infection is usually expected by the referring doctor.
   B. Cardiac surgery not involving prosthetic material requires no routine preoperative oral surgical consultation (e.g., coronary artery bypass graft surgery).
II. Review of the patient's record. Key elements affecting oral surgical management include:
   A. Hemodynamic instability—a fragile patient, especially one confined to an intensive care unit, might not be able to tolerate oral surgical manipulation before cardiac surgery to correct the instability.
   B. Unstable angina—if chest pain is steadily increasing in frequency and severity and is harder to control, it might be triggered by oral surgical procedures. When hemodynamic instability or unstable angina exists, it might be necessary to allow cardiac surgery to proceed without the (optimal) removal of potential sources of infection. In this case the risks from an unstable cardiac condition would outweigh the risk of endocarditis.

C. Arrhythmias—if an arrhythmia is difficult to control or refractory to medication, any local anesthetic agent used should be free of epinephrine. An intravenous injection of epinephrine must then be avoided if aspiration fails to reveal intravenous placement of the needle. Well-controlled arrhythmias should not require this restriction.

D. Stable angina—epinephrine can be used in local anesthetic agents if care is taken, by aspiration, to avoid an intravascular injection. Some practitioners believe that the anesthesia obtained is more profound and prolonged when epinephrine is in the local anesthetic, and that angina will be less likely during the procedure because of less discomfort and accompanying anxiety. Oxygen and 0.3 mg of trinitroglycerin (TNG) in the form of sublingual tablets must be available should angina occur. If angina does occur, start oxygen at 5–8 L/min by nasal prongs, nasal mask, or face mask; give one TNG tablet sublingually and repeat in 2–3 min if the angina is unrelieved; monitor blood pressure; obtain a 12-lead ECG if angina persists; and call the patient's physician.

E. Anticoagulants

   1. Warfarin (Coumadin)—if the prothrombin time (PT) is ≤1½ times the control value, carry out the prophylaxis, restorative care, and minor oral surgical procedures as possible. If it is ≥1½ times the control value or if extensive oral surgery is needed, check with the patient's physician about reducing or holding the warfarin until the PT is in line. If this is inadvisable, attempt to change from warfarin to intravenous heparin (5000 U in an IV loading dose, 500–1200 U/hr in an IV drip to keep the PTT between 37 and 60). Heparin is stopped 4 hr before oral surgery and restarted immediately afterward, switching back to warfarin over the next 1–3 da until the PT is in the appropriate therapeutic range.

   2. Heparin—manage this as described above, in concert with the patient's physician.

   3. Aspirin (and other antiplatelet medications)—check the bleeding time. If it is abnormal, consult with the patient's physician on the possibility of eliminating the medication for 2 wk before oral surgery. If time does not allow and oral surgery is urgent, consider infusing 10–20 U of platelets immediately before the operation.

F. Heart murmurs—these will require antibiotic prophylaxis as follows*:

---

*Adapted from a statement for health professionals by the Committee of Rheumatic Fever and Infective Endocarditis: *Prevention of bacterial endocarditis, Circulation* 70:1123A, 1984. Also excerpted in *J Am Dent Assoc* 110:98, 1985.

Refer to these joint American Heart Association–American Dental Association recommendations for more complete information regarding which patients and which procedures require prophylaxis.

For dental procedures and surgery of upper respiratory tract

1. For most patients
   Oral amoxicillin

   Adults: 3.0 g of amoxicillin 1 hr before the procedure, then 1.5 g of amoxicillin 6 hr after the initial dose.

   Children <60 lb: 1.0 g of penicillin V 1 hr before the procedure, then 500 mg 6 hr after the initial dose.

2. For patients allergic to penicillin (may also be selected for those receiving oral penicillin as continuous rheumatic fever prophylaxis)
   Erythromycin

   Adults: 1.0 g of erythromycin orally 1 hr before the procedure, then 500 mg 6 hr after the initial dose.

   Children: 20 mg/kg 1 hr before the procedure, then 10 mg/kg 6 hr after the initial dose.

3. For patients at higher risk of infective endocarditis (especially those with prosthetic heart valves) who are not allergic to penicillin
   Ampicillin plus gentamicin

   Adults: 1.0–2.0 g of ampicillin plus 1.5 mg/kg of gentamicin IM or IV, both given 30 min before the procedure, then 1.0 g of penicillin V (500 mg for children <60 lb) orally 6 hr after the initial dose.

   Children: Timing of doses is same as for adults. Doses are 50 mg/kg of ampicillin and 2.0 mg/kg of gentamicin.

4. For higher risk patients (especially those with prosthetic heart valves) who are allergic to penicillin
   Vancomycin

   Adults: 1.0 g of vancomycin IV over 60 min begun 60 min before the procedure; no repeat dose is necessary.

   Children: 20 mg/kg IV over 60 min, begun 60 min before the procedure; no repeat dose is necessary.

For gastrointestinal and genitourinary tract surgery and instrumentation

1. For most patients
   Ampicillin plus gentamicin

   Adults: 2.0 g of ampicillin IM or IV plus 1.5 mg/kg of gentamicin IM or IV given 30 min before the procedure. May repeat once 8 hr later.

   Children: Same timing of medications as adult schedule. Doses are 50 mg/kg of ampicillin and 2.0 mg/kg of gentamicin.

2. For patients allergic to penicillin
   Vancomycin plus gentamicin

   Adults: 1.0 g of vancomycin IV given over 60 min plus 1.5 mg/kg of gentamicin IM or IV, each given 60 min before the procedure. Doses may be repeated once 8–12 hr later.

NOTE: In patients with compromised renal function, it may be necessary to modify or omit the second dose of antibiotics. Intramuscular injections may be contraindicated in patients receiving anticoagulants. Children's doses should not exceed adult doses.

	Children: Timing as above. Doses are 20 mg/kg of vancomycin and 2.0 mg/kg of gentamicin.
3. Oral regimen for minor or repetitive procedures in low-risk patients *Amoxicillin*	**Adults:** 3.0 g of amoxicillin 1 hr before the procedure and 1.5 g 6 hr after the initial dose. **Children:** Same timing of doses: 50 mg/kg initial dose and 25 mg/kg follow-up dose.

III. Patient history—note any complaints of swelling, foul taste, drainage, bleeding gingivae, or teeth that are sensitive to pressure or thermal change.

IV. Patient examination—note the periodontal condition, recording any fluctuant or draining areas, carious lesions, tender or mobile teeth, and mucosal lesions and irritations.

V. Additional studies
   A. Panoramic radiographs—these are obtained to help identify lesions of the jaw. They are not generally sufficient alone for accurate periodontal and periapical examination.
   B. Full-mouth periapical series (dentulous areas)—note the periodontal condition, depth of caries, and radiolucencies, along with any indications of active infection or conditions likely to result in infection.

VI. Response
   A. If time and patient stability permit, oral hygiene should be optimized, restorable teeth restored, and nonrestorable teeth removed before cardiac surgery. Severely periodontally involved teeth should also be removed. Teeth likely to need endodontic therapy postoperatively should probably be removed, although some controversy exists over this. If permanent restorations are not possible, control caries and place temporary restorations. If cardiac surgery is not urgent, attempt to postpone it until oral health is optimized.
   B. If the patient is unstable or needs cardiac surgery on a more urgent basis, necessary oral surgery may need to be deferred. If the physician will permit oral surgery on a fragile patient preoperatively, it should be done with continuous vital sign and ECG monitoring with local anesthesia and light intravenous sedation. The operating room is a good place for this, with an anesthesiologist performing the sedation and monitoring the patient. An awake patient can effectively communicate when chest pain first occurs so it can be dealt with immediately. If this is not possible, any needed oral surgical care will have to wait until approximately 6 mo after cardiac surgery. Any teeth that become symptomatic before then can be treated individually, with careful vital sign monitoring and antibiotic prophylaxis as indicated.
   C. When the patient is deemed free of orofacial sources of infection, it should be so stated in the record, clearing the patient for cardiac surgery from the oral surgical standpoint.

VII. Follow-up
   A. The patient's own dentist needs to be advised of the results of the oral surgical consultation.
   B. If prosthetic material was used in cardiac surgery or if murmurs exist, details of prophylactic antibiotic regimens for dental care should be sent to the dentist.

Assessment after cardiac surgery

   I. The general scheme is the same as that outlined for patient assessment before cardiac surgery.
   II. Often consultation is requested because the patient has a fever, and bacterial endocarditis is suspected.
   A. Signs include fever of unknown origin, diaphoresis, malaise, splinter hemorrhages of the nail beds, and sometimes hemodynamic instability. An echocardiogram may show bacterial vegetations on, or dysfunction of, a natural or prosthetic valve. Blood cultures, held for 2 wk and numbering at least six sets (one at each fever spike), are an additional study that, together with a careful history and examination, may support an oral source.
   B. If such a source exists, 2,000,000 U of IV penicillin G q2–4h, or 500 mg of IV vancomycin q6h, should be started. Streptomycin, 1 g IM q8h, should be added if a prosthetic valve is in place. Abscesses should be drained and offending teeth removed under such coverage.
   C. Data on antibiotic sensitivities of bacteria in the cultured blood or drainage will guide further therapy.

Assessment before radiation therapy

   I. Purpose—consultation may be sought to identify and eliminate existing and potential sources of orofacial infection in a patient about to undergo radiation therapy for head and neck cancer. Poor oral hygiene, periodontitis, and nonrestorable or abscessed teeth can cause osteomyelitis in irradiated bone, whose resistance to infection is low because of radiation-induced vascular compromise.
   II. Review of the record
   A. One must note the location and area of planned irradiation. Diseased or nonrestorable teeth in this area will have to be removed at least 1 wk before irradiation to allow some healing to occur before radiation begins. Restorable teeth will also need removal if the radiation is to be directed at the periodontium.
   B. Restorable teeth in other areas of the mouth will need repair before radiation therapy begins so that progression of abscesses into irradiated areas does not occur.
   III. Patient history and examination
   A. Symptomatic and diseased teeth are identified.
   B. Oral hygiene habits are analyzed. In the patient who has undergone radiotherapy, oral hygiene must be meticulous.

IV. Additional studies
   A. Radiographs (panoramic and periapical)
      1. One must look for teeth in need of removal or repair based on caries or periodontal condition.
      2. One must also check for invasion of tumor into bone, which will alter the general treatment plan.
   B. Vitality testing of questionable teeth, electrically or thermally
V. Response
   A. Careful dental prophylaxis and restoration or removal of teeth that are infected, nonrestorable, or located in the radiation field must be performed before radiation.
   B. The patient must be taught assiduous brushing and flossing techniques, as well as the use of daily topical fluoride application. Gels with trays can be used.
VI. Follow-up
   A. Oral examination with prophylaxis should be scheduled every 6 mo, or more often if oral hygiene is a problem. Any teeth that become carious will need early restoration. Any prosthesis that is constructed must not irritate or abrade the mucosa. Oral examinations must include careful checks for recurrent or new lesions, with early biopsy.
   B. A neck examination should be conducted to assess for the development of adenopathy.
   C. Multidisciplinary follow-up (surgical, oral surgical, radiation, oncologic) in an organized setting is advisable.

Assessment after radiation therapy

I. Purpose
   A. Any new lesions are discovered and evaluated.
   B. Symptomatic teeth or periodontal tissues in or near an irradiated field are treated.
   C. Oral mucosal irritation from irradiation is treated.
II. Review of the record
   A. One must carefully determine whether the area under study is within the irradiated field.
   B. If it is, the patient should be started on a regimen of daily antibiotics before oral surgery. This will help prevent serious infections that might ensue when oral flora are introduced into irradiated tissue.
III. Patient history, examination, and additional studies
   A. These are the same as for preradiation patients.
   B. Radiographic studies can usually be limited to the symptomatic area.
IV. Response
   A. The oral surgeon should submit any suspicious lesions to biopsy, drain abscesses, and remove nonrestorable teeth.
   B. Lesions strongly suspected of being caused by irritation from a prosthesis can be treated by removing the prosthesis, starting saline or half-strength hydrogen peroxide rinses, and reex-

amining the patient in 1 wk. If unimproved, the lesion should then be biopsied.

C. Mucosal irritations and dryness, in the absence of lesions, may be managed with artificial saliva, saline rinses, or 2% viscous lidocaine (xylocaine) rinses. Lemon-flavored lozenges can be used to try to stimulate more salivary flow. This additional moisture may soothe the mucosa.

D. Suggested antibiotic coverage for oral surgery in irradiated areas is:
   1. Potassium penicillin, 2 g PO 1 hr before the procedure and then 500 mg PO q6h for 5 da after the procedure
   2. In the presence of penicillin allergy, erythromycin, 1 g PO 1 hr before the procedure and then 500 mg PO q6h for 5 da after the procedure
   3. As an alternative, IV or IM penicillin G or clindamycin

Assessment of oral lesions

I. Purpose—the oral surgeon is often asked to diagnose oral lesions and to determine whether they are cancerous.

II. Review of the record—the surgeon should note any history of previous lesions and their diagnoses.

III. Patient history
   A. The acuteness or chronicity of a lesion is noted. An acute lesion, especially with a concurrent viral-type syndrome, may not require biopsy unless it persists unimproved for 1 wk to 10 da.
   B. Pain, bleeding, the presence of other lesions intraorally or extraorally, and any irritation from prostheses are noted.
   C. A history of smoking, alcohol abuse, or habits traumatic to the mucosa is important.
   D. Any systemic symptoms indicative of a nutritional, infective, or allergy syndrome that might have accompanying oral lesions must be treated.

IV. Patient examination
   A. One must accurately describe the lesion and note other lesions or irritations.
   B. The neck must be examined for adenopathy.
   C. Bimanual palpation of the floor of the mouth will reveal submaxillary or submental adenopathy.

V. Additional studies—lesions that cannot be explained on the basis of systemic illness and lesions that are suspicious because of their chronicity, a smoking history, adenopathy, or the lack of obvious local irritation should be submitted to biopsy.

VI. Response
   A. The definitive diagnosis of a suspicious area is by biopsy. Any lesion observed should be biopsied if it is not clearly improving after 7–10 da of treatment.
      1. If irritation is thought to be the cause, its source is eliminated (including leaving out the prosthesis), and the lesion is biopsied if the condition does not improve in 7–10 da.

2. To clean areas of suspected irritation, the patient must start saline or half-strength hydrogen peroxide mouth rinses qid.

B. When the biopsy is done, excision with a margin of normal-appearing tissue is advisable if the size of the lesion so permits. Thus, biopsy can be the definitive and curative procedure.

VII. Follow-up

A. Treatment planning relative to excision, radiation, or chemotherapy is needed for lesions shown to be cancerous and incompletely removed at biopsy. A multidisciplinary approach is best, especially in a clinic organized for this purpose. All patients should be observed for healing and recurrence.

B. Recurrence of a suspicious lesion requires biopsy.

Assessment for iatrogenic dentoalveolar trauma

I. Purpose

A. The oral surgeon is often called to the operating room to replant avulsed teeth and to repair lacerations that at times may occur when a patient is intubated for general anesthesia.

B. Elapsed time is critical if a subluxated or avulsed tooth is to survive reduction and reimplantation.

II. Patient examination

A. Vertical fracture of a tooth or teeth and roots fractured in the cervical half are nonrestorable. A root fractured at the cervical margin may be retained, the pulp extirpated, and the tooth later reconstructed.

B. Any cleanly subluxated or avulsed teeth are reimplanted.

III. Response

A. Using adequate light and suction, the oral surgeon must:

1. Stop any active bleeding.
2. Pack the pharynx if the patient is intubated.
3. Remove any nonsalvageable teeth.
4. Extirpate the pulps of salvageable roots and teeth with class III fractures, plugging the canals with cotton pellets and a temporary sealer and administering antibiotics.
5. Reduce and splint any subluxated teeth and replant and splint-avulsed teeth. Root canal therapy "in hand" might be necessary for avulsed teeth that have been out longer than 30 min. (See Chapter 7, Replantation and Transplantation of Teeth, page 183 on treatment of dentoalveolar trauma.)
6. Administer antibiotics and remove the pharyngeal pack.

B. Because these cases may involve litigation, care must be taken to document in the record the exact anatomic details of the injury.

IV. Follow-up

A. The oral surgeon assesses the patient for evidence of infection or developing nonvitality of the teeth. Signs include new pain, mobility, and darkening of the teeth. The patient's dentist will also need to watch for these signs.

B. Reduced and replanted teeth may eventually require endodontic therapy. Restorative care is usually coordinated through the patient's dentist.

Assessment before chemotherapy

I. Purpose—many chemotherapeutic agents cause oral problems, either through a direct toxic effect on the tissues or by effects on the bone marrow (making the tissues less resistant to bleeding or infection).

   A. Common oral problems in chemotherapy patients include xerostomia, angular cheilitis, mucositis (bacterial, viral, or fungal), mucosal bleeding, and odontogenic infection.

   B. When the patient becomes myelosuppressed, there is a predisposition to rampant infection and uncontrollable bleeding from sources not usually problematic.

II. Patient history

   A. The oral surgeon can ascertain the agent to be used and discuss with the physician the experience with oral problems from that agent. Predicted effects on blood counts need to be considered.

   B. The level of the patient's prior oral care and his or her motivation to maintain rigorous oral hygiene must be assessed. One must determine whether any teeth have been symptomatic and whether bleeding in the oral cavity is an existing problem. A history of previous mucositis consistent with bacterial, viral, or fungal infection is important.

   C. A check is made to see whether the patient received prior radiation therapy.

III. Patient examination

   A. Odontogenic infection is carefully sought. Deeply carious teeth must be considered as potential sources of infection.

   B. The periodontal condition is carefully assessed, especially for deep pockets that cannot be kept clean. Friable tissues are noted as potential sources of bleeding. Irritating factors (e.g., sharp edges of teeth, restorations, or prostheses) can also cause bleeding. The condition of the mucosa is evaluated for ulcerations or lacerations that might break down when myelosuppression occurs.

IV. Additional studies—a panoramic and full-mouth periapical series with particular attention to depth of caries, periapical disease, and periodontal condition should be obtained.

V. Response

   A. Restorable teeth should be restored. Endodontic therapy is not contraindicated.

   B. Thorough prophylaxis should be done, and home care with brushing, flossing, and topical fluoride application taught.

   C. Lips can be kept moist with lanolin or nonpetrolatum lubricants to reduce mucosal irritation.

   D. Nonrestorable teeth and hopelessly periodontally involved teeth should be removed. Ideally this will be done 10-14 da before chemotherapy to allow adequate healing before any myelosuppression occurs. If the chemotherapeutic agent causes myelosuppression late in its course, oral surgical treatment can be performed closer to the scheduled start of therapy.

E. If the patient has received prior radiation therapy, treatment will proceed as described earlier.

VI. Follow-up

A. The patient should be examined several times during the course of chemotherapy and afterward. Any oral disease that becomes manifest should be dealt with swiftly.

B. Examination and prophylaxis should be done every 6 mo thereafter, if the WBC and platelet counts permit.

Assessment during or after chemotherapy

I. Purpose

A. Usually the clinician requests treatment of an acute oral problem in a patient debilitated by chemotherapy or by the disease for which it is being used. The chemotherapy or the underlying disease may prevent immediate necessary treatment of the oral problem. In some cases there is no specific treatment other than to await the passing of the side effects from chemotherapy.

B. Sometimes a patient will have a fever of uncertain origin while undergoing chemotherapy. Then, the oral surgeon is called on to identify and treat any likely oral sources of the fever.

II. Patient history

A. For mucosal lesions a prior history consistent with herpes labialis, acute necrotizing ulcerative gingivitis (ANUG), or fungal infection of the mouth should be sought.

B. The oral surgeon must determine whether the patient is myelosuppressed and if special precautions are needed. Thorough hand washing and use of gowns, gloves, and masks may be necessary just to examine the patient. Such patients are often in isolation.

III. Patient examination

A. Topical anesthetic agents may be required to make the patient's irritated mouth comfortable during treatment. Key elements include:

1. Xerostomia—thickened saliva, difficulty with speech
2. Angular cheilitis or mucositis—cracking, bleeding, exudates, broad irregular ulcerations with necrotic centers and surrounding erythema, hemorrhage
3. Mucosal bleeding—usually slow oozing; may indicate a coagulopathy, especially if spontaneous; a surgically controllable bleeding point is sought
4. ANUG—necrotic gingival papillae, bleeding, adenopathy, fetor oris
5. Candidiasis—white plaques, organisms on smears

6. Herpes labialis—crops of vesicles on the mucosa or beyond the mucocutaneous border; viral inclusion bodies on smears of cells taken from the base of a vesicle

B. Odontogenic infection may be accompanied by tenderness or mobility of the teeth involved. Often, because of poly-morphonuclear leukocyte (PMN) suppression, there is no pu-rulence.

IV. Additional studies

A. The following tests may be performed:
1. Panoramic radiographs and specific periapical films if the problem relates to the teeth
2. White blood cell count with differential
3. Bleeding time, PT, PTT
4. Platelet count

B. The pattern of recent WBC counts and coagulation studies should be noted to see whether there is a worsening or im-proving trend. This will help determine the timing of oral surgery and any necessary hematologic replacement therapy.

V. Response

A. Oral hygiene needs to be optimized. If the WBCs are <2000, with <10% PMNs, prophylaxis should not be done and brush-ing and flossing should be discontinued. This is necessary also if the platelet count is <25,000/mm³ or if spontaneous bleeding is a problem. At that point the teeth and tissues should be gently cleaned with gauze or cotton swabs. Rinses of peroxide mixed 1:5 with water can be used, as well. If this is irritating, a solution of table salt (¼ tsp) and baking soda (¼ tsp) to one 8-oz glass of water can be used instead. The baking soda may be eliminated if it is irritating.

B. Xerostomia can be palliated by glycerin swabs, artificially sweetened gum or candy, or artificial saliva.

C. Mucositis is palliated with Kaopectate rinses, often mixed with diphenhydramine (Benadryl). Orabase, with or without benzocaine, can be used. Viscous lidocaine (2%) is helpful but often must be mixed with water (1:2–1:5) to prevent the common irritation encountered at full strength. Dyclonine rinses can also be tried for more refractory cases (but not in patients taking monoamine oxidase inhibitors (MAOIs)). Sys-temic analgesic agents are sometimes necessary. Angular cheilitis can usually be palliated with lanolin or nonpetrola-tum lubricants. In myelosuppressed patients, steroid-contain-ing ointments are generally not advisable.

D. Mucosal bleeding is treated with topical thrombin soaked into sponges or a topical hemostatic (e.g., Avitene) or ε-amino-caproic acid if the PT or PTT is abnormal. If thrombocytope-nia is present, 10–20 U of platelets are transfused. Brushing and flossing are discontinued. A specific bleeding point can be treated surgically with cautery (electrocautery or silver ni-trate sticks) or with a suture.

E. ANUG is treated with parenteral antibiotics, especially penicillin. Gram-negative coverage to prevent opportunistic infections, common in these patients, should be considered. Debridement can be performed if the platelet count allows, but this is usually not the case.

F. Candidiasis is treated with a nystatin swish and swallow or vaginal suppositories held in the mouth. Nystatin ointment is often more adherent to the mucosa than is the rinse. Amphotericin B may be used systemically if systemic candidiasis has been diagnosed or is suspected or when the pharynx and esophagus are involved.

G. Herpes labialis is palliated with lubricating ointments or topical anesthetics. If healing does not occur in 10–14 da, acyclovir (Zovirax) may be required in the sick patient.

H. Odontogenic infection is treated by extraction and, if necessary, drainage. Neutropenia may result in the absence of purulence. A single extraction can usually be safely done if the WBC count is 1500 and the platelet count 25,000/mm^3; otherwise, transfusions of WBCs and platelets are necessary. Coverage with parenteral antibiotic is needed. Aqueous penicillin G (2,000,000 U q4h) is usually chosen, but clindamycin can be used in penicillin-allergic patients (400–600 mg IV q4h).

I. In any oral infection in patients in whom bacterial involvement is likely, therapy needs to include coverage for gram-negative opportunistic organisms in addition to the usual oral flora. Broad-spectrum antibiotics are used.

VI. Follow-up—hemostasis and the development or worsening of infection need to be carefully monitored, especially after oral surgical manipulation.

Assessment of a bleeding patient

I. Purpose

A. Spontaneous oral bleeding necessitates referral to disclose a possible surgically correctable cause. Often an underlying coagulopathy is known or suspected, and only its correction results in definitive hemostasis.

B. Sometimes a patient is referred for severe bleeding after an oral surgical procedure. There may be a sense of alarm that the procedure has unmasked a coagulopathy. More often, the bleeding is from a specific surgically correctable point that was not discovered. Even so, the possibility of a coagulopathy must be borne in mind.

II. Patient history

A. One must elicit information concerning known coagulopathies in the patient or family and must inquire whether hemostasis has been a problem for the patient.

B. It is also necessary to determine whether anticoagulants are in use and to list medications that might induce thrombocytopenia (e.g., quinidine or chemotherapy) or inhibit platelet function (e.g., aspirin).

III. Patient examination
  A. One must search for a specific bleeding point, which will usually be the result of trauma or surgery rather than a coagulopathy. The presence of slow, generalized oozing from tissues often indicates a coagulopathy.
  B. If petechiae are present, thrombocytopenia is likely. Ecchymosis in untraumatized areas may indicate a problem in the extrinsic or intrinsic coagulation pathway.

IV. Additional studies
  A. In the presence of a bleeding point and without a history of coagulopathies, no additional studies are needed as long as the bleeding is effectively controlled.
  B. If a coagulopathy is suspected or if bleeding is refractory despite measures that usually provide adequate control, the bleeding time, PT, PTT, and platelet count should be obtained as a start.

V. Response
  A. Surgical bleeding—"snaps" with the electrocautery needle or sutures with deep "bites" into tissue around the bleeding vessel can be tried if biting on a gauze or tea bag does not work. A figure-8 suture placed through the tissue around the bleeding vessel usually works. If bleeding is related to a fracture, reduction may cause it to stop. If exploration is needed to identify the source of bleeding deep in the tissues, it is usually best done in the operating room with red cell and plasma replacement available.
  B. Coagulopathies
    1. Hemophilia A—normal bleeding time and PT and an elevated PTT (VIII lowered—levels between 5% and 25% in mild cases and 0.25% and 5% in severe cases), the treatment is factor VIII replacement, specifically cryoprecipitate enriched in factor VIII (prepared from plasma [risk of hepatitis]); ε-aminocaproic acid can be used prophylactically (100 mg/kg preoperatively and 100 mg/kg q6h. 10 da postoperatively).
    2. Von Willebrand's disease—for an elevated bleeding time and PTT and a normal PT (impaired platelet adhesiveness) (type I vWF [von Willebrand factor] lowered; type II vWF absent), treatment is cryoprecipitate.
    3. Hemophilia B—for a normal bleeding time and PT and an elevated PTT (factor IX lowered), treatment is factor IX ánd fresh frozen plasma.

VI. Follow-up—close monitoring for continued recurrent bleeding is necessary. Note: tight suturing of the injured tongue or floor of the mouth in a patient with a coagulopathy can lead to massive bleeding in the tissue planes and airway obstruction. A few relatively loosely placed sutures will approximate the tissues while allowing any low-grade oozing to come out of the wound.

General References

American Heart Association: Prevention of bacterial endocarditis, *Statement for health professionals by the Committee on Rheumatic Fever and Ineffective Endocarditis of the Council on Cardiovascular Disease in the Young*, Dallas, 1984, American Heart Association.

Braunwald E et al: *Harrison's principles of internal medicine*, ed 7, New York, 1985, McGraw-Hill.

Judge RD et al: *Clinical diagnosis: a physiologic approach*, ed 5, Boston, 1989, Little, Brown.

Wyngarden JB, Smith LH: *Cecil's textbook of medicine*, ed 19, Philadelphia, 1992, WB Saunders.

Management Considerations in the Medically Compromised Patient

EDWARD B. SELDIN

PREOPERATIVE CONSIDERATIONS

In this chapter we outline considerations that arise in providing oral surgical care for patients with a variety of medical disorders. The conditions selected for discussion were chosen because they occur frequently or because they demand significant alteration of the way in which oral surgical care is delivered. Because this is a chapter on management, we discuss initial diagnosis and treatment only sparingly and assume that we are dealing with patients who have one or more established diagnoses. The disorders discussed in this chapter are:

Cardiac dysfunction
Pulmonary dysfunction
Hypertension
Renal dysfunction
Hepatic dysfunction and alcoholism
Coagulation and bleeding disorders
Seizure disorders
Endocrine dysfunction
Diabetes mellitus
Thyroid dysfunction
Adrenal dysfunction and patients taking corticosteroids
Dysfunction of the immune system, HIV infection, and AIDS

GENERAL CONSIDERATIONS

The initial contact with any new patient should be carefully orchestrated to achieve five specific goals:

1. Assessment of the patient's oral surgical needs
2. Identification of potential management problems
3. Establishment of a good working rapport with the patient
4. Formulation of a treatment plan in light of the patient's oral and medical status
5. Preparation of the patient for indicated procedures

Assessment of the patient's needs

I. The patient visits the doctor "on his own," or is referred by a physician or dentist, usually with a specific goal in mind:

Removal of a tooth
Alleviation of pain
Biopsy of a lesion
Treatment of an infection
Correction of a deformity

II. Sometimes the patient requires a general evaluation and "treatment as necessary."

III. It is essential to recognize that in all but the most straightforward circumstances (and even in some apparently straightforward circumstances), the patient, his or her physician and the consulting oral and maxillofacial surgeon may each have a different perception of the clinical entity in need of attention. The oral surgeon should be aware of the potential for misunderstanding in this setting and should strive to make sure that all parties are in agreement regarding the diagnosis and treatment options.

IV. Having formed an impression of the patient's needs based on history, physical examination, radiographs, and other studies, as required, the oral surgeon should be prepared to assume an active role in communicating with the other participants in the patient's management, including the actual patient, in the interest of reaching a consensus.

Identification of potential management problems

I. Few things are more important than acquiring the habit of taking a brief medical history from all patients. A reasonably complete screening history can be obtained from a well patient in less than 2 min. The further elucidation of positive findings also need not be a lengthy procedure.

II. From a practical point of view, a medical illness may predispose to either or both of two kinds of problems: 1) acute physiologic decompensation under stress, as may occur in the perioperative period, and 2) failure to do well postoperatively because of an infection or impaired hemostasis or wound healing.

III. Circumventing such problems depends in large part on being aware of the potential for their occurrence and then taking adequate precautions. To this end, historic points of special significance, regardless of the specific illness, include:

A. Acuteness versus chronicity of symptoms—It is important to document the stability of the patient's medical condition. If questioning reveals a pattern of increasing symptoms, upgrading the patient's medical regimen may take priority over oral surgical needs. The oral and maxillofacial surgeon may play a vital role in identifying the decompensating patient and placing him or her in proper hands.

B. Physiologic reserve of the patient—It is important also to know something about the patient's capacity for handling physical or emotional stress. Inquiry may be made into the issue of exercise tolerance, response to anxiety-provoking situations, and response to a similar operation in the past. Such information may help determine how much to do at any one time and in what setting to do it (e.g., inpatient versus outpatient, clinic versus operating room).

C. Current medications—Some patients may be unable to state their exact diagnosis. In the absence of medical records, medications can then be a useful indication of what condition(s) the patient is being treated for.

Establishment of a good working rapport with the patient

I. Most routine oral surgical procedures are not inherently physiologically stressful; however, any surgical procedure, especially one to be performed on an awake patient, may be the psychological equivalent of an assault and thus evoke fear, anxiety, and even anger. Such emotional responses are accompanied by the release of endogenous catecholamines and are therefore physiologically taxing, especially to the medically compromised patient with reduced reserve.

II. A major psychological objective is to reduce the assaultive aspect of impending surgery. Toward this end, the value of good rapport with the patient can hardly be overestimated; next to good luck, it is possibly the single most important ingredient in the uneventful management of sick patients.

III. Good rapport markedly reduces anxiety and the need for sedation by pharmacologic means. There are no medications that can compensate for lack of patient confidence in the surgeon. Good rapport flows naturally from a genuine concern for the well-being of the patient. Most patients can immediately sense this quality in those doctors who possess it.

IV. One factor that helps reduce anxiety is attention to choice of language. The manner in which the doctor speaks to the patient should be calculated to optimize communication of essential information rather than to impress the patient with expertise. Terms that have threatening connotations should be avoided, but at the same time, honesty with the patient is essential. The doctrine of informed consent demands, and most patients appreciate, a thorough explanation of a proposed surgical procedure. Taking the time to explain things fully and comprehensibly helps establish rapport and builds trust.

V. A major cause of anxiety for patients is the feeling of loss of control that comes from having to submit to invasions of privacy, not to mention physical intervention. Once again, a full explanation of proposed procedures increases the patient's feeling of participation and allows him or her to maintain a sense of control.

Especially in performing surgery on awake patients, anything that can be done to help preserve this sense of control will make the procedure less stressful. For instance, assure the patient that he or she can call for a pause during a procedure if he or she needs to rest. Also assure him or her that you will stop immediately if he or she reports any pain.

Formulation of a treatment plan

I. Starting from an assessment of the patient's dental needs, the goal of the oral surgeon is to determine the appropriate treatment in light of the patient's medical status. For example, a full course of periodontal therapy, endodontics, and a "roundhouse" splint might be ideal therapy for the patient with advanced periodontal disease and no medical contraindications, but appropriate treatment for the same dental findings in the patient with infective endocarditis who is facing valve replacement might be multiple extractions and full denture prostheses.

II. Having established a treatment plan, the oral surgeon then determines the best setting for carrying it out.

    A. Based on the nature and extent of treatment and the patient's condition and state of mind, a decision is made as to whether to proceed on an inpatient or outpatient basis (if the patient is not already in the hospital when seen) and whether treatment should be carried out in an outpatient unit or in the operating room. These decisions are based, in turn, on the requirements for anesthesia, monitoring, and postoperative care and are best made in consultation with the patient's attending physician and with an anesthesia consultant when a general anesthetic agent is contemplated.

    B. Patient preference is an important factor in the choice of setting and type of anesthesia, as is an objective assessment of anesthetic risk. An anxious patient may express strong preference for a general anesthetic. For many medically compromised patients, general anesthesia has an increased element of risk, but for some of these patients, a well-managed general anesthetic with careful monitoring may be safer than an anxiety-provoking procedure under local anesthesia.

    C. The need for a general anesthetic may be a contraindication to elective surgery in some compromised patients and is an important consideration in treatment planning.

    D. Again, the ability to establish a good working rapport with the patient and to reduce anxiety by nonpharmacologic means extends the range of procedures that can be successfully performed under local anesthesia.

Preparation of the patient for indicated procedures

I. Patients frequently dread oral surgery and other manipulation of their teeth more than they fear a major procedure such as heart surgery.

II. When oral surgery must be performed before other treatment can commence (e.g., before immunosuppression for organ transplantation or before prosthetic valve replacement), the patient may be referred for evaluation and treatment with little or no explanation as to why the oral surgical consultation has been requested. The oral surgeon may be placed in the position of having to inform the patient that before he or she can undergo the procedure for which he or she was admitted, he or she must first submit to the removal of teeth or other oral surgical procedures. In these circumstances the quality of the relationship established with the patient during the evaluation is all important in getting the patient to accept the clinically indicated oral procedure.

SPECIFIC MEDICAL DISORDERS AND ORAL SURGICAL MANAGEMENT
Cardiac dysfunction

I. The term "cardiac dysfunction" is inclusive of numerous clinical entities. Problems of concern to the oral surgeon include:

Angina pectoris and coronary artery occlusive disease
Congestive heart failure
Cardiac arrhythmias
Cardiac valvular disease, especially mitral and aortic stenosis
    and/or regurgitation, and corrected and uncorrected
    congenital heart conditions
Myocardial infarction
Infective endocarditis

II. General considerations
  A. Positioning the awake patient for surgery
    1. Under local anesthesia, the most desirable position for operating may be unsatisfactory for patient comfort.
    2. In the patient with congestive failure, the so-called *cardiac position,* with head and feet elevated, may be optimal. This promotes venous return from the extremities, relieves neck vein engorgement, and eases respiration.
  B. Use of sedative agents
    1. In skilled hands, conscious sedation may be useful in the outpatient care of selected cardiac patients. Nitrous oxide and oxygen are advocated by some, as are a variety of intravenously administered agents, some of which are new, that are in routine use for ASA class I patients.
    2. However, the need for sedation for a given procedure may be taken as an indication to treat the patient in the operating room, where careful monitoring by an anesthesiologist is possible while the surgeon devotes himself or herself fully to the operative procedure and to maintaining verbal contact with the patient. A good argument can be made for monitoring an unstable patient undergoing a procedure under local anesthesia without sedation.

If sedation is to be used, the need for monitoring is absolute because even the most innocuous of agents may have an exaggerated effect on a failing or unstable myocardium.

C. Value of oxygen—In many cardiac patients, oxygen administered by nasal prongs is recommended for various reasons:

1. Breathing air with elevated proportions of oxygen is known to produce a mild euphoria independent of its other physiologic effects.
2. Increasing the oxygen content of inspired air provides better tissue perfusion with no increase in cardiac output, heart rate, or work of the heart.
3. When myocardial oxygenation is improved, ischemic events are less likely, as are arrhythmias.
4. Should cardiopulmonary resuscitation become necessary, an initially well-oxygenated patient is at an advantage from the standpoint of both cerebral ischemia and metabolic acidosis.

D. Local anesthesia

1. 2% Lidocaine (Xylocaine) with 1:100,000 epinephrine is a reasonable choice of agent for the majority of cardiac patients; however, epinephrine should be used with caution or not at all in patients with a history of:
   a. Palpitations or ventricular arrhythmias
   b. Aortic stenosis with symptoms, especially a history of syncope
   c. Angina provoked by minimal exertion or stress
   d. Prior adverse reactions to epinephrine
2. In these cases 4% prilocaine (Citanest) is a useful alternative, as is 3% mepivacaine (Carbocaine).

E. Trinitroglycerin (TNG)—In patients with frequent attacks of angina, especially those whose attacks are triggered by situational anxiety, it may be useful to administer sublingual nitroglycerin just before injection of the local anesthetic agent. Such injections frequently are the most stressful point of an outpatient oral surgery visit. Patients often are more comfortable knowing that TNG is available should they need it.

III. Under stressful circumstances, patients with the following conditions are the most worrisome:

A. Aortic stenosis with a history of syncope

1. Patients with tight aortic stenosis with syncope and/or angina are of great concern because the chances of performing a successful resuscitation in the event of cardiac arrest are extremely poor. This is because closed-chest cardiac massage provides inadequate perfusion in the face of a stenotic valve. In aortic stenosis the heart is essentially contracting isometrically in generating an enormous transvalvular pressure gradient. This kind of pressure work, in contradistinction to volume work, requires

especially high myocardial oxygen consumption and predisposes to ischemia (Fig. 4-1).

  2. The following suggestions may be helpful in treating a patient with aortic stenosis:

    a. Oxygen by nasal prongs is advisable for reasons already discussed.

    b. Epinephrine-containing local anesthetic agents should be avoided. These patients definitely do not need the chronotropic effect of this agent.

    c. Sedation—The operating room is appropriate for patients with symptomatic aortic stenosis.

    d. Monitoring the heart rate is important, as is continuous monitoring of the ECG pattern for ST-segment depression or other signs of ischemia.

    e. Intravenous propranolol (Inderal) may be indicated for the control of heart rate but should be used only in a setting in which intensive monitoring is available.

B. Mitral stenosis or mitral regurgitation with congestive heart failure

  1. Unlike patients with aortic stenosis, this group of patients tends to decompensate more slowly and with more warning. Under stress they may develop congestive symptoms.

  2. The preemptive use of oxygen and sedation is indicated.

C. Coronary artery disease with angina or congestive heart failure. In such patients prophylactic use of nitroglycerin is important, epinephrine should be avoided, and oxygen therapy should be employed.

D. Recent myocardial infarction

  1. Conventional wisdom, backed by clinical studies, suggests that stressful surgery be avoided for 3 and preferably 6 mo after a myocardial infarction. The basis for this is that some of these patients are physiologically more

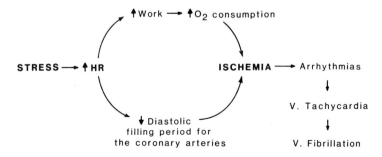

Fig. 4-1 Relationship between work and oxygen consumption. Stress increases the heart rate (*HR*), which in a diseased heart can cause ischemia by both the greater need of the coronary arteries for O_2 and the reduced time available for them to get it.

stable after they have had a chance to recover from the infarction.

2. Some of the more unstable postmyocardial infarction patients exclude themselves by having a second infarction, the likelihood of which decreases with increasing time since the initial infarct.

3. However, if symptomatic teeth cannot be palliated by the use of antibiotics, then emergency treatment (extraction or endodontic therapy) is indicated even in the relatively immediate postinfarction period. The operating room is the safest setting for treatment of these patients (with careful monitoring, oxygen, and sedation), although a suitably equipped and staffed ambulatory facility is satisfactory in most cases.

E. Unstable arrhythmias, ventricular irritability, complete heart block, Stokes-Adams attacks—The need for monitoring makes the operating room mandatory for the performance of surgery on these patients. Use of transvenous pacing during anesthesia is a controversial subject but may be indicated in some circumstances.

IV. Infective endocarditis

A. Infective endocarditis is a rare but potentially devastating disease. It arises when causative organisms infect an area of damaged endothelium on which a platelet thrombus has formed. Such endothelial damage is principally associated with turbulent blood flow produced by regurgitant or stenotic valves, septal defects and other lesions. Thus, the majority of patients at risk for endocarditis are found to have a murmur on physical examination. Exceptions to this rule include patients with recent subendocardial infarction and patients in atrial fibrillation with a clot in the atrial appendage. Bacterial seeding of such lesions is known to occur, although infrequently. It should also be noted that acute bacterial endocarditis, caused by organisms of high pathogenicity that may gain access to the blood stream in the setting of IV drug abuse, can arise in patients with no prior murmur.

B. In patients with a murmur and an unexplained fever, a diagnosis of endocarditis should be considered until definitively ruled out. In this setting, a change in the character of a preexistent murmur is considered to be a highly significant finding, possibly indicating the formation of bacterial vegetations.

C. The onset of endocarditis may be insidious or abrupt, and the course prolonged or fulminant, depending on the virulence of the causative organism.

D. Untreated infective endocarditis is fatal.

E. Defects with which endocarditis and analogous infections are associated include congenital and acquired cardiac and noncardiac lesions.

1. Congenital lesions
   a. Ventricular septal defect
   b. Patent ductus arteriosus
   c. Bicuspid aortic valve
   d. Tetralogy of Fallot
   e. Atrial septal defect (low incidence)
   f. Prolapsing mitral valve (click murmur syndrome)
2. Acquired lesions
   a. Rheumatic valvular lesions
   b. Syphilitic and/or atherosclerotic aortic lesions
   c. Mural thrombi adjacent to subendocardial infarction
   d. Clots in the atrial appendage in atrial fibrillation
3. Foreign bodies
   a. Valve prostheses
   b. Indwelling catheters
   c. Vascular prostheses
   d. Pacing wires (probably *not,* because they endothelialize rapidly)
   e. *Streptococcus viridans* accounts for 70%–80% of infective endocarditis.
   f. Principal manifestations include:
4. Organisms of high pathogenicity *(Staphylococcus)* may destroy the chordae and valve leaflets, leading to valvular insufficiency and fulminant congestive failure.
5. Organisms of low pathogenicity in combination with platelets and fibrin produce vegetations associated with a change in the character of the patient's murmur and with embolization.
6. Embolic phenomena may occur:
   a. Pulmonary embolization from ventricular septal defect, patent ductus, or pulmonic and tricuspid valvular lesions to the lungs leads to pulmonary infarction. The first sign of this may be hemoptysis.
   b. Systemic embolization to:
      (1) Brain (stroke)
      (2) Retinal vessels (blindness or visual field defects)
      (3) Spleen (friction rub, with right upper quadrant abdominal pain)
      (4) Kidneys (hematuria, flank pain, renal infarction, glomerulonephritis)
      (5) GI tract (abdominal pain, ileus, melena)
      (6) Skin and mucous membranes (mucocutaneous petechiae, painful nodules)
      (7) Extremities (Osler's nodes, gangrene)
      (8) Coronary vessels (myocardial infarction)
      (9) Bone (osteomyelitis)
      (10) Vasa vasorum (mycotic aneurysms)

7. Persistent bacteremia produces ongoing fevers with evening temperature spikes. Chills are uncommon in infective endocarditis.

8. Filtration of bacteria and immune complexes by the reticuloendothelial system leads to:
   a. Splenomegaly (usually nontender)
   b. Anemia
   c. Increased bilirubin from sequestration and destruction of RBCs, producing jaundice
   d. Immune complex nephritis, arthritis, or arthralgia resembling that occurring with acute rheumatic fever, vasculitis, petechiae (Roth's spots in the eye)

F. Laboratory findings include:
   1. Increased WBC count and neutrophilia
   2. Anemia (normocytic, normochromic)
   3. Histiocytes seen on peripheral smears
   4. Increased sedimentation rate
   5. Increased immunoglobulins
   6. Mild bilirubinemia
   7. Urinalysis: proteinuria and microscopic hematuria
   8. Positive blood cultures in 85% of cases (when organisms are recovered, they are found in one of three culture bottles 98% of the time)

G. Because endocardial vegetations contain anoxic slow-growing organisms, bactericidal levels of antibiotics at dilutions of 1:8 or better are usually maintained for 4–6 wk. Defervescence usually occurs 3–7 da after commencement of appropriate therapy. If symptoms recur during treatment, superinfection with a resistant organism must be ruled out.

H. Prognosis
   1. Untreated endocarditis has a fatal outcome.
   2. Treated infective endocarditis has an overall survival rate of 70%.
   3. When penicillin-sensitive streptococcal organisms are cultured, survival is 90%.
   4. A poor prognosis is associated with:
      a. Congestive heart failure
      b. Culture-negative endocarditis
      c. Resistant organisms
      d. Delayed treatment
      e. Prosthetic valve endocarditis (about 50% survival for plastic and metal valves, somewhat better for porcine heterografts)

I. Prophylaxis
   1. The majority of organisms implicated in infective endocarditis are constituents of the normal oral flora. It has been well established that professional manipulation of the teeth, home hygiene activities, and even chewing produce transient bacteremias, the magnitude of which re-

flect the individual's state of dental and periodontal health. Equally well established is the role of transient bacteremias in the pathogenesis of endocarditis.

2. Based on the foregoing, there are two main concerns in providing prophylaxis: protection of the patient from bacteremias induced by professional manipulation, and protection from bacteremias caused by underlying dental and periodontal disease.

3. The American Heart Association (AHA) updates its published guidelines for prophylactic coverage for invasive dental therapy at regular intervals (refer to Appendix III). Copies of these guidelines can be obtained by writing to the AHA or to the journal *Circulation.* Similar documents are available from the American Dental Association. All dentists and oral and maxillofacial surgeons should be familiar with this material.

4. Because, according to the Surgeon General, the average American goes to a dentist twice a year, the antibiotics given during invasive procedures work only for those bacteremias that occur in the context of professional care. These professionally induced transient bacteremias are numerically insignificant when compared with the thousands that occur annually in conjunction with home hygiene activities such as brushing and flossing and with chewing. It is also not clear that bacteremias induced by professional care are necessarily of greater magnitude than those produced at home.

5. The efficacy of prophylactic antibiotics has never been established in a satisfactory clinical study. Their use is based on good intentions, disseminated advice from the AHA, and medicolegal considerations.

6. Because chronic administration of antibiotics to at-risk individuals is unreasonable and probably not efficacious, the best way of protecting these patients is to reduce the magnitude of transient bacteremias by minimizing dental disease as much as possible. Pathologically mobile teeth should be eliminated, and active periapical and periodontal disease should be treated either by extraction or by more conservative means consistent with the restorability of the dentition and with the patient's motivation to establish and maintain a satisfactory level of dental health. This applies particularly to patients with prosthetic valves, for whom endocarditis carries a 50–50 chance of mortality. It is similarly important for patients with prior episodes of infective endocarditis. These patients must be presumed to be uniquely susceptible and liable to have additional episodes of endocarditis.

7. The hospital-based oral and maxillofacial surgeon should be available to screen prosthetic valve and endocarditis

patients and to actively confer with cardiologists, internists, or cardiac surgeons regarding the management of such patients.

Pulmonary dysfunction

I. General considerations
  A. The respiratory apparatus, including the lungs, pulmonary tree, pulmonary vasculature, and thoracic musculoskeletal system, adds oxygen to and recovers carbon dioxide from the bloodstream.
  B. Carbon dioxide, produced by oxidative metabolism, forms carbonic acid and thus contributes hydrogen ions to the blood. Thus, retention of carbon dioxide produces respiratory acidosis.
  C. Conversely, hyperventilation, which emits carbon dioxide, produces a respiratory alkalosis. When hyperventilation is chronic, the resultant respiratory acidosis is normally balanced by a compensatory metabolic alkalosis, maintaining the normal pH. Therefore, the lungs, in addition to providing oxygen and recovering carbon dioxide, are intimately involved, along with the kidneys, in the maintenance of the acid-base balance.
II. Diagnosis
  A. The analysis of arterial blood gases (ABGs) reveals whether the respiratory apparatus is functioning properly. The interpretation of blood gases is discussed in Chapter 6.
  B. In addition to ABGs, a thorough evaluation of pulmonary function includes pulmonary function tests (PFTs), which measure the mechanics of respiration (breathing), ventilation (gas exchange at the alveolar level), and oxygenation (delivery of O_2 to the hemoglobin in the blood).
    1. Mechanics of respiration
      a. When one takes a full breath and exhales as fully as possible, the volume of air exhaled is the vital capacity (VC) (average 4.8 L in men, 3.1 L in women). Total lung capacity includes vital capacity plus a residual volume of air that is still present in the lungs after full exhalation.
      b. At rest one normally inhales and exhales only a fraction of vital capacity; this volume (0.5 L) is called tidal volume (V_T). The volume of air that can be inspired above the V_T is called inspiratory reserve volume (IRV), and the volume of air that can be exhaled below V_T is called expiratory reserve volume (ERV). These are shown diagrammatically in Fig. 4-2.
      c. Dead space volume (V_D) is the volume of air in the pulmonary tree that does not come in contact with alveolar surfaces and thus does not participate in gas exchange. Residual volume (RV) plus ERV is called the functional residual capacity (FRC).

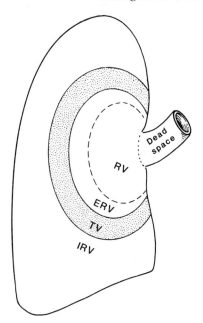

VC = TV + ERV + IRV

FRC = RV + ERV

Fig. 4-2   Vital capacity.

d. Respiratory mechanics are measured by having the patient blow through a spirometer, which measures both volumes and flows and graphically displays these in a spirogram (Fig. 4-3).

   (1) Modern spirometers incorporate computers that allow an automatic comparison to be made between observed values and predicted values based on age, gender, height, and weight. Some of these devices will also print out an interpretation of differences between observed and predicted values.

   (2) Parameters typically measured include:

   First sec of VC (L)
   VC (L)
   First sec of VC/VC%
   Peak expiratory flow rate (L/sec)
   Expiratory flow at 50% of VC (L/sec)
   Peak inspiratory flow rate (L/sec)
   Maximal breathing capacity (L/min)

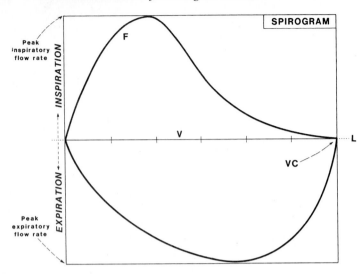

Fig. 4-3 Typical spirogram.

(3) Different pulmonary diseases produce characteristic changes in the spirogram and parameters.
  a) For example, decreased expiratory flow at
  25% of VC suggests abnormality of the small
  airways.
  b) Parenchymal disease of the lung is associated
  with diminished VC.
  c) Bronchitis and emphysema typically reduce
  expiratory peak flow and maximal breathing
  capacity. In emphysema, RV and FRC are increased in proportion to VC.
2. Ventilation
  a. Alveolar membranes are exposed to a mixture of freshly
  inspired air plus previously expired air occupying dead
  space in the tracheobronchial tree and pharynx.
  b. V_T is calculated by dividing the minute volume (measured using an expiratory spirometer) by the respiratory rate. When it is small, a larger proportion of dead
  space air is rebreathed and the percentage of O_2 in the
  mixture reaching the alveolar surface is decreased.
  The ratio of dead space ventilation to total ventilation
  (V_D/V_T) is determined by measuring expired CO_2
  (Pe_{CO_2}) and arterial CO_2 (Pa_{CO_2}):

$$\frac{V_D}{V_T} = \frac{Pa_{CO_2} - Pe_{CO_2}}{Pa_{CO_2}}$$

  c. Occasionally, dead space is deliberately added to increase the retention of CO_2 when a patient is hyper-

ventilating. This is the reason for having a patient with carpopedal spasm who is hyperventilating breathe into a paper bag. Similarly, dead space may be added during mechanical ventilation by inserting a tube or rebreathing vessel into the system.

3. Oxygenation
   a. Oxygen content of the blood is measured as a part of arterial blood gases. How well oxygenated the blood is when it enters the aorta, however, depends on the percentage of pulmonary blood flow that actually circulates through the capillaries in the walls of well-ventilated alveoli.
   b. Normally about 2% of cardiac output consists of blood not exposed to pulmonary exchange surfaces. This includes blood passing through the bronchial vessels and also the venous outflow from the coronary arteries. It is called the physiologic shunt.
   c. Various disease states lead to pathologic shunting of blood and decreased oxygenation. These include a number of irreversible parenchymal diseases of the lungs plus some potentially reversible conditions (e.g., atelectasis). In atelectasis, blood flowing through the atelectic segments contributes to the shunt but can be corrected by good pulmonary toilet and ventilatory assistance. The quantity of shunt (Q_S/Q_T) can be calculated from the measured alveolar-arterial oxygen difference ($AaDO_2$) after breathing 100% oxygen long enough to reach a steady state (usually 20 min). Because this calculation is undertaken principally in the setting of intensive care, we will not elaborate further. Even when breathing 100% oxygen, the oxygenation can vary greatly as a function of the quantity of shunt present.

III. Management
   A. Only the most severe respiratory compromise is a contraindication to routine outpatient oral surgical care.
   B. Asthma, principally an allergic phenomenon, may also be brought on by emotional factors (e.g., stress). Thus, in at least some patients with asthma, management of stress related to oral surgery is essential. Sedative agents may be useful. Establishment of a good doctor–patient relationship is very helpful. During treatment of asthmatics in the outpatient setting, oxygen should be available, and it should be possible to establish an intravenous line on short notice for hydration and administration of a bronchodilator.
   C. The patient with significant respiratory disease who requires general anesthesia will usually be managed on an inpatient basis. PFTs may be important to quantify the patient's degree of compromise, and a preoperative anesthesia consultation may be advisable.

D. The presence of severe degrees of respiratory compromise is a contraindication to the use of intermaxillary fixation (IMF), because IMF increases upper airway resistance and makes pulmonary function difficult to maintain. In this setting, rigid fixation is indicated for both fractures and osteotomies. If IMF is unavoidable, consideration should be given to elective tracheostomy.

E. Pulmonary complications of multiple trauma, including lung shock, may delay definitive repair of facial injuries. It is therefore essential to make every effort to evaluate facial fractures immediately and to treat these as completely as possible while other members of the trauma team carry out the emergency repair of other injuries. In discussions with other members of the trauma team, the oral surgeon should be prepared to make the case for early treatment of facial injuries in order to spare the patient the potential adverse sequelae of delayed treatment of oral and facial injuries, which may include unnecessary loss of teeth, diminished function, malocclusion and compromised facial aesthetics.

F. Under normal circumstances homeostatic control of respiratory activity is keyed to blood levels of carbon dioxide detected by sense organs in the carotid bodies. However, in patients with chronic obstructive pulmonary disease (COPD) and retention of carbon dioxide, the respiratory response to carbon dioxide is diminished or absent and hypoxemia becomes the stimulus to respiration. Thus, in patients with COPD, the sudden exposure to oxygen in high concentration may eliminate the hypoxic stimulus, leading to hypoventilation and even apnea. Therefore, 100% oxygen is inappropriate for patients with COPD who are breathing spontaneously.

G. Various CNS diseases (e.g., stroke, coma, seizure disorders, brain tumors, intoxication), certain medications, and old age diminish the reflex protection of the airway. The risk of aspiration increases in proportion to the degree of debilitation.

  1. In severely debilitated patients, unless appropriate measures are taken, the risk of aspiration is heightened by poor oral hygiene, increasing dental disease, and the accumulation of bacteria-laden oral debris.

  2. Oral surgical consultation on such patients should stress the importance of good oral hygiene. In some instances, especially when periodontal disease is severe, prophylactic extraction of teeth may be appropriate.

H. In many of the above settings, pulse oximetry has become an essential component of patient management and can be lifesaving for patients sent back to a hospital room with IMF.

Hypertension

I. Hypertension is defined as a persistent elevation of blood pressure above values normal for age, measured during repeated examinations.

A. As a disease entity, hypertension denotes mainly the elevation of diastolic pressure; 90 mm Hg is considered the upper level of normal for young adults. Blood pressure tends to increase with age; thus, a given elevation of diastolic pressure is considered more significant in a young person than in an older one. Diastolic pressures in the ranges of 90–110, 110–130, and >130 define mild, moderate, and severe hypertension, respectively.

B. When diastolic pressure is normal, systolic hypertension generally denotes the loss of elasticity of arterial vessel walls, as seen in atherosclerosis. It can also be seen when cardiac output is elevated above normal (as in exercise, fever, anemia, thyrotoxicosis, or the presence of large atrioventricular [AV] fistulas).

II. The principal cause of diastolic hypertension is elevated total peripheral resistance, arterioles being the major resistive element in the vascular bed. Hypertension may be asymptomatic for long periods, and early manifestations (e.g., headache, palpitations, dizziness) can be vague. Epistaxis, hematuria, and proteinuria may also occur.

III. The principal consequences of uncorrected hypertension are renal failure, accelerated cardiovascular disease (including coronary artery disease and congestive failure), and cerebral vascular disease. Examination of the retinal vessels (funduscopic examination) is a useful means of assessing the damage caused by hypertension. Typical changes include compression of venules by arterioles (AV nicking), segmental constriction of arterioles, flame-shaped hemorrhages, and white exudative patches. Papilledema (seen as blurring of the disc margins and due to swelling that alters the visual plane of the optic disc) is suggestive of advanced disease and is a poor prognostic sign, as is elevation of blood urea nitrogen (BUN) secondary to hypertensive renal disease.

IV. The workup for hypertension includes the following:

A. Documentation of the presence of hypertension. Because situational anxiety associated with medical visits can elevate blood pressure, the documentation of mild to moderate hypertension can be difficult, requiring multiple determinations on separate visits or during a hospital admission. Elevation of blood pressure under general anesthesia is a significant finding.

B. Attempts to identify surgically correctable causes:
1. Pheochromocytoma of the adrenal cortex
2. Renal arterial occlusion
3. Renal parenchymal disease
4. Coarctation of the aorta

C. Assessment of damage already done by the condition, especially with regards to:
1. Renal function
2. Cardiovascular status

V. When surgically correctable causes have been ruled out, treatment of hypertension consists of drug therapy and dietary control.

A. Because obesity is a contributing factor, weight reduction is part of the therapy for hypertension.

B. Sodium restriction is another dietary approach to therapy. In restricting sodium, the goal is presumably to cause a fluid volume contraction and thus a fall in cardiac output and blood pressure.

C. Drugs used in hypertensive therapy are:

1. Diuretics (including the thiazides and aldosterone antagonists)

2. Ganglionic-blocking agents, which reduce autonomic vasoconstriction

3. Norepinephrine antagonists, which block production or compete for receptor sites

4. Smooth muscle relaxants

5. Beta-adrenergic blocking agents, which work at the receptor sites (propranolol, atenolol, etc.)

6. CNS agents, which work on spinal or thalamic vasomotor centers

7. Tranquilizers, which work on the psychogenic component of hypertension

8. Calcium-channel blocking agents (nifedipine, Procardia, etc.), which relax smooth muscle in vessel walls, promote peripheral pooling and decrease the preload of the heart

9. Angiotensin-converting enzyme (ACE) inhibiters (Capoten, etc.), which work by competitive inhibition of ACE, which controls conversion of angiotensin I to angiotensin II

D. Except in mild forms of hypertension, multiple drug therapy is used both to capitalize on drug synergy and to lower the required dosage for each agent, thereby reducing undesirable side effects.

E. Management considerations in hypertensive patients include:

1. Mild to moderate hypertension in adults is not a contraindication to oral surgical procedures under local anesthesia.

2. Severe hypertension, if suspected on the basis of patient evaluation for elective surgery, should be fully worked up and treated before elective surgery.

3. A diastolic pressure >150 mm Hg is grounds for admission to the hospital for workup and immediate treatment.

4. Emergency surgery in the patient discovered to be hypertensive may be undertaken with caution. If the degree of hypertension warrants it, parenteral therapy may be instituted in conjunction with the general anesthesia, as required.

5. In the patient with long-standing hypertension and associated vascular disease, adequate perfusion of brain and

myocardium may require elevated blood pressure. Then "normal" blood pressure can predispose to ischemia and damage to vital organs.

6. Because psychogenic factors play a significant role in hypertension, sedative techniques may prove useful. Once again, the value of a good doctor–patient relationship cannot be overemphasized as an aid to the control of such factors.

7. Some antihypertensive medications complicate the administration of general anesthesia.

   a. The issue of whether to discontinue antihypertensive medications in anticipation of elective surgery under general anesthesia engenders much discussion. The oral surgeon should raise the issue with the patient's physician and also with an anesthesia consultant in advance of surgery.

   b. Generally one would like to eliminate long-acting drugs that inhibit homeostatic cardiovascular reflexes from the patient's therapeutic regimen. However, in a severely hypertensive patient, the need for control of blood pressure may preclude discontinuation of therapy.

      (1) Special care must be exercised in the case of beta-blocking agents such as propranolol, which is in wide use today. When such medications are stopped abruptly, blood pressure may rebound to levels exceeding those before therapy was instituted. Beta blockade must therefore be withdrawn gradually. Some anesthesiologists prefer to continue beta blockers in the perioperative period.

      (2) The advisability of timely anesthesia consultation cannot be overemphasized.

8. Preoperative evaluation of the hypertensive patient must include an assessment of renal and cardiac function. Chest radiograph, ECG, BUN, creatinine, and electrolytes are appropriate baseline studies, with further work-up as may be dictated by historic and physical findings.

9. Hemostasis requires special attention in hypertensive patients. Not only may it be more difficult to achieve intraoperatively, but there is an increased risk of postoperative bleeding if the blood pressure, well-controlled during general anesthesia, increases significantly after the patient reaches the recovery room. Postoperative orders must both stress the careful monitoring of blood pressure and specify the level of pressure above which the house officer, surgeon, or attending physician should be called.

10. Conversely, because of the risk of ischemia in tissues fed by vessels adapted to high blood pressure, all parties concerned should be vigilant about hypotension.

11. The patient with both hypertension and ischemic heart disease merits special attention. Blood pressure must be high enough to perfuse myocardial tissues through partially occluded coronary vessels. However, the work required of the heart to maintain elevated pressures leads to increased myocardial oxygen consumption and augments the likelihood of ischemia. Thus, in such a patient, the range of acceptable blood pressures is much narrower than normal, and careful monitoring is required.

Renal disease

I. There are many causes and manifestations of renal disease.

II. Renal insufficiency may be acute or chronic.

A. In the acute condition, independent of etiology, the principal manifestations are oliguria and progressive azotemia.

1. Acute renal failure may occur for reasons extrinsic to the kidneys (prerenal azotemia):
   a. Hypotension (shock)
   b. Congestive heart failure
   c. Extracellular fluid volume contraction, as occurs in dehydration, blood loss, or long-term uncompensated nasogastric suction

2. Intrinsic causes of acute renal failure include:
   a. Acute glomerulonephritis
   b. Acute vasculitis
   c. Acute urinary tract obstruction

3. Acute renal failure is also a feature of the hepatorenal syndrome, which is seen in some patients with advanced liver disease and portal hypertension. The hepatorenal syndrome typically occurs after massive gastrointestinal bleeding from varices and associated therapeutic measures.

B. Chronic renal failure is associated with an irreversible loss of functioning nephrons. Decreased size of the kidneys is demonstrated by appropriate radiographic or ultrasound studies.

C. Renal disease may advance insidiously until the patient is in severe failure. The workup of such a patient must distinguish between acute renal failure and chronic renal insufficiency.

III. Laboratory measurements in renal failure include the following:

A. Glomerular filtration rate (GFR)

1. The GFR is the principal index of renal function. Normal values are 100–150 ml/min, which is the volume of plasma removed from the approximately 1250 ml of blood passing through the two kidneys per minute. (Renal blood flow is about 25% of cardiac output.) Patients with renal disease generally remain free of symptoms until the GFR falls below 10 ml/min.

2. In clinical practice the GFR is not measured directly but is estimated by measuring the clearance of various sub-

stances from the plasma. The clearance of endogenous creatinine is considered to be a good indicator of glomerular function.

    a. Creatinine clearance is measured by assaying creatinine in a 24-hr collection of urine and by measuring the serum creatinine once during that period.

$$\text{Clearance} = \frac{\text{mg/ml urine} \times \text{ml urine/min}}{\text{mg/ml plasma}}$$

    b. Normal creatinine clearances
        (1) Men: 97–140 ml/min
        (2) Women: 85–125 ml/min
  3. The GFR, as approximated from creatinine clearance, is the rate of passive filtration by the glomeruli. It tells nothing about active secretion and resorption of substances by the renal tubules.

B. Blood urea nitrogen
  1. The BUN is another important measurement in renal failure. However, it reflects renal function only indirectly.
    a. It rises when renal function is severely compromised, but an increase in protein degradation (as occurs with gastrointestinal bleeding) will also increase the BUN.
    b. Conversely, a BUN elevated by renal disease will fall when dietary protein is restricted, but this fall need not reflect any improvement in renal function.
  2. The normal BUN is 8–25 mg/dl. Symptoms of uremia do not generally appear until the BUN exceeds 75–100 mg/dl. The BUN is a measure only of renal function under steady state conditions. In these circumstances a reading of 100 suggests a GFR <10 ml/min.

C. Renal tubular function
  1. The renal tubules concentrate the urine and maintain normal hydration.
  2. They regulate the acid-base balance through active secretion of hydrogen ions and resorption of bicarbonate and other bases.
  3. They also maintain normal mineral and electrolyte balance and retrieve glucose and other essential substances from the glomerular filtrate.

D. In renal failure there are disturbances of the above functions that reflect both the variety and the severity of the renal disease responsible. Most of these disturbances are correctable by measures that range from dietary control to renal dialysis and renal transplantation.

E. In addition to serum creatinine, creatinine clearance, and BUN, a work-up of renal function involves determination of plasma and urine electrolytes, glucose, protein, calcium, and phosphorus, as well as serum osmolarity and urine specific gravity and H+ concentration. Microscopic examination of the urine is performed to detect RBCs, WBCs, bacteria, crystalline and amorphous solids, and tubular casts, each of which has diagnostic significance.

IV. Management considerations include the following:

A. Compensated renal disease is not a contraindication to routine oral surgery or dental care.

B. It is fair to say that the patient with acute renal failure is not a candidate for routine dental care. Dental problems arising in this setting are treated emergently, and the goal is to palliate dental pain and treat dental infection with antibiotics (incision and drainage if indicated) until the renal problem is stabilized and more definitive dental treatment can be carried out.

C. The choice of medications for the patient in renal failure must be made with reference to the mode of excretion or degradation and with consideration of possible renal toxicity. A renal route of excretion is not necessarily a contraindication to drug use, but adjustment of the dosage is called for. Such therapy should be instituted in consultation with the patient's primary physician.

D. Severe uremia may interfere with normal hemostatic mechanisms, particularly platelet function. Wound healing may also be compromised. However, the patient who has compensated renal disease (with a BUN <75 mg/dl) and who is not in a negative nitrogen balance from a protein-wasting nephropathy will generally heal normally. The patient with chronic renal failure is prone to hypocalcemia and hyperphosphatemia, which, along with other factors, may lead to secondary hyperparathyroidism. Osteomalacia and osteitis fibrosa may develop, and the possibility of such disorders of bone metabolism should be taken into account when a patient with renal failure is being evaluated for surgery involving the facial bones.

E. Moderate renal disease, not producing symptoms by itself, may become significant in the face of other medical problems (e.g., heart disease). Thus, the patient who has a failing myocardium and renal insufficiency may go into congestive failure at an early stage owing to hypoperfusion of intrinsically damaged kidneys and resultant fluid retention. Similarly, a patient prone to arrhythmias may be very sensitive to disturbances of electrolyte balance produced by renal disease, such as hypokalemia or hypercalcemia.

F. Compensated renal disease is not necessarily a contraindication to general anesthesia, but such patients deserve very careful preoperative evaluation to assess the level of renal function and to detect and correct electrolyte and other imbalances. The presence of renal disease may contraindicate some anesthetic agents and favor others. An anesthesia consultation before surgery is appropriate for the patient with significant renal disease.

G. Patients receiving dialysis are closely monitored by the attending physician or nephrologist. When oral surgical care is called for, it is usually necessitated by a dental emergency, and in these cases treatment is usually palliative.

   1. Simple outpatient procedures (e.g., extraction of teeth) are not generally a problem under local anesthesia, and the use of lidocaine (Xylocaine) with epinephrine is not contraindicated.

   2. Special considerations in the dialysis patient include:

      a. Choice of medications and regulation of dose. The medications for such a patient should be selected in consultation with the patient's physician. Penicillin is not contraindicated, but the dose will be regulated on the basis of residual renal function and the patient's frequency of dialysis. Given the difficulty of eliminating potassium by dialysis, sodium may be substituted for the more usual potassium penicillin.

      b. Anticoagulation—because a dialysis patient is anticoagulated during dialysis runs, surgical procedures are best performed midway between runs, if possible.

      c. Elevated risk of hepatitis—the strict adherence to universal precautions pays dividends in this setting, as does the prior immunization of all staff with direct contact with patients. It may be reasonable to institute hepatitis precautions for dialysis patients.

      d. Long-term management—when a dialysis patient is seen, it is worthwhile to discuss long-term management with the attending physician, especially as it relates to possible renal transplantation.

      e. The chronic dialysis patient will usually have a surgically created AV shunt (radial artery to cephalic vein) to facilitate arterial and venous cannulation during dialysis runs. These shunts have the potential to become infected by transient bacteremias. Thus, it is appropriate to eliminate dental foci of infection and to use prophylactic antibiotic coverage for invasive dental treatment.

H. Under favorable circumstances the renal transplant patient will maintain essentially normal renal function. Unless the donor kidney came from an identical twin or other individual with identical histocompatibility antigens, the patient will require chronic immunosuppressive therapy. Such therapy reduces the capacity to fight infection. Therefore, it is essential that the patient be maintained in an optimal state of dental health. The best time for evaluating and providing for such a patient's dental needs is before the start of immunosuppression. Setting up a program for routine preoperative screening of prospective renal transplant patients is worthwhile.

Hepatic dysfunction and alcoholism

I. The liver is the largest gland in the body and performs many functions:

    A. It secretes bile.

        1. Bile salts are essential to the emulsification and absorption of fatty substances from the intestines.

        2. Bile contains pigmented substances, bilirubin, and related compounds that are excreted with conjugated glucuronic acid. These pigments are breakdown products of hemoglobin from the lysis of RBCs.

        3. Bile contains substances deactivated, conjugated, and excreted by the liver (e.g., drugs, endogenous substances such as adrenal and gonadal steroid hormones, and toxic substances ingested as part of the diet).

    B. The liver plays an essential role in the metabolism of carbohydrates and fats, and it stores carbohydrates as glycogen.

    C. It is central to protein metabolism, including degradation of amino acids and formation of urea.

    D. It manufactures plasma proteins, including albumin.

    E. It produces many specialized substances (e.g., proteins active in the immune system and clotting factors such as II, VII, IX, and X).

    F. It has a dual blood supply. In addition to arterial flow, from which it derives oxygen, the liver also receives the venous outflow from the gastrointestinal tract via the portal circulation. All substances absorbed through the GI tract must therefore traverse the liver before entering the general circulation.

II. Categories of liver disease of greatest interest to the oral and maxillofacial surgeon are hepatitis and cirrhosis.

    A. Hepatitis denotes any acute inflammatory condition of the liver. There are many kinds, ranging from hepatitis caused by toxic chemicals such as carbon tetrachloride and chloroform to hepatitis caused by infectious agents, including bacteria and viruses.

        1. Hepatotoxicity sets the upper limits on safe dosage for many medications, including some anesthetic agents, anticonvulsants, many antibiotics, thiazide diuretics, and oral contraceptives.

        2. Of concern to the oral surgeon is the patient with acute viral hepatitis or chronic active hepatitis (carrier state), because of the risk of acquiring the disease through inadvertent inoculation with contaminated instruments.

            a. There are several types of viral hepatitis, including A, B, non-A, and non-B (now referred to as hepatitis C).

Hepatitis is also a feature of mononucleosis in about 5% of cases.

b. Of the viral hepatitides, types B and C are the biggest concern because both can be transmitted percutaneously, and because fulminant disease has a significant rate of mortality (up to 15% in some series). In addition, 10% of patients develop chronic liver disease (chronic active hepatitis), and patients with a history of hepatitis have a risk of liver cancer exceeding that of nonhepatitis patients.

3. Measures to prevent hepatitis include the following:

a. An effective and safe vaccine produced by recombinant biotechnology is currently available for the prevention of type B hepatitis. Fears attached to the use of the first of the hepatitis B vaccines, that inoculation might place the recipient at risk for AIDS, are now groundless. Many hospitals make vaccination available to at-risk personnel. Oral and maxillofacial surgeons and surgical support staff are well advised to seek vaccination if they do not already have antibodies. It is appropriate to be tested for antibodies not only before but also after vaccination to confirm that protection has been conferred, because the vaccine does not induce antibody formation in every individual.

b. A vaccination for hepatitis A is now available. Recommendations for its administration to health care workers are not fully formulated as yet but will become available as experience is gathered. A vaccine for hepatitis C is not yet a practical reality but is greatly desired because the prevalence of hepatitis C is increasing and because it is emerging as a significant cause of severe liver disease.

c. Hepatitis B–specific immune globulin reduces the likelihood of contracting hepatitis B after percutaneous exposure by a factor of 3 to 10. However, pooled gamma globulin is not effective against type B and is only somewhat effective against type C hepatitis. These measures are, at best, a poor substitute for vaccination in the prevention of hepatitis B.

d. Other prophylactic measures include proper isolation, proper sterilization of instruments, and proper disposal of needles and contaminated materials (drapes, sponges, and sutures). The oral and maxillofacial surgeon should be thoroughly familiar with institutional protocols for dealing with known or suspected hepatitis patients, including instructions on the proper handling, containment, and identification of laboratory specimens for the protection of other hospital personnel.

e. Universal precautions—it is important to bear in mind that the greatest risk of exposure to hepatitis comes not from known or suspected cases but from unknown cases, as is also true for HIV infection. Therefore, one's routine sterile technique, use of biologic barriers, and other practices should be fastidious enough to confer a high degree of protection from infectious agents that may be bourne by any patient. Inoculation can occur through the conjunctiva, and proper eye protection tends to be underutilized. All institutions have infection control policies, and private offices should as well. Most such policies are based on Centers for Disease Control (CDC) recommendations as well as Occupational Safety & Health Administration (OSHA) regulations. It is important that all individuals at risk by virtue of contact with patients familiarize themselves with institutional guidelines and requirements.

4. Whether or not a person with an occupational risk of hepatitis elects to be vaccinated, he or she should be tested for antibodies, because 5%–15% of the population has hepatitis B antibodies.

   a. In the event of accidental inoculation when the status of the source is unknown, it is appropriate to test the source for hepatitis B surface antigen (HBsAg), antibody (anti-HBs), and also SGPT (alanine aminotransferase) as an index of hepatocellular inflammation. Testing for HIV antibodies may also be indicated.

   b. Accidental inoculation from patients in the following groups merits heightened concern:
      (1) Those with acute viral hepatitis of an unknown type
      (2) Those institutionalized with Down's syndrome
      (3) Those receiving hemodialysis
      (4) Patients of (recent) Asian origin
      (5) Male homosexuals
      (6) Known drug abusers

5. Signs and symptoms of acute viral hepatitis include jaundice preceded by a variable period of other nonspecific constitutional and GI symptoms including dark urine (94% of patients), fatigue (91%), anorexia (90%), nausea (87%), and fever (76%). The onset of jaundice is usually accompanied by hepatic enlargement and right upper quadrant tenderness. Symptoms noted in the preicteric phase tend to increase in severity as the jaundice becomes manifest and tend to abate as the jaundice subsides.

6. The following are some management considerations in hepatitis:

    a. No elective procedure should be undertaken in a patient with acute viral hepatitis.

    b. Any emergency procedure in a patient with acute viral hepatitis should be undertaken only with full precautions, as noted above.

    c. When a choice exists, local anesthesia is preferable to general anesthesia. Many agents used for or in conjunction with general anesthesia have a degree of hepatotoxicity or are metabolized in the liver and may be poorly tolerated by the patient with acute viral hepatitis.

    d. All drugs for use by hepatitis patients should be selected with reference to possible hepatotoxicity.

B. Cirrhosis

  1. This term denotes a fibrosis disrupting the lobular architecture, on which normal hepatic function depends. If the ongoing disease process is arrested at an early stage, excellent healing may occur with preservation of normal function. When the disease process has been long-standing, some healing may occur, but widespread disruption of the lobular architecture may prevent the return of normal liver function.

  2. Cirrhosis is seen in the 10% of patients whose viral hepatitis (type B) goes on to become chronic active hepatitis.

  3. The most common cause of cirrhosis in the United States is chronic alcoholism. Malnutrition is thought to be a contributing factor in this setting but does not independently lead to cirrhosis in the absence of alcoholism.

  4. Because of the liver's remarkable regenerative capacity and built-in redundancy, the onset of cirrhosis is insidious. Early presenting symptoms can be nonspecific and tend to be masked by the symptoms of alcoholism and malnutrition. The two primary manifestations of cirrhosis are hepatocellular dysfunction and portal hypertension.

    a. Hepatocellular dysfunction

      (1) Active hepatocellular disease is suggested by elevation of liver enzymes in the blood including SGOT (aspartate aminotransferase) and LDH (lactic dehydrogenase). Alkaline phosphatase also tends to be elevated, especially when there is obstruction of biliary drainage. As hepatocellular disease progresses, serum albumin falls while globulin levels are selectively maintained. Thus, total protein tends to fall and the A/G ratio reverses.

      (2) As noted previously, clotting factors VII, IX, and X, along with prothrombin, are manufactured in the liver. The PT increases in response to decreased production of these factors; however,

prolongation of the PT is a late sign of liver disease and denotes severe hepatocellular dysfunction.

(3) Carbohydrate metabolism may become disordered, with loss of glycogen stores and an increasing tendency toward hypoglycemia.

(4) Ammonia, a product of the action of bacterial deaminases on amino acids in the intestines, is normally removed from the portal circulation by the liver and converted to urea. In liver failure, ammonia accumulates in the bloodstream, leading to hyperreflexia, a characteristic tremor (asterixis, or "liver flap"), and hepatic encephalopathy (marked by confusion, drowsiness, and inappropriate behavior). Uncorrected ammonia intoxication can eventually cause hepatic coma and death.

(5) The principal mode of treatment for hepatic encephalopathy is to decrease ammonia production by sharply limiting dietary intake of protein and by administering, orally or by enema, an antibiotic (e.g., neomycin) that kills intestinal bacteria but is poorly absorbed by the GI tract.

b. Portal hypertension

(1) Portal hypertension is a manifestation of advanced destruction of the hepatic lobules, such that the normal flow of portal blood is partially obstructed. In this setting, portosystemic venous collateral channels become dilated, shunting blood from the portal to the systemic circulation and bypassing the liver. This contributes to hepatic encephalopathy, because substances absorbed by the intestines enter the general circulation without being processed by the liver.

(2) The most significant consequence of portal hypertension is GI bleeding from esophageal varices. Such bleeding may be catastrophic in its own right, but, secondarily, the breakdown of blood in the intestines leads to additional ammonia production and can precipitate hepatic encephalopathy and coma. Nasogastric suctioning, cleansing enemas, and other measures are used to eliminate blood from the GI tract. Endoscopic identification and control of esophageal bleeding sites is an important modality.

(3) The hypoalbuminemia that is a feature of hepatocellular dysfunction lowers the colloid osmotic pressure of blood and predisposes to edema. This tendency, coupled with portal hyperten-

sion, leads to weeping of serum from serosal surfaces in the abdomen, resulting in ascites. By a similar mechanism, pleural effusions are also seen in liver failure. Infection of these fluid accumulations is a significant problem.

III. Alcoholism is responsible for numerous sociologic and medical problems:

A. Alcoholic intoxication is a major factor in the occurrence of automotive and other forms of trauma. Alcohol is a CNS depressant, adversely affecting both mentation and motor skills.

B. Chronic alcohol ingestion is a factor in the occurrence of several diseases of the nervous system, including:

1. Wernicke-Korsakoff syndrome (encephalopathy)
2. Alcoholic polyneuropathy
3. Pellagra
4. Cerebellar degeneration

C. Alcohol ingestion leads to pancreatitis in some persons, which may present as an acute abdominal catastrophe with autolysis of the pancreas, pseudocyst formation, and widespread damage to the abdominal viscera.

D. Abstinence from alcohol after long periods of intoxication produces serious medical consequences jointly referred to as the alcohol withdrawal syndrome. The principal features of the syndrome are:

1. Tremulousness—the earliest and most universal manifestation of alcohol withdrawal, appearing even after short periods of abstinence
2. Auditory or visual hallucinations—occurring in at least 25% of tremulous patients during alcohol withdrawal
3. Alcoholic seizures—usually of the grand mal type, usually self-limited, and tending to occur within 48 hr of the cessation of drinking; as a rule the EEGs of such patients are normal at times removed from periods of seizure activity
4. Delirium tremens (DTs)—having a fatal outcome in at least 10% of cases; the most serious feature of alcohol withdrawal

a. Onset typically occurs several days after cessation of alcohol consumption, when other symptoms of withdrawal (tremulousness, hallucinations, and seizures) may already have resolved.

b. DT is variable in severity.

(1) It is mild and not life threatening in the majority of cases. When mild, it may present as restlessness, agitation, and insomnia of several days' duration.

(2) Full-blown DTs is characterized by profound confusion and disorientation, agitation, tremors, insomnia, and symptoms of autonomic system hyperactivity and hypermetabolic state—profuse

diaphoresis, tachycardia, dilated pupils, temperature elevation. Large fluid and electrolyte shifts can occur, and patients may require many liters of fluid replacement every day, along with careful monitoring of electrolytes to prevent hypotension and cardiovascular collapse, especially in individuals with preexisting cardiac disease. The patient may also require active cooling to prevent hyperpyrexic damage to vital organs such as the brain and kidneys.

(3) Agitation in DTs is treated with sedative agents, of which chlordiazepoxide (Librium) is preferred. Cumulative doses up to 400 mg/da may be required, and care must be taken that the dose is tapered to prevent overmedication as the delirium resolves.

IV. Management issues in cirrhosis and alcoholism include:

A. A typical setting for the occurrence of DT is the alcoholic patient admitted with trauma who becomes acutely and involuntarily abstinent as a consequence of the hospitalization. Because the likelihood and severity of DTs reflect the extent and duration of alcohol consumption, a careful history of alcohol intake should be obtained. Patients tend to downplay their actual consumption, sometimes flagrantly. Furthermore, many alcoholics do not conform to the stereotype. Thus, it is easy to be fooled.

B. Maxillomandibular fixation for facial fractures combines poorly with full-blown DTs in the convalescent period. Fixation is not well tolerated by the agitated and disoriented patient. Fixation may be disrupted by the seizure activity that sometimes occurs early in withdrawal, and the increased respiratory demands of the patient in a hypermetabolic state may be poorly met because of the increased upper airway resistance imposed by fixation. In the known or suspected alcoholic with a risk of DTs, there is a premium on early operative intervention so that fracture repair will not be postponed by acute withdrawal symptoms. Furthermore, avoidance of IMF through the use of rigid fixation deserves strong consideration.

C. The patient with end-stage liver disease, as manifested by portal hypertension, a history of GI bleeding, and chronic elevation of the PT, is a poor candidate for elective oral and maxillofacial surgery. Malnutrition, including compromised protein metabolism frequently seen in this setting, may interfere with healing after procedures such as fracture repair.

1. The patient with an elevated PT >18 sec (>1.5 × control) who requires surgery with a risk of significant blood loss (e.g., multiple extractions) will need special preoper-

ative attention. This is a setting in which vitamin K administration may be appropriate.

2. Depending on the preoperative hematocrit, either fresh whole blood or fresh frozen plasma may be transfused preoperatively to replace deficient clotting factors. This therapy also increases the level of plasma proteins, which may reduce the tendency to form edema and also provide a measure of nutritional support. If the patient has a history of GI bleeding with multiple transfusions, the presence of unusual antibodies may make cross-matching difficult. Therefore, it is appropriate to have several units of blood available for such patients in advance of surgery, should unusual blood loss occur.

D. When a severely alcoholic patient is admitted with traumatic injuries or with other problems, his or her dietary intake is likely to improve rather suddenly in the hospital environment. In a malnourished individual deficient in thiamine, a sudden increase in carbohydrate intake may precipitate Wernicke's encephalopathy unless the deficiency is corrected. Thus, admitting orders for severe alcoholics should specify multiple vitamins, including thiamine 50–200 mg IM.

E. Admitting orders for severe alcoholics should also specify the frequent recording of vital signs, with attention to onset of tremulousness, for which appropriate doses of diazepoxide (Librium) or other sedative agent should be prescribed.

F. Signs of intoxication or delirium in known or suspected alcoholics may mask or confuse the identification of other serious problems (e.g., hyperglycemia or hypoglycemia, an expanding subdural hematoma due to head trauma [which is not uncommon in severe alcoholism]).

G. Some chronic alcoholics may have a long history of repetitive facial trauma. This can complicate the physical examination of the patient and also the interpretation of radiographs. For example, a patient with evidence of a new periorbital swelling and flattening of the malar eminence may have an old untreated fracture underlying a new soft-tissue injury.

1. Careful inspection of the radiograph should help in judging the age of the injury, but it is easy to be fooled, especially from suboptimal radiographs obtained from an uncooperative patient.

2. The distinction between old and new injuries is important because of their markedly different operative requirements. One may elect not to treat an old zygomatic fracture despite some cosmetic impairment, as long as ocular function has remained normal. Alternatively, if the patient, upon sober reflection, elects to have an old injury repaired, one must be ready to do the several osteotomies that this may require.

H. Patients with a history of heavy alcohol use may detoxify barbiturates and other agents more rapidly than normal. This has a bearing on anesthesia management, because the effective dose for such agents is likely to be increased.

I. The hyperemia induced by alcohol rapidly dissipates and reduces the effectiveness of local anesthetic agents, even those containing a vasoconstrictor. Therefore, larger amounts than usual may be required in performing emergency procedures on an intoxicated patient.

J. Given the current concern over informed consent, some thought is warranted on the subject of elective surgery for intoxicated patients. Intoxication compromises the validity of consent; thus, there may be legal as well as medical grounds for refusing to perform elective surgery on an intoxicated individual.

K. Some chronic users of alcohol lead well-regulated lives in which a physical dependence is not manifest until something happens, such as a period of hospitalization, that interrupts their access to a steady supply of alcohol. Management problems associated with alcohol withdrawal may be avoided by providing selected at-risk individuals with a daily ration of an alcoholic beverage as part of their hospital diet. This practice need not be viewed as aiding and abetting the patient's dependency, which may be addressed more effectively at a time removed from that of a hospital admission for a surgical problem.

Coagulation and bleeding disorders

I. Bleeding and clotting disorders may be either inherited or acquired. In the majority of instances such disorders are known to the patient. When a patient is unaware of a problem with bleeding or coagulation, it is likely to be an acquired defect of recent onset, perhaps secondary to an intercurrent medical problem or its treatment.

II. It is nearly impossible to discuss coagulation and bleeding disorders without offering a depiction of the clotting cascade (Fig. 4–4). Such diagrams suggest the complexity of the clotting mechanisms but fail to do justice to the dynamic nature of a system that can seal breaches in the vascular bed without allowing disseminated clot formation. Although they help explain a systematic approach to the clinical evaluation of bleeding problems, there is little clinical utility in memorizing such a diagram in detail. It is worth noting, however, that concentrates are available for the replacement of all factors whose lack produces serious bleeding, and also that techniques exist for assaying specific factor deficiencies.

III. Because most patients with inherited coagulopathies have a previously established diagnosis, the management of such patients involves confirmatory factor assay and planning for replacement

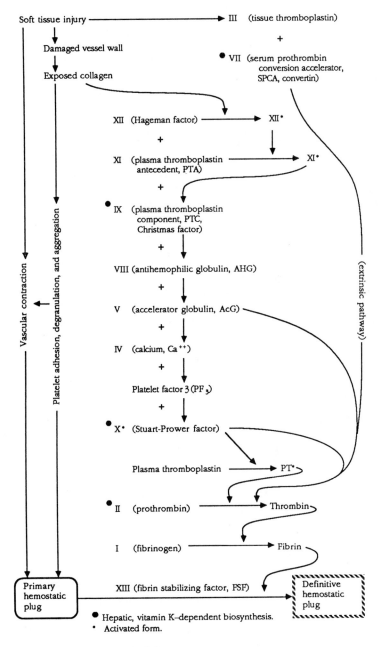

Fig. 4-4 Coagulation cascade.

therapy. In most hospitals this is undertaken in consultation with a member of the hematology department and/or transfusion service.

A. The advent of agents that help stabilize clots by inhibiting fibrinolysis has simplified the management of many patients with inherited coagulopathies, especially classic hemophiliacs (factor VIII deficiency, and sex-linked, recessive inheritance).

B. ε-Aminocaproic acid (EACA) (Amicar) is such an agent, and its use has significantly reduced the requirement for factor VIII infusion and also the length of hospital stay for elective surgical procedures.

C. Another agent of interest is desmopressin acetate (DDAVP), which is an antidiuretic hormone. DDAVP has been shown to increase factor VIII levels in patients with mild classic hemophilia (>5% factor VIII) and with Von Willebrand's disease.

D. Synthetic factor VIII is now available. Its use eliminates the infectious disease risk associated with use of pooled human factor VIII.

E. The clinical characteristics of the inherited coagulopathies are variable from patient to patient with the same disorder, and some patients will produce enough of a deficient factor to suppress clinical symptoms. For example, a patient with classic hemophilia A might remain symptom free (no spontaneous hemorrhage) with factor VIII levels between 3% and 5% and need factor replacement only in the event of trauma or for surgical procedures.

IV. A screening history for any new patient should include questions about bleeding:

Family history of bleeding
Unusual bleeding associated with previous surgical procedures, lacerations, or venipuncture
Epistaxis
Easy bruising
Ingestion of aspirin or aspirin-containing compounds
Anticoagulant therapy
Liver disease or other major medical illness
Chronic use of oral antibiotics

Because significant amounts of vitamin K are produced by the intestinal flora, chronic ingestion of broad-spectrum antibiotics, especially in the nutritionally compromised person, is known to contribute to a deficiency of vitamin K, upon which the synthesis in the liver of clotting factors II, VII, IX, and X depends.

V. Any patient with a positive or a suggestive history deserves further evaluation, especially if a significant surgical procedure is anticipated. Approaches to the evaluation of a patient with an undiagnosed bleeding disorder include:

A. Simply referring the patient with a positive history to a hematologist. This is the "easy way out," but may be required as a matter of policy in some institutions. However, this approach conflicts with a philosophy of care for the whole patient, and is intellectually dissatisfying.

B. Ordering a large battery of tests—this "shotgun" approach may lead to a diagnosis but is very wasteful.

C. The most efficient approach to the workup of an undiagnosed bleeding disorder starts with the patient's history:

  1. The character of bleeding that has occurred in the past is an important aid to diagnosis.

    a. Easy bruisability, bleeding into the integument (including skin and mucous membranes), and prolonged bleeding from cuts and venipuncture sites all suggest a problem with platelets or with the blood vessels themselves (e.g., capillary fragility or a defect in vascular contraction).

    b. Spontaneous bleeding into joints (hemarthrosis) or visceral organs and muscle tissue suggests a congenital or acquired clotting factor deficiency.

  2. Because systemic disease is the basis for many acquired coagulopathies, the following should be ruled out by taking a history and by laboratory studies, as may be suggested by historic findings:

    a. Renal failure

    b. Hepatic dysfunction

    c. Leukemia and related disorders (megakaryocytes in the marrow replaced by tumor cells)

    d. Polycythemia (excessive RBCs mechanically interfering with clot formation)

    e. Severe infections, especially gram-negative ones (may lead to a consumption coagulopathy or disseminated intravascular coagulation [DIC])

D. In the absence of evidence of organic disease, routine screening studies consist of PT, (PTT), and platelet count.

  1. If the platelet count is decreased, the causes of thrombocytopenia are sought:

    a. Idiopathic thrombocytopenic purpura (ITP) (a diagnosis invoked with ever-decreasing frequency as factors that influence platelet number and function are elucidated.)

    b. Hypersplenism of various etiologies with sequestration of platelets

    c. Leukemia

    d. Aplastic anemia

    e. Drug reaction (thiazide diuretics, sulfonamides, antimalarial drugs, etc.)

    f. Viral illness (thrombocytopenia, a feature of mononucleosis in about 5% of cases; a bone marrow biopsy may be required as part of the work up for thrombocytopenia).

2. A platelet count of <40,000 is an emergency situation because of the risk of intracranial bleeding. Medical admission is appropriate.

3. If the platelet count is normal, the PT and PTT are determined:

   a. In patients not on heparin, an elevated PTT is indicative of an inherited coagulopathy such as hemophilia A or B. It would be highly unusual for such a diagnosis to go undetected after taking a history.

   b. An elevated PT suggests an acquired coagulopathy, i.e., interference with the vitamin K–dependent hepatic biosynthesis of factors II, VII, IX, and X, such as is seen in end-stage liver disease or with warfarin anticoagulation.

4. Platelets may be adequate in number but functionally deficient in a number of disorders such as:

   a. Von Willebrand's disease

   b. Qualitative platelet disorders such as Glansman's thrombasthenia, Portsmouth syndrome and aspirin use.

VI. Management of the anticoagulated patient

A. Indications for anticoagulation include:

1. Thrombophlebitis and phlebothrombosis

2. Embolic cerebral vascular accidents and transient ischemic attacks

3. Prevention of mural thrombus formation following a subendocardial MI

4. Atrial fibrillation, to prevent clot formation in the atrial appendage

5. Coronary artery bypass graft surgery

6. Cardiac valve replacement

7. Vascular reconstruction and microvascular surgery

8. Hemodialysis for renal failure

9. History of pulmonary emboli

10. Congenital or acquired hypercoagulable states

B. Anticoagulants

1. Heparin is a naturally occurring substance found in mast cells. It blocks the conversion of fibrinogen to fibrin and retards the formation of thrombin from prothrombin by interfering with the activity of thromboplastin. It also decreases platelet adhesiveness. Heparin activity is assayed via the PTT or by clotting time.

   a. Heparin administered intravenously has a rapid onset of action and is rapidly metabolized. Therefore, its anticoagulant effect is easy to regulate but requires close monitoring.

    b. The action of heparin is rapidly reversed by protamine sulfate.

    c. Heparin anticoagulation is used almost exclusively in a hospital setting. Given the indications for its use, it is likely that oral surgery to be performed on heparinized patients will be of an emergent nature. The degree of urgency of the procedure must be balanced against the risk of transiently discontinuing heparin therapy. Heparin should be discontinued only an hour or so before an intended procedure, if approved by the patient's physician. Patients requiring longer term anticoagulant therapy are switched to warfarin sodium.

2. Warfarin sodium (Coumadin) is a structural analogue of vitamin K and competitively inhibits the vitamin K–dependent biosynthesis of factors II (prothrombin), VII, IX, and X in the liver.

    a. The action of warfarin is assayed via the PT. Its therapeutic range is between 1.5 and 2 times the normal control time. Thus, if control is 12 sec, the therapeutic range of warfarin is 18–24 sec.

    b. In contradistinction to heparin, warfarin (taken by mouth) is used on an outpatient basis, and many patients are chronically anticoagulated with this agent. Therefore, it is not unusual for elective surgery to be performed on a patient taking warfarin. To manage such a patient successfully, it is necessary to consider the following:

        (1) The patient receiving warfarin may be anticoagulated for therapeutic or prophylactic reasons. The strength of the indication for anticoagulation will vary from patient to patient, and thus consultation with the patient's physician is appropriate to determine the extent to which anticoagulant therapy can be downregulated during the perioperative period.

        (2) When a dose of warfarin is given, its peak effect occurs approximately 48 hr later. Thus, there is a latency period before an alteration in dose will have an appreciable effect. Most patients take the warfarin once a day, at bedtime.

        (3) Elective oral surgery can be performed with a PT of 18 sec or less. There is a growing body of experience suggesting that some dental and minor oral surgical procedures can be safely carried out at even higher levels of anticoagulation if rigorous local hemostatic measures are applied. Patients should be told to expect some oozing of blood.

(4) It is appropriate to check the patient's PT on the day of an elective procedure. When this represents a hardship for the patient, the more removed the last PT is from the time of surgery, the more important it is to review the last several readings to see how much variation there has been. The greater the range of fluctuation, the more important it becomes to check the PT on the day of surgery.

(5) If the PT is 18 sec or less, no alteration in warfarin dose is called for, nor is it required to omit a dose.

(6) If the PT is substantially <18 sec, the patient's physician should be notified so he or she can review the patient's status and adjust the warfarin dose as necessary.

(7) If the PT is >18 sec, the patient should be rescheduled, warfarin discontinued 48 hr before surgery, and the PT checked once again before surgery to confirm an acceptable value for surgery and as a basis for advising the patient regarding when to resume taking the medication.

(8) After most minor procedures, especially if there is a strong indication for anticoagulation, warfarin is appropriately restarted on the evening of surgery. It should be bourne in mind, however, that the PT will probably continue to fall toward normal during the first 12–24 hr after surgery if the patient has been instructed to omit the previous one or two doses.

(9) A PT >2×control should be reported to the patient's physician, so he or she can more closely regulate warfarin administration.

(10) Although vitamin K reverses the effect of warfarin, its use should be avoided in patients with an indication for anticoagulation. Vitamin K can produce what has been termed *rebound hypercoagulability*, and it should be reserved for use in bleeding emergencies or to correct a deficiency state (e.g., malnutrition, severe liver disease).

(11) Physicians vary in their willingness to permit manipulation of anticoagulation in their patients. The oral surgeon will need to establish an understanding about this with each physician.

3. Aspirin is frequently used for its negative effect on platelet adhesiveness as a means of preventing platelet thrombi, which are precursors to definitive clot formation. Aspirin also decreases the hepatic biosynthesis of factors II and VII, and therefore potentiates the effects of warfarin.

The patient taking warfarin is instructed to avoid all aspirin-containing medications. This can be difficult owing to the large number of analgesic preparations that contain aspirin but are not clearly labeled as such. Occasionally a patient will have an unusual sensitivity to aspirin, and a single tablet can wipe out the adhesiveness of an entire cohort of platelets.

4. Low-molecular-weight dextrans are used intravenously as anticoagulants, especially to maintain the patency of vascular grafts.

5. In nonanticoagulated patients, elevation of the PT is a sign of severe hepatocellular disease, usually secondary to alcohol-induced cirrhosis or to chronic active hepatitis. Alcohol also decreases both platelet count and platelet function in some persons. When aspirin-containing compounds are used for a "hangover," their effect with alcohol may be additive.

VII. The following locally applied measures may be useful in the management of bleeding:

A. Fastidious suturing technique

B. Use of the smallest flaps possible consistent with good surgical technique (i.e., smallest incisions and minimal stripping of periosteum)

C. Use of absorbable gelatin sponges, oxycellulose, and other agents to provide a matrix for clot formation

D. Topical thrombin to control bleeding from denuded surfaces

E. Adhesives such as those used for attaching ostomy bags to control mucosal bleeding

F. Small pledgets of gauze or cotton tied in an embrasure space with silk suture material or dental floss to tamponade spontaneous bleeding from interdental papillae

G. Silver nitrate sticks

VIII. The International Normalization Rate (INR) is now widely in use as an alternative to PT. Oral and maxillofacial surgeons should be familiar with this method of measuring anticoagulation and with institutional standards.

Seizure disorders

I. A seizure may be defined as uncontrolled motor activity, sensation, behavior, consciousness, or a combination of these, produced by abnormal electrical activity in the brain.

A. The most dramatic type is grand mal, or major motor seizure. Generally a single episode in an otherwise healthy person is not a life-threatening event, especially if it is observed and supportive care can be rendered.

B. Status epilepticus, defined as repetitive seizures without intervening return of consciousness, can be life threatening, mainly because of hypoxic brain damage. It may occur secondary to:

    1. Loss of control of the thoracic respiratory muscles
    2. Upper airway obstruction by foreign bodies (e.g., dentures or food)

Aspiration of gastric contents

I. The history of a seizure disorder should come to light during the evaluation of any new patient.

  A. The oral surgeon must document the frequency of seizures, their duration and type, any premonitory signs and postictal sequelae, any precipitating factors, and the antiseizure medications taken (including dosage).

  B. Well-controlled epileptic patients withstand routine oral surgery as well as the average patient. Anxiety may be a precipitating factor in unstable or poorly controlled epileptics but is not a major factor in well-controlled patients. Sedation may be a useful adjunct to therapy for the same indications as would apply in normal patients. However, consideration should be given to the additive effect of agents used for sedation in combination with antiseizure medications already being taken.

  C. Syncopal episodes occur in many nonepileptic patients and may be accompanied at times by short bursts of seizure-like tonic or clonic movement of the extremities. Seizure patients also experience syncope, and this may occur without provoking a seizure. However, transient hypotension and cerebral hypoxia, which account for loss of consciousness in syncope, may initiate seizure activity, especially in the poorly controlled epileptic patient.

    1. Most syncopal episodes occur after an injection of a local anesthetic agent or venipuncture. Careful observation of the patient will normally reveal premonitory signs before syncope occurs—dizziness, diaphoresis, slowing of the pulse, sudden thirst, blurring of vision.

    2. Raising the feet, lowering the head, use of spirits of ammonia, and inhalation of O_2, if rapidly available, may help abort a syncopal episode and are particularly useful in epileptics.

  D. Many epileptic patients experience an aura and know when a seizure is imminent; some may be able to give warning.

II. When a seizure occurs, most of the care applied is supportive.

  A. The patient is placed in a position that minimizes the potential for physical injury from unrestrained motor activity.

  B. He or she is observed for airway obstruction, and measures are taken to relieve it should it occur. This is usually a simple matter of correctly positioning the head and neck so the tongue does not obstruct the pharynx. An oral airway is seldom necessary, and its use may damage the teeth. Dentures are removed whenever possible.

  C. For an isolated single seizure no medication is needed immediately. If the patient has been taking phenytoin (Dilantin) or other assayable agents, blood may be drawn to ascertain whether the drug level is within the therapeutic range.

D. The patient's physician or neurologist should be informed so he or she can review the patient's therapeutic regimen.

E. After the seizure the patient may be able to go home but should be accompanied by an adult.

F. If the patient has no previous history of seizures, it is appropriate that he or she be conveyed to an emergency facility for evaluation. A careful description of the seizure will be helpful to any neurologist who subsequently sees him or her. The patient's posture and head, eye, and limb position, the laterality of motor activity, and the character of movements are diagnostically significant.

III. Status epilepticus requires aggressive management.

A. The major priority is to establish an adequate airway. If this cannot be secured by positioning the patient properly or by use of an oral airway, then endotracheal intubation is required. Endotracheal intubation has the advantage of allowing mechanical ventilation, and it prevents aspiration of gastric contents.

B. An IV line should be established, but before infusion of any medications is started, a blood sample should be drawn for determination of antiseizure medication and serum glucose levels (hypoglycemia being a precipitating factor that is easily correctable). A glucose infusion (50 ml of 50% solution) can be given immediately after the blood sample is drawn.

C. Drug therapy is started.

1. Diazepam (Valium) is a rapid-acting and effective agent in all forms of epilepsy. It has less of a respiratory depressant effect than do the barbiturates, which are also used for acute management.

2. Phenytoin (Dilantin) is used but is less effective than diazepam acutely. It has the advantage of minimal respiratory depressant and sedative effect. Given the short duration of diazepam's antiseizure effect, phenytoin may be given adjunctively for long-term seizure control.

3. On occasion, general anesthesia is called for in the attempt to break status epilepticus, and it has the advantage of allowing use of muscle relaxants. This helps prevent physical exhaustion from persistent violent muscular activity. It also allows good control of respiration.

D. Especially if the patient has no prior history of seizure activity, an aggressive effort must be made to establish the cause. Typical causes or exacerbating factors include:

1. Inflammatory lesions: meningitis, encephalitis (either bacterial or viral)

2. Traumatic lesions (subdural, epidural, or subarachnoid hemorrhage)

3. Electrolyte imbalances (hyponatremia, hyperkalemia, hypocalcemia, hypomagnesemia)

    4. Hypoglycemia

    5. Uremia

    6. Expanding intracranial tumors and other space-occupying lesions (e.g., aneurysm)

    7. Increased CSF pressure

    8. Inappropriate discontinuation of antiseizure medication, especially in combination with alcohol withdrawal

    9. Ingestion of toxic substances

IV. Some additional considerations in the management of the patient with seizures include:

    A. General anesthesia is not contraindicated. For unstable patients a hospital setting or day care unit may be the preferable site. An epileptic patient is probably less likely to have a seizure during general anesthesia than at any other time. An IV dose of phenytoin may be given intraoperatively to ensure that postanesthetic excitement does not initiate seizure activity. The preoperative evaluation of such a patient should include assay of blood levels of antiseizure medications.

    B. IMF increases the risk of upper airway obstruction and aspiration of gastric contents. Strong consideration should be given to the use of rigid fixation for fractures, osteotomies or bone grafts to avoid IMF in any patient with a history of a seizure disorder.

    C. Careful monitoring of antiseizure medication blood levels is indicated. It may be worth discussing with the patient's physician a temporary increase in dosage during a period of unavoidable IMF.

    D. When such a patient is hospitalized, there may be a real benefit in seeing that he or she is assigned to a multiple-bed room. Surveillance by other patients can provide added safety in the event of a seizure that might otherwise go unobserved in a single-bed room.

    E. Pulse oximetry should be considered mandatory for any patient with a seizure disorder and the potential for upper airway obstruction.

Endocrine dysfunction
Diabetes mellitus

I. Diabetes is a disease in which a defect of insulin production or secretion leads to difficulty in maintaining a normal range of serum glucose levels. Diabetics may experience hyperglycemia or hypoglycemia, either of which can have fatal consequences.

    A. This disease varies widely in severity and mode of presentation—from mild, adult onset (type II) controllable by diet alone, to severe, juvenile onset (type I) requiring lifetime insulin injections and careful monitoring of urinary or (preferably) serum glucose levels.

B. Brittle diabetics have metabolic disease that is unstable and difficult to regulate. They are usually thin, with juvenile onset of symptoms.

II. The complications of diabetes include retinopathy, nephropathy, neuropathy, and accelerated occlusive vascular disease. These are variable in presentation relative to the onset of symptoms of the metabolic imbalance.

III. In providing care for diabetics, one is concerned with the issue of metabolic control in the perioperative period and also with issues of wound healing and risk of infection.

A. Metabolic control

1. This is not a major management issue in most adult-onset diabetics whose condition is controlled by diet, especially for outpatient procedures under local anesthesia.

2. Diabetics taking insulin under good metabolic control generally do well in the outpatient setting as long as they are able to maintain their usual dietary habits and insulin dosage in the face of surgery.

3. Some patients must be admitted for inpatient management before surgery under general anesthesia.

   a. The following information is important preoperatively:

   (1) Answers to questions about usual insulin doses and results of urine testing give an index of the patient's education about diabetic control and his or her reliability, and they may also be a predictor of compliance with postoperative instructions.

   (2) Fasting blood sugar obtained the morning before ingestion of food, institution of an IV line, or administration of insulin establishes a baseline.

   (3) A glucose tolerance test (GTT) establishes the patient's response to a known bolus of glucose and reflects the dynamics of his or her homeostatic mechanisms.

   b. The preoperative routine includes:

   (1) Writing orders for an American Diabetics Association diet with an appropriate number of calories

   (2) Keeping the patient NPO after midnight

   (3) In the morning, giving half the patient's usual dose of insulin and starting an IV line with 5% dextrose in water to be run at 100 ml/hr initially

   c. The intraoperative routine includes:

   (1) Continuing the glucose infusion

   (2) For long cases, checking the serum glucose and acetone levels intraoperatively

   d. Postoperative care involves the following instructions:

   (1) Continue the glucose infusion.

(2) Check serum glucose and acetone levels.

(3) Write orders for a sliding scale indicating the amount of crystalline zinc insulin (CZI) to be given for specific serum glucose levels (with an additional 5–10 U for acetone). The availability of a glucometer on the ward or in the recovery room facilitates patient management.

10 to 20 U of CZI for serum glucose in excess of 400 mg%

10 to 15 U of CZI for serum glucose in the 300 to 400 range

5 to 10 U of CZI for serum glucose in the 200 to 300 range

A sliding scale must be customized to the individual patient based on his or her known daily insulin requirement and responsiveness to insulin.

(4) Resume the patient's usual morning neutral protamine Hagedorn insulin only if he or she seems likely to resume normal dietary intake.

(5) Obtain a dietary consultation prior to discharge, especially if the surgical procedure is likely to alter the patient's ability to adhere to his or her usual diet.

B. Other considerations in diabetic patients

1. Wound healing—compromise of the microvasculature and atherosclerosis may impair wound healing in some diabetics, but this is seen most significantly in the distal extremities. The soft tissues of the face and the facial skeleton, having a generally good blood supply, do not usually manifest wound-healing problems in well-controlled diabetics.

2. Infection

a. The risk of postoperative infection in a well-controlled patient is probably not significantly elevated compared to that in a normal patient undergoing the same surgery.

b. Poorly controlled diabetics are more prone to infectious complications of surgery than are well-controlled or nondiabetic patients.

c. The consequences of infection may be significant in a diabetic patient in terms of the effect on diabetic control. Because of metabolic stress, insulin requirements can significantly increase. Thus, in a patient who is well controlled by diet alone, a transient requirement for insulin may develop to prevent hyperglycemia and even ketoacidosis caused by an infection.

d. The diabetic patient, especially when poorly controlled, may be at risk of unusual infections not generally seen in nondiabetic patients. Mucormycosis, a systemic fungal infection occasionally seen in the head and neck, may involve the soft tissues or sinuses and spread to the CNS and cranial cavity, with fatal consequences. There is also reason to believe that the poorly controlled diabetic experiences an accelerated form of periodontal disease.

 e. Because of the detrimental effect of infection on diabetic control, a good argument can be made for the prophylactic use of antibiotics in the perioperative period.

Thyroid dysfunction

 I. Thyroid hormone regulates tissue metabolism, the consumption of oxygen and nutrients (carbohydrates and lipids), and the production of heat in the maintenance of body temperature. In early life and childhood, it is required for normal development and maturation.

  A. The production and release of thyroid hormone are under the control of thyroid-stimulating hormone (TSH), secreted by the pituitary, which in turn responds to circulating thyroid hormone levels in a negative feedback loop.

  B. This feedback loop is further regulated by hypothalamic neurosecretory mechanisms, wherein a tripeptide, thyrotropin-releasing hormone (TRH), has the effect of stimulating TSH secretion by the anterior lobe of the pituitary.

 II. In the absence of sufficient thyroid hormone there is cold intolerance, a general slowing of mental and physical processes, and weight gain. Symptoms of hypothyroidism are frequently nondescript and may go undiagnosed for protracted periods.

 III. An excess of thyroid hormone produces a constellation of overt physical and emotional symptoms that can suggest the correct diagnosis in advance of confirmatory laboratory tests—tremors, nervousness, insomnia, heat intolerance, increased body temperature, muscle wasting, weight loss, and tachycardia.

  A. A distinction must be made between "thyrotoxicosis," which the above symptoms denote, and "hyperthyroidism," which is properly applied only to thyrotoxicosis produced by oversecretion of hormone by the thyroid gland itself. There are numerous other causes of thyrotoxicosis, including secretion of TSH by a pituitary adenoma, thyroid hormone secretion by a variety of tumors (e.g., choriocarcinoma), and inappropriate ingestion of thyroid hormone.

  B. Thyroid storm is the most severe form of thyrotoxicosis. It is a life-threatening emergency characterized by fever, diaphoresis, agitation, confusion, tachyarrhythmias, heart failure, nausea, vomiting, diarrhea, gross tremors, and hyperreflexia. It can be brought on, in the face of thyrotoxicosis, by sources of metabolic stress including infection, trauma, and general anesthesia in an inadequately prepared patient.

C. The most common form of hyperthyroidism is Graves' disease, or diffuse toxic goiter, which is caused by an abnormal immunoglobulin interacting with the TSH receptor site on the thyroid cell membrane. It is frequently accompanied by exophthalmos.

IV. Cellular metabolism is responsive to both thyroxine (T_4) and triiodothyronine (T_3). In the assessment of thyroid function, T_4 is usually measured by a radioimmunoassay. Thyroid hormone in plasma binds to proteins, including thyroxine-binding globulin (TBG), prealbumin, and albumin. A T_3 resin uptake test may also be obtained to determine whether abnormalities in the T_4 level may be due to a disturbance in protein binding (as could occur, for example, when protein metabolism is altered or when binding is altered by drugs such as salicylates and phenytoin).

V. Management considerations include the following:

A. The patient most in need of assessment of thyroid function is the one with overt physical symptoms suggestive of thyrotoxicosis or severe hypothyroidism. It is also appropriate to check the status of any patient previously treated for hyperthyroidism before attempting major elective oral surgery under general anesthesia. This is best done in consultation with an endocrinologist, especially if treatment is necessary.

B. Thyroid hormone is one of the most indiscriminately prescribed medicines. It is frequently given in the treatment of obesity without laboratory assessment of thyroid function, and even without the presumption of hypothyroidism.

C. In the absence of physical symptoms, a patient generally is unlikely to be suffering from significant thyrotoxicosis. However, hypothyroidism is a more elusive diagnosis.

D. Infection, trauma, and surgery under general anesthesia may be poorly tolerated by patients at either end of the spectrum of thyroid dysfunction. A patient should be made euthyroid before any major elective procedure is undertaken.

E. Minor oral surgical procedures under local anesthesia should be well tolerated by the patient who does not have overt symptoms.

F. Hyperthyroid patients exhibit exaggerated responses to vasoactive drugs and catecholamines and may be prone to cardiac arrhythmias.

G. Hypothyroid patients may respond in an exaggerated manner to sedative and narcotic medications, necessitating, in extreme instances, respiratory support until such drugs are metabolized or eliminated.

Adrenal dysfunction and patients taking steroids

I. Each adrenal gland actually consists of two separate endocrine glands: the medulla and the cortex.

A. The adrenal medulla, part of the sympathetic nervous system, secretes epinephrine and norepinephrine and participates in the marshaling of physiologic resources in "fight or flight" emergencies.

B. The adrenal cortex secretes numerous steroid hormones including sex hormones, mineralocorticoids, and glucocorticoids.

   1. Adrenal sex hormones are important in sexual maturation and development but play a relatively minor role in adult reproductive function.

   2. Mineralocorticoid activity is essential to the maintenance of sodium balance and the regulation of extracellular fluid volume.

   3. Glucocorticoid activity is essential to carbohydrate and protein metabolism and resistance to stress.

   4. In the absence of mineralocorticoids and glucocorticoids, cardiovascular collapse and death occur.

II. Hyposecretion and hypersecretion of each of the adrenal hormones are associated with a classically described clinical condition. Although these disease entities are, for the most part, rare (Table 4-1), the oral and maxillofacial surgeon should nevertheless be acquainted with them. A discussion of their diagnosis and treatment is beyond the scope of this chapter.

III. Glucocorticoid therapy

A. Glucocorticoid hormones in normal physiologic quantities have numerous biologic effects, including:

   1. Increased protein catabolism in the liver and periphery as part of gluconeogenesis. Through this mechanism, glucocorticoid hormones elevate serum glucose and produce a glucose tolerance curve suggestive of diabetes mellitus. (Conversely, when glucocorticoid hormones are deficient, normal blood glucose levels are maintained only when food intake occurs at regular intervals. Fasting in the face of glucocorticoid deficiency leads to hypoglycemia and collapse.)

   2. Glucocorticoids have a permissive action in a variety of physiologic mechanisms. The hormones do not produce these effects but allow them to occur. Thus, small amounts of glucocorticoids are required for both glucagon and catecholamines to produce an increase in serum glucose. Glucocorticoids are also necessary for vascular smooth muscle to contract in response to norepinephrine and epinephrine. This mechanism is important in the cardiovascular compensation for hypovolemia.

   3. Whereas mineralocorticoids regulate Na metabolism, glucocorticoid deficiency leads to an inability to excrete excess body water.

B. In high doses a different spectrum of activities is observed, including the classic stigmata of Cushing's syndrome:

Table 4-1 ADRENAL DYSFUNCTION

Hormone	Hyposecretion	Hypersecretion
Epinephrine-norepinephrine	Very rare (hypoglycemia)	Pheochromocytoma, hypertension
Mineralocorticoids	Rare (salt wasting)	Conn's syndrome (primary aldosteronism)
Glucocorticoids	Addison's disease	Cushing's syndrome
Adrenal androgens	Rare	Adrenogenital syndrome

1. Somatic changes:

   Moon face
   Red cheeks
   Cervical fat deposition (buffalo hump)
   Muscle wasting
   Easy bruisability, capillary fragility with ecchymoses
   Pendulous abdomen, purple abdominal striae
   Inhibition of hair growth
   Poor wound healing

2. Osteoporosis
   a. This occurs because excessive protein catabolism inhibits new bone formation, while at the same time glucocorticoids inhibit the activity of vitamin D and increase glomerular filtration.
   b. These activities lead to a loss of calcium and demineralization of bone. Clinically, there may be collapse of vertebrae, pathologic hip fracture, and skeletal deformities.
3. Inhibition of the inflammatory response to tissue injury and infection
4. Inhibition of the manifestations of allergic and autoimmune disease
5. Exacerbation of hypertension, diabetes mellitus, and peptic ulcer disease
6. Production of characteristic psychologic disturbances and mood changes
7. Reduction of host defenses against a variety of infections, including tuberculosis and viral illnesses

C. It is important to recognize that the desirable antiinflammatory and antiallergic effects of glucocorticoids are seen only at dosage levels that also produce undesirable stigmata of Cushing's disease, especially if treatment is continued for a protracted period. Some undesirable effects are reduced by alternate-day drug therapy. Short courses of glucocorticoids with rapid tapering of dose produce minimal side effects.

D. Conditions for which glucocorticoid therapy may be useful include severe rheumatoid arthritis, systemic lupus erythematosus, severe asthma, and other allergic or autoimmune entities. Such therapy is also used to suppress the rejection of transplanted organs. The subject of steroids for reduction of postoperative swelling in oral and maxillofacial surgery is controversial, because they have been implicated in cases of Bell's palsy.

IV. Management of the patient receiving steroid therapy includes:
A. The principal source of concern is that high-dose glucocorticoid therapy, if extended for more than a short period, suppresses both the secretion of corticotropin by the pituitary gland and the ability of the adrenal glands to secrete hor-

mones in response to stress. In long-term glucocorticoid therapy, profound suppression occurs and the adrenal glands become atrophied. The time it takes for the adrenal glands to
return to a normal level of activity is a function of the duration of suppression. In a patient chronically suppressed for a
long time, there are grounds for concern about his or her ability to respond to stress a year after cessation of therapy, and
perhaps even longer.

B. The concern over adrenal suppression is moot when the patient is receiving glucocorticoids in excess of the daily physiologic requirement. It is only when steroids have been discontinued or the dosage has been tapered to a low level that
the risk of an addisonian crisis in the face of stress becomes
real.

C. It is possible to assay adrenal function, but it is much easier
simply to provide a patient with supplemental glucocorticoid
in the perioperative period if a stressful surgical procedure is
to be undertaken. The steroids can be rapidly tapered to the
previous maintenance dose or to zero.

D. The definition of *stress* is important. From the standpoint of
adrenal physiology the term refers to noxious stimuli of sufficient impact to lead to an increase in corticotropin secretion
and, in turn, an increase in the release of glucocorticoids into
the circulation. In fact, the term stress is wrongfully applied
to most dental or outpatient oral surgical procedures. These
procedures may be "stressful" in the colloquial sense in that
they evoke nervousness, but when a decision about steroid
dosage in the perioperative period has to be made, stress
probably should be considered to be an attribute of more protracted invasive procedures under general anesthesia. However, given the innocuous nature of a short course of steroid
therapy, it is advisable to overtreat rather than to undertreat
when in doubt.

Dysfunction of the immune system, HIV infection, and AIDS

I. General considerations

A. The oral and maxillofacial surgeon is privileged to work in an
area of the body where host defenses are strongly marshaled
against infection and allow the healing of wounds that frequently prove troublesome elsewhere in the body. On the
other hand, the oral cavity is often the first area to become
symptomatic when the immune system is malfunctioning. For
example, the presenting symptoms in acute leukemia may be
painful hemorrhagic swelling of inflamed gingival tissues.
Biopsy will typically show a leukemic infiltrate, which is the
response of a compromised immune system to the presence
of oral flora. Such organisms, usually benign, become pathogenic when host defenses are inadequate.

B. The science of immunology is one of the most rapidly evolving areas in medicine. It is an active front in the battle to understand and rationally treat cancer, and a growing number of diseases are now identified as being caused by autoimmune phenomena. Progress in the realm of organ transplantation is based on evolution of surgical technique, but even more so on our growing ability to manipulate some of the immunologic factors underlying histocompatibility.

C. The oral and maxillofacial surgeon is likely to encounter patients with dysfunction of the immune system in the following contexts:

1. Malignancy—marrow replacement by tumor cells, leukemic or metastatic, leads to neutropenia and immunologic compromise.

2. Chemotherapy for tumor—in addition to killing or suppressing the growth of rapidly dividing tumor cells, chemotherapy also kills or suppresses rapidly dividing normal cells (e.g., marrow cells). Thus, along with other forms of toxicity, immunosuppression sets a limit to the use of such drugs.

3. Immunosuppressive therapy—such therapy is used in organ transplantation to prevent rejection. It is also employed in the management of a broad spectrum of autoimmune disorders, including severe rheumatoid arthritis, systemic lupus erythematosus, and pemphigus vulgaris.

4. Marrow suppression and immunologic compromise—these result from whole body radiation, which may be employed therapeutically before marrow transplantation or which might occur in the event of a thermonuclear war or an accident at a nuclear facility.

5. Aplastic anemia or pancytopenia—these occur idiopathically, as a consequence of an overdose of marrow suppressive agents, as a result of exposure to industrial chemicals, or as an idiosyncratic reaction to medications such as chloramphenicol, antihistamines, and phenylbutazone.

D. HIV Infection and AIDS

Within the last two decades, a new disease entity known as the acquired immunodeficiency syndrome (AIDS) has appeared and caused great alarm. First described in 1981 and initially thought to be a disease unique to sexually active male homosexuals, it soon became apparent that the disease is transmissible hematogenously as well as by sexual intercourse. AIDS is on the rise in heterosexuals as a consequence of sexual transmission and intravenous drug abuse.

1. As of mid-1984, there were fewer than 5000 cases of AIDS reported in the United States, but the number has been doubling roughly every 6 mo. The U.S. Public Health Service estimates that between one and two million Americans may have HIV by the mid-1990s. Worldwide, 13 mil-

lion (1 in 250) adults are estimated to be infected with HIV. About two-thirds of the total cases have occurred in sub-Saharan Africa.

2. HIV, the causative agent for AIDS, is a retrovirus. It was first isolated and identified in 1983. Initial infection with HIV produces no signs or symptoms in the majority of cases and is indicated only by the presence of antibodies. The mean interval between infection with HIV and the development of AIDS is currently thought to be about 10 years, but there is great variation from case to case. Survival after the onset of severe illness is currently about 2 years in developed countries and about 6 months in developing countries. Although progress has been made in delaying the progression of this disease, to date there are no documented instances of recovery from AIDS.

3. AIDS is characterized by lymphadenopathy, multiple opportunistic infections, and multifocal Kaposi's sarcoma. Oral lesions are a prominent feature of AIDS. Characteristic oral lesions have prognostic significance in the progression of HIV infection to full-blown AIDS, and their appearance correlates well with CD4+ T-lymphocyte counts. Typical lesions include:

Oral Kaposi's sarcoma
Oral candidiasis
Herpes simplex
Giant aphthous ulcers
HIV-associated gingivitis
HIV-associated periodontitis
HIV-associated salivary gland disease
Hairy leukoplakia

4. In the absence of a vaccine, the prevention of transmission of HIV infection to health care workers depends on the strict adherence to universal precautions and on the cultivation of work habits calculated to reduce the incidence of needle sticks, injuries from sharp instruments, and other forms of inadvertent exposure. A safe work environment cannot be created by decree. Each individual with potential exposure to blood-borne pathogens must make a conscious effort to continually refine their work habits and routines in the interest of personal safety and the safety of others.

5. To place the risk of occupational exposure to HIV in perspective, it is worth taking note of the following:

   a. The likelihood of acquiring HIV infection from a single accidental puncture with an HIV-contaminated needle is currently estimated to be <0.5%.

   b. As of 1995, the CDC had 32 reports of health care workers with documented seroconversion following occupational exposure to HIV. Of these, none were dental personnel. Six of 69 health care workers with "possible" occupational acquisition of HIV infection were dental health care providers. It seems probable that documentation of occupational HIV infection of dental and oral surgical providers will emerge as the HIV pandemic expands, but to date the number of documented cases remains small.

II. General management considerations for all forms of immunosuppression

   A. When immunosuppressive treatment can be anticipated, patients should be screened in advance of therapy and any potential oral sources of sepsis treated preemptively. For example, in a renal patient with a history of recurrent episodes of pericoronitis, one would tend to remove the wisdom teeth to prevent such an episode from escalating into a major problem after the start of immunosuppression. Similarly, patients should be screened for dental disease before the start of chemotherapy for malignant disease.

   B. During immunosuppression, oral care is likely to be supportive or palliative in the event of a dental emergency.

   C. Immunosuppressed patients are prone to opportunistic oral infections such as candidiasis and are also subject to reactivation of viral illnesses such as herpes simplex. Oral candidiasis maybe controlled by topical nystatin and other antifungal agents, although in patients with AIDS, *Candida* has proved to be remarkably capable of developing drug resistance. Despite the growing value of antiviral agents, viral stomatitis is amenable mainly to palliative measures (e.g., institution of a bland diet, use of topical anesthetic mouth rinses, various oral coating agents, and, in severe cases, intravenous nutritional and fluid support).

   D. The maintenance of hygiene is difficult in a patient with viral or another form of stomatitis. Half-strength peroxide rinses, or peroxide mixed with saline, can be useful when tooth brushing is too painful. The use of topical anesthetic agents (e.g., viscous lidocaine [Xylocaine] or 0.25%–0.5% dyclonine solution) may be useful before hygiene activities or before meals.

   E. The best time to undertake an elective or semielective oral surgical procedure in a patient receiving chemotherapy is midway between cycles of treatment, when blood counts are presumably on the rise.

   F. Perioperative antibiotics may be appropriate, but their use carries the risk of selecting out resistant organisms or opening various ecologic niches for colonization by nosocomial organisms that may be hard to eradicate and pathogenic in a compromised host.

   G. Wound healing may be impeded in the patient receiving aggressive chemotherapy. Currently available chemotherapeutic drugs do not distinguish between one rapidly growing tissue and another; thus, both tumor neoplasia and normal proliferation of tissues in a healing wound may be affected.

H. Because immunosuppressed patients are vulnerable to infection, they are frequently placed on precautions whose details are part of a standardized hospital protocol. It is appropriate to continue to observe these precautions for the protection of the patient when he or she is transferred to an outpatient facility for oral surgical treatment.

III. Special management considerations in patients with HIV infection and AIDS

A. Universal precautions (see also the discussion of universal precautions in the section **Hepatic dysfunction and alcoholism** in this chapter)—in as much as health care workers are more at risk from unidentified carriers of the AIDS virus (the same is true for hepatitis and other infectious diseases), it is deemed appropriate to assume that all patients carry such viruses and to rigorously adhere to universal precautions. The precautions advised by the CDC are essentially the same as those applied to hepatitis:

1. Instruments contaminated with blood, saliva, or other secretions from accidental wounds must be carefully avoided, as should exposure of open skin wounds or lesions on AIDS patients.

2. Gloves should be worn at all times when handling blood- or saliva-contaminated instruments or surgical specimens.

3. When the possibility of contaminating clothing with blood or secretions exists, gowns should be worn and disposed of properly.

4. All laboratory specimens should be properly bagged and labeled for the protection of transport and laboratory personnel.

5. All blood spills should be promptly cleaned with a disinfectant (1:10 dilution of 5.25% sodium hypochlorite and water).

6. Masks and protective glasses should be worn in all clinical encounters in which aerosolization of blood and saliva is a possibility.

7. Use of disposable instruments is encouraged.

8. Needles should *not* be bent or resheathed after use. This is a common cause of needle injury. Needles and other disposable sharp materials should be placed in a puncture-resistant container for proper disposal as hazardous medical waste material.

9. Proper hand washing before and after treatment and after cleaning of instruments is mandatory.

10. Pregnant women should avoid direct contact with AIDS patients, because many of these patients excrete cytomegalovirus or other viruses.

B. Unlike the care of patients with other causes of compromise of the immune system, the care of patients with AIDS is complicated in many instances by fear, prejudice, misinformation, and lack of knowledge on the part of health care providers. Many patients with HIV or AIDS are overtly or covertly treated as if their disease were punishment for activities proscribed by God, or as if homosexuality and drug addiction are contagious. For these reasons, patients with HIV positivity and AIDS find it difficult to find providers willing to care for them.

C. Patients with HIV who have CD4+ T-lymphocyte counts of 500/μl or more and no history of an AIDS-defining illness have no contraindications to routine dental care.

D. An oral and maxillofacial surgeon or dentist should be familiar with the clinical appearance of various AIDS-defining oral lesions such as Kaposi's sarcoma, hairy leukoplakia, oral candidiasis, herpes simplex, giant aphthae, and HIV-associated gingivitis and periodontitis. One or more of these lesions may be the first sign of HIV infection or AIDS in an otherwise asymptomatic individual with no prior history of illness. The surgeon should be prepared to:

   Institute appropriate therapies for the presenting lesions.
   Discuss with the patient the possible significance of clinical findings
   Take a comprehensive medical history, including a sexual history and a history of IV drug use or exposure to transfused blood products
   Discuss, encourage, and initiate confidential testing for HIV
   Assist the patient in finding a primary care provider to coordinate overall management

E. The management of the oral manifestations of AIDS and the provision of regular dental care for patients with HIV infection is rapidly evolving as a subspecialty of dentistry. A considerable debate is ongoing as to the optimal setting for meeting the needs of patients with HIV infection and AIDS. There are proponents for care in private offices and also for care in dedicated facilities. Underlying concerns in this debate have to do with not stigmatizing patients by separating them from the general population on the one hand, and providing highly specialized care in a sympathetic environment on the other. Both approaches to care delivery have positive and negative features, and there is no reason why both approaches can not coexist.

F. The reader may wish to refer to source material noted at the end of this chapter for information on the diagnosis and treatment of oral manifestations of HIV infection that is beyond the scope of this chapter.

G. Treatment planning for patients with AIDS should aim at limiting the negative impact of oral lesions on the quality of life.

Communication and cooperation with primary care providers is essential. Appropriate care must anticipate evolving problems with hemostasis and the progressive loss of the ability to fight infection.

GENERAL REFERENCES

Campbell JW, Frisse M, eds: *Manual of medical therapeutics, Washington University, St. Louis, School of Medicine*, ed 28, Boston, 1995, Little, Brown.

Condon RE, Nyhus LM, eds: *University of Illinois, Department of Surgery, Manual of surgical therapeutics*, ed 9, Boston, 1996, Little, Brown.

Ganong WF: *Review of medical physiology*, ed 17, Los Altos, Calif, 1995, Lange Medical Publications.

Glick M: *Dental management of patients with HIV*, Carol Stream, Ill, 1994, Quintessence Books.

Greenspan JS, Greenspan D, eds: *Oral manifestations of HIV infection,* Carol Stream, Ill, 1995, Quintessence Books.

Isselbacher KJ, et al, eds: *Harrison's principles of internal medicine*, ed 13, New York, 1994, McGraw-Hill.

Nora PF: *Operative surgery: Principles and techniques*, ed 2, Philadelphia, 1980, Lea & Febiger.

Sonis ST, et al: *Principles and practice of oral medicine,* ed 2, Philadelphia, 1995, WB Saunders.

Local Anesthesia and Sedation in Oral and Maxillofacial Surgery

5

EARL G. FREYMILLER

LOCAL ANESTHESIA

I. Classification of anesthetic agents
   A. Amides and esters constitute the major categories of local anesthetic agents. These designations refer to the molecular linkage between constituent hydrophilic and lipophilic groups. Because of their increased effectiveness and fewer hypersensitivity reactions, amides have largely supplanted esters; however, ester-linked agents remain an appropriate alternative for patients with amide allergies.
   B. Metabolism of amide anesthetic agents occurs in the liver; ester-linked agents are hydrolyzed in the plasma by pseudocholinesterases. Water-soluble products are excreted by the kidneys. Knowledge of the metabolic and elimination mechanisms is important when choosing appropriate local anesthetics and dosages for certain patients.

II. Dissociation constants
   A. The pH of anesthetic solutions is low (typically 3.3–5.5). Such solutions contain hydrochloride salts of anesthetic bases and exist in the form of uncharged base (RN) and cation (RNH+).
      1. An equilibrium between charged and uncharged forms is expressed by the equation

      $$RNH^+ \rightleftharpoons RN + H^+$$

      The proportion of RN and RHN+ at a given instant depends on pH and the anesthetic molecule's dissociation constant (pKa).
      2. For a given molecule, pKa is characteristic and constant; it is defined as the pH at which half of the molecular species are ionized (RNH+) and half are nonionized (RN) (Table 5-1).
   B. This is of clinical significance, because after injection, anesthetic molecules are exposed to the pH of the injection-site tissues. When tissue pH is low (i.e., in an area of active infection), excess H+ is present and the reaction is driven to the left. The proportion of RN correspondingly declines. Because the anesthetic diffuses into nerve membranes in the RN

Table 5-1   INJECTABLE LOCAL ANESTHETICS

	Classification	pKa	Maximum dose of local anesthesia (mg)*	Vasoconstrictor	Cartridges†		Duration (hr)	
					Healthy	CV impaired	Pulpal	Soft tissue
Procaine HCl, 4%	Ester	9.1	1000	Phenylephrine, 1:2,500	5.3	2.1	0.5	1.5–2.0
Lidocaine HCl, 2%	Amide	7.9	300	None	8.3	8.3	0.1	1.0–2.0
Lidocaine HCl, 2%	Amide	7.9	300	Epinephrine, 1:50,000	5.5	1.0	1.0–1.5	3.0–4.0
Lidocaine HCl, 2%	Amide	7.9	300	Epinephrine, 1:100,000	8.3	2.0	1.0–1.5	3.0–4.0
Mepivacaine HCl, 3%	Amide	7.6	400	None	7.2	7.2	0.3–0.7	2.0–3.0
Mepivacaine HCl, 2%	Amide	7.6	400	Levonordefrin, 1:20,000	5.5	2.2	1.0–1.5	3.0–4.0
Prilocaine HCl, 4%‡	Amide	7.9	600	None	8.3	8.3	0.2–1.0	2.0–4.0
Prilocaine HCl, 4%‡	Amide	7.9	600	Epinephrine, 1:200,000	8.3	4.4	1.0–1.5	2.0–4.0
Propoxycaine HCl, 0.4% and procaine HCl, 2%	Ester		400 Total	Levonordefrin, 1:20,000	5.5	2.2	0.5–1.0	2.0–3.0
Propoxycaine HCl, 0.4% and procaine HCl, 2%	Ester		400 Total	Levarterenol, 1:30,000	5.7	2.3	0.5–1.0	2.0–3.0

Bupivacaine HCl, 0.5%	Amide	8.1	140	None	15.5	15.5		
Bupivacaine HCl, 0.5%	Amide	8.1	140	Epinephrine, 1:200,000	15.5	4.4	1.5–3.0	4.0–9.0
Bupivacaine HCl, 0.75%	Amide	8.1	140	None	10.4	10.4		
Bupivacaine HCl, 0.75%	Amide	8.1	140	Epinephrine, 1:200,000	10.4	4.4		4.0–9.0
Etidocaine HCl, 0.5%	Amide	7.7	300	None	33.3	33.3		
Etidocaine HCl, 0.5%	Amide	7.7	300	Epinephrine, 1:200,000	22.2	4.4	1.5–3.0	4.0–9.0
Etidocaine HCl, 1.0%	Amide	7.7	300	None	16.6	16.6		
Etidocaine HCl, 1.0%	Amide	7.7	300	Epinephrine, 1:200,000	16.6	4.4	1.5–3.0	4.0–9.0

*Maximum doses are based on maximum recommended doses of local anesthetic agent alone for a healthy 70-kg adult per appointment.

†Maximum volumes are established on the basis of the most toxic constituent (which may be either the anesthetic or the vasoconstrictor) for a 70-kg adult. *Cartridges* refers to standard 1.89-ml dental cartridges.

‡Contraindicated in patients with methemoglobinemia and in those taking medications known to produce methemoglobinemia (e.g., acetaminophen, phenacetin).

form, anesthetic effectiveness also decreases. Because the pH of infected tissues is low, anesthetic agents with a high pKa offer a smaller proportion of RN for diffusion through nerve sheaths, and local anesthetic effect declines.

III. Composition of local anesthetic solutions

    A. Several local anesthetics are available (see Table 5-1). Anesthetic concentrations are expressed as percentages. Knowing the volume of a standard U.S. dental cartridge to be 1.8 ml, it is possible to compute the anesthetic content (see section V. C., p. 135).

    B. Vasoconstrictors are frequently added to prolong the effect of the local anesthetic, reduce peak plasma concentrations, and control bleeding. Several vasoconstrictors are available (Table 5-2). Vasoconstrictor concentrations are given as ratios, making it possible to compute the total dose as described below (see section V. C., p. 135).

    C. Preservatives of various types may be incorporated into anesthetic solutions.

        1. Dental cartridges formerly contained the preservative methylparaben (1 mg/ml), but a significant incidence of paraben reactions caused confusion over whether the patient was allergic to the anesthetic or to the preservative. Because genuine allergies to amide anesthetic agents are extraordinarily rare, most hypersensitivity reactions have been attributed to methylparaben. This preservative is now omitted from most dental cartridges, but may still be included in multidose vials.

        2. For anesthetic solutions containing a sympathomimetic vasoconstrictor, 0.5 mg/ml of sodium metabisulfite may be present as an antioxidant.

    D. Drug doses are expressed either by stating the amount of each drug in milligrams (e.g., 36 mg of lidocaine with 0.018 mg of epinephrine) or by giving the concentration and volume (e.g., 1.8 ml of a solution containing 2% lidocaine and 1:100,000 epinephrine).

IV. Representative local anesthetic solutions

    A. Injectable agents are summarized in Table 5-1.

    B. Topical anesthetics decrease the pain and anxiety of anesthetic injections. Although they do not readily penetrate intact skin, they do provide superficial anesthesia for abraded skin and intact mucosa; deep tissues are not anesthetized. Topical agents are not completely innocuous, since application to intraoral mucosa permits rapid absorption and leads to significant blood levels. Representative topical anesthetic preparations include the following:

        1. Benzocaine—this ester-linked, water-insoluble agent is poorly absorbed. Overdose reactions are virtually nonexistent.

        2. Lidocaine—this agent is the only amide-linked anesthetic with clinically important topical properties. The base

form (5% lidocaine) is poorly soluble in water. The salt form (2% lidocaine HCl), which is water soluble, is potentially more toxic.

3. Dyclonine—this agent represents the only ketone-linked local anesthetic. Its low water solubility accounts for a low systemic toxicity. It is available as a 0.5% solution; the maximum recommended dose is 200 mg (40 ml).

4. Butacaine sulfate—this ester is more potent and toxic than cocaine. It is available as a 4% ointment; the maximum recommended dose is 200 mg (5 ml).

5. Tetracaine—this highly water-soluble ester is more than five times as potent as cocaine and has a relatively high potential for systemic toxicity. It is used as a 2% solution; the maximum recommended dose is 2 mg (1 ml).

6. Cocaine—the main use for this agent in oral and maxillofacial surgery is as a nasal mucosal vasoconstrictor before nasal endotracheal intubation, reduction of nasal fractures, and rhinoplasty procedures. Because it is highly water soluble, it is absorbed rapidly and eliminated slowly. It is available in 2%–10% solutions; the recommended dose for topical application is 4%. Its lack of stability in solution and potential for psychic dependence and tolerance militate against its routine intraoral use as a topical anesthetic.

V. Vasoconstrictors

   A. Vasoconstrictors in local anesthetic solutions enhance the duration of anesthesia, reduce the peak plasma concentrations of anesthetic, and control local hemorrhage. However, sufficient dosages of all sympathomimetic vasoconstrictors can cause adverse reactions, particularly in the presence of predisposing conditions.

   B. Representative vasoconstrictors are listed in Table 5-2. Epinephrine is the most widely used vasoconstrictor in oral and maxillofacial surgery. It stimulates both alpha and beta receptors, but its value in dentistry as a vasoconstrictor is based on the predominance of alpha receptors in the oral mucosa, submucosa, and periodontium. When it is used to enhance pain control, no distinction exists between 1:100,000 and 1:50,000 concentrations. The more dilute solution (1:100,000) is therefore recommended.

   C. Healthy adults may receive up to 0.2 mg of epinephrine per appointment. This translates into 20 ml of a 1:100,000 solution (approximately 11 local anesthetic cartridges). However, the fact that anesthetic solutions contain multiple constituents must be recognized when determining the maximum permissible volume of an anesthetic to be administered at a single sitting. Maximum doses for multicomponent solutions should be based on the most toxic constituent. Although the maximum allowable dose of epinephrine for a healthy patient is 0.2 mg (11 carpules of a 1:100,000 solution), the maximum dose of lidocaine is only 300 mg (see Table 5-1). Therefore,

Table 5-2   VASOCONSTRICTORS

	Maximum adult doses (mg)		
	Healthy	CV impaired	Concentration*
Epinephrine	0.20	0.04	1:50,000; 1:100,000; 1:200,000
Levarterenol	0.34	0.14	1:30,000
Levonordefrin	0.5	0.2	1:20,000
Phenylephrine	4.00	1.60	1:2,500

*Ratios represent concentrations of vasoconstrictors commonly used in oral and maxillofacial surgery.

the actual number of 1.8-ml cartridges permitted for 2% lidocaine with 1:100,000 epinephrine is only eight, based on the toxic levels of lidocaine. The anesthetic and vasoconstrictor content of dental cartridges is shown below.

Anesthetic concentration (%)*	Anesthetic content (mg) per cartridge†
0.05	0.9
0.40	7.2
1.00	18.0
2.00	36.0
3.00	54.0
4.00	72.0

Vasoconstrictor concentration‡	Vasoconstrictor content (mg) per cartridge†
1:2500	0.75
1:20,000	0.09
1:30,000	0.06
1:50,000	0.036
1:100,000	0.018
1:200,000	0.009

D. Cardiovascular impairment, when clinically significant, may render the patient "epinephrine sensitive." The maximum epinephrine dose for such a patient is controversial. Published

---

*A1% solution = 1 g anesthetic per 100 ml solution.

† Based on a standard 1.8-ml dental cartridge.

‡ Expressed as ratios by weight; 1:100,000 = 1 gm vasoconstrictor per 100,000-g solution = 1 mg vasoconstrictor per 100-g solution = 1 mg vasoconstrictor per 100-ml solution (1-g solution = 1 ml).

recommendations have been divergent and inconsistent. Based on an extrapolation from guidelines promulgated by the New York Heart Association in 1955, a dose of epinephrine one fifth that permitted for a normal adult is suitable for use in a sensitive individual. This translates into 0.04 mg of epinephrine per appointment (only two carpules of a 1:100,000 solution; see Table 5-1). In fact, such a low level of epinephrine (and other vasoconstrictors) can probably be used safely in any patient with mild to moderate cardiovascular disease. However, the development of effective local anesthetics that do not contain sympathomimetic amines (3% mepivacaine, 4% prilocaine) often makes this decision unnecessary. When a vasoconstrictor is considered desirable, solutions containing 1:200,000 epinephrine can be used.

E. Vasoconstrictors may interact with other medications the patient may be taking. Previously it was recommended that patients taking monoamine oxidase (MAO) inhibitors for depression should not receive local anesthetics with epinephrine. This concept has been well disputed. However, patients taking the more commonly prescribed tricyclic antidepressants have been shown to exhibit an increased sensitivity to the pressor and arrhythmogenic effects of vasoconstrictors used in local anesthetics. For patients taking nonspecific beta blockers such as propranolol, an exaggerated increase in vascular resistance may occur with the administration of epinephrine, resulting in an increase in systemic blood pressure with a reflex bradycardia. It has been reported that patients chronically taking nonspecific beta blockers are more likely to develop mycardial ischemia if local anesthesia with epinephrine is used.

F. Vasoconstrictor use during general anesthesia may be complicated by the tendency of certain inhalation general anesthetics to sensitize the heart to the arrhythmogenic effects of the vasoconstrictor. Halothane and cyclopropane are considered sensitizing; fluroxene, methoxyflurane, and isoflurane are not. Anesthetics (e.g., enflurane) may sensitize specific subsets of patients, so limitation of sympathomimetic amine dosage is advised.

VI. Selection of local anesthetic. Although 2% lidocaine with 1:100,000 epinephrine is the most commonly used local anesthetic, certain medical conditions may warrant selecting another agent or decreasing the dosage of the anesthetic, or both.

Because both amide and ester local anesthetic agents are eventually eliminated by the kidneys, lower dosages of both should be used in patients with severe end-stage renal disease to avoid toxicity.

Because amide local anesthetic agents are metabolized by the liver, for patients with severe hepatic insufficiency, consideration should be given to using an ester anesthetic (or lower doses of amides) to avoid toxic reactions.

In patients with known or suspected pseudocholinesterase deficiency (prolonged paralysis after succinylcholine administration for general anesthesia induction), ester anesthetics should be avoided.

In patients suspected of having a true allergy to a local anesthetic of a given class (either amide or ester), an agent of the opposite class should be chosen to avoid allergic cross reactivity. Although rare, a malignant hyperthermal reaction can be fatal. Amide local anesthetics have been implicated as agents capable of triggering a malignant hyperthermal reaction, and esters have been recommended for patients suspected of having malignant hyperthermia. (Some investigators have challenged this concept.)

Avoid local anesthetics with a vasoconstrictor in patients with significant coronary artery disease, cardiac arrhythmias, severe or uncontrolled hypertension, uncontrolled hyperthyroidism, pheochromocytomas, and other cardiac conditions. Plain mepivacaine or prilocaine is recommended when vasoconstrictors are to be avoided, owing to their increased duration of action when compared with plain lidocaine.

Epinephrine can interact with other medications a patient may be taking (see section V. E., p. 137). For patients on tricyclic antidepressants or nonspecific beta blockers, the need for epinephrine should be carefully evaluated.

Although not related to the anesthetic, patients with bleeding dyscrasias (hemophilia, coumadin therapy, etc.) should not receive a deep injection likely to cause bleeding.

In cases where prolonged anesthesia is desired, a longer acting agent (e.g., bupivacaine or etidocaine) should be considered.

To safely treat all patients, in addition to lidocaine with epinephrine, the oral and maxillofacial surgeon should have an effective anesthetic without a vasoconstrictor (e.g., plain mepivacaine or prilocaine) and a local anesthetic of long duration (e.g., bupivacaine or etidocaine). Access to an ester anesthetic (e.g., procaine or chlorprocaine) may be needed on rare occasions.

VII. Techniques of regional anesthesia—thorough knowledge of relevant anatomy is necessary for reliable success in regional anesthesia. Details of specific anesthetic techniques are available in standard textbooks and review papers; however, several alternative approaches for block anesthesia are beneficial for the oral and maxillofacial surgeon, and will be considered in detail:

A. Gow-Gates technique—advantages: greater area of mandibular anesthesia with a single injection.

1. The nerves anesthetized are the inferior alveolar, mental, incisive, lingual, mylohyoid, auriculotemporal, and buccal.
2. Needle—25 gauge and long (1⅝ in.)
3. The site of penetration is the oral mucosa along the medial border of the mandibular ramus lateral to the pterygomandibular depression, but medial to the temporalis muscle tendon. With the patient's mouth wide open, the nee-

dle is inserted along a line extending from the corner of the mouth opposite the side of injection to the lower border of the tragus on the same side as the injection. The alignment of the needle should be parallel to the angulation of the ear to the face of injection.

4. Depth of penetration—the needle should be advanced until bone (neck of condyle) is contacted and then withdrawn 1 mm. Anesthetic solution is deposited after negative aspiration.

B. Tuberosity (Akinosi) approach—the advantage is the ability to anesthetize a patient with significant trismus.

1. Nerves anesthetized are the inferior alveolar, mental, incisive, lingual, long buccal, and mylohyoid.
2. Needle—25 gauge and long (1⅝ in)
3. The site of penetration is the oral mucosa along the medial border of the mandibular ramus. The mouth is kept closed (teeth in occlusion) with the cheek and muscles of mastication relaxed. The syringe is aligned parallel to the occlusal plane, positioned at the mucogingival junction in the region of the maxillary third molar. The needle penetrates the oral mucosa just medial to the ramus.
4. Depth of penetration—the needle should be advanced 1½ in.

C. V-2 block—the advantage is the greater area of maxillary anesthesia with a single injection.

1. The nerves anesthetized are the second division of the trigeminal nerve, including the anterior, middle and posterior superior alveolar nerves, infraorbital nerve, and the greater and lesser palatine nerves.
2. Needle—25 gauge and long (1⅝ in)
3. The site of penetration is through the palatal mucosa adjacent to the maxillary second molar, at the junction of the vertical and horizontal hard palate, advancing through the greater palatine foramen.
4. Depth of penetration—the needle should be advanced 1¼ in.

VIII. Complications

A. Local

1. Needle breakage is rare and usually occurs because of unexpected movement by the patient or because of the (unjustifiable) iatrogenic practice of intentionally bending the needle. Broken needles seldom migrate within tissues; they become encapsulated by fibrous connective tissue and remain stationary until delayed recovery is feasible.
2. Persistent anesthesia and paresthesia are caused by direct needle trauma to nerve trunks or by anesthetic solutions contaminated with alcohol or cold sterilization media. Abnormal sensation is usually temporary but may be permanent. Persistent sensory deficit may require surgical explo-

ration, anastomosis of severed nerve ends, or anastomosis after removal of a damaged nerve segment.

3. Trismus (spasm of the muscles of mastication) is common after local anesthetic injections and results from trauma, hemorrhage, or infection. Treatment includes heat therapy, analgesics, muscle relaxants, and opening-closing exercises.

4. Hematomas are caused by extravasation of blood after needle damage to a blood vessel. Resulting swelling may develop rapidly or slowly depending on the consistency of the surrounding tissue and whether an artery or vein is involved. Swelling and ecchymosis resolve over the ensuing weeks, and no specific treatment is needed. In the case of immediate swelling, application of pressure to the injection site may minimize hematoma formation.

5. Infection after injections is uncommon. When it does occur, management is the same as for any other intraoral infection (i.e., systemic antibiotics and drainage of fluctuant abscesses).

6. Lip chewing is most common in children and the mentally handicapped. Prevention requires use of shorter acting agents, placement of protective gauze or cotton rolls between the lips, and careful instructions for parents or guardians.

7. Facial nerve paralysis may arise from introducing anesthetic solution into the substance of the parotid gland. This blocks the propagation of impulses along facial nerve branches that innervate the muscles of facial expression. Cessation of nerve transmission is temporary and no specific treatment is required, but closure of the eye on the involved side may not be complete. Retention of the corneal reflex is usually sufficient for normal eye lubrication until complete muscle function returns.

B. Systemic

1. Adverse drug reactions to anesthetic solutions (i.e., local anesthetic agent, vasoconstrictor, preservatives, or other components) may result from direct extension of the agent's pharmacologic effects, altered physiology, or allergy. Toxicity resulting from an extension of pharmacologic properties includes side effects, overdosage, and local toxic effects.

2. Intravascular injection is not a systemic reaction in itself, but it greatly increases the possibility of an adverse occurrence. The probability of an intravascular injection is diminished (but not eliminated) by preinjection aspiration.

3. An authentic allergic reaction to a local anesthetic may range from a minor skin reaction to life-threatening anaphylaxis.

   a. Prevention of allergic reactions requires a detailed medical history. Allergy to amide local anesthetics is uncommon; nonetheless, assertions by patients of "Novocain" reactions should be taken seriously. To many patients, Novocain is synonymous with local anesthetics. This makes it difficult to know whether the patient experienced a reaction to an ester (e.g., Novocain) or to an amide anesthetic. If the category of anesthetic can be definitively established, the alternate class can be used with confidence.

(1) The possibility of previous overdosage or of reactions to vasoconstrictors or other agents must be considered. Inquiry should be made into whether the patient has been taking other medications, whether hyperventilation or syncope provides a more realistic description of the previous incident, how the reaction was managed, and whether the patient required hospitalization.

(2) An attempt should be made to contact the previous oral and maxillofacial surgeon or dentist for an objective appraisal of the event and for positive identification of the anesthetic class. Elective therapy should be postponed until the nature of the occurrence is discerned.

b. Management can be difficult for patients in pain who require emergency treatment and who allege a history of local anesthetic allergy. Use of general anesthesia can be considered. Alternatively, the local anesthetic effect of injected antihistamines can be exploited. A1% solution of Benadryl (diphenhydramine) with 1:100,000 epinephrine is relatively effective. Management of anaphylaxis and other allergic reactions is discussed elsewhere in this manual.

SEDATION
I. Definition
   A. No completely satisfactory definition of sedation in oral and maxillofacial surgery has been devised, but generally, sedation produces a minimally depressed level of consciousness that retains the patient's ability to maintain an airway independently and continuously and to respond appropriately to physical stimulation and verbal command. By contrast, general anesthesia produces a controlled state of depressed consciousness or unconsciousness, a partial or total loss of protective reflexes, and an inability to maintain an airway independently or respond purposefully to physical stimulation or verbal command.
   B. Detailed consideration of the applications of sedation and ambulatory general anesthesia in oral and maxillofacial surgery cannot be adequately covered in this brief descriptive outline. The present section will therefore provide a general

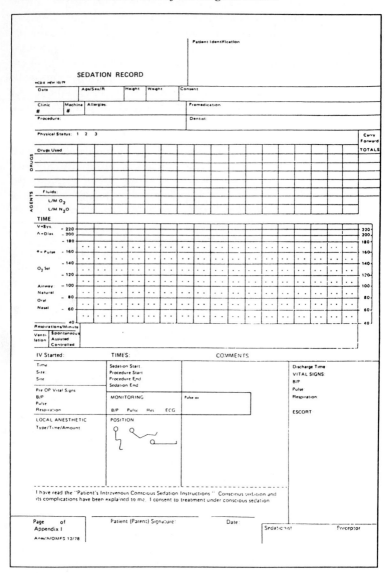

Fig. 5-1   Sedation monitoring record.

summary of commonly employed techniques. Application of such methods should be limited to individuals who have undergone appropriate hospital-based clinical training in general anesthesia and who are in compliance with state licensing requirements for sedation or general anesthesia.

II. Techniques of conscious sedation
    A. Routes of administration for sedative agents may be inhalational, oral (PO), intravenous (IV), intramuscular (IM), or

rectal (PR). Inhalation sedation using nitrous oxide–oxygen (N_2O–O_2) and IV sedation has gained wide popularity. It should be noted, however, that sedation techniques should in no way diminish the need for excellent local anesthetic technique.

B. Patient monitoring is required whenever conscious sedation is employed. Monitoring involves measuring and recording blood pressure, pulse, oxygen saturation, and respiratory rate before sedation, and at least every 15 min during the procedure. A recording of postsedation values is also required (Fig. 5-1). A precordial stethoscope, pulse oximeter, and automatic blood pressure cuff allow the surgeon to continuously monitor the patient without interfering with the ability to safely perform the surgical procedure. ECG monitoring also allows for the early diagnosis of aberrant arrhythmias.

C. N_2O–O_2 sedation requires O_2 (supplied as a compressed gas) and N_2O (provided in cylinders as a liquid that vaporizes during use). This distinction in physical state is clinically significant because the vapor pressure within N_2O cylinders is maintained at roughly 750 lb/in^2 until the cylinder is virtually empty. By contrast, as O_2 is depleted, a proportionate decrease in O_2 pressure occurs.

	Tank color	Tank size	Volume (gal)	Pressure (lb/in^2)
N_2O	Blue	E	420	750
	Blue	H	3665	750
O_2	Green	E	65	2100
	Green	G	1400	2100

1. Flow is measured as liters per minute and expressed as a percentage; for instance, 2 L of N_2O/min and 4 L of O_2/min is expressed as

$$\frac{2\ L\ of\ N_2O/min}{(2\ L\ of\ N_2O/min + 4\ L\ of\ O_2/min)}$$

   or

$$33.3\%\ N_2O;\ 66.7\%\ O_2$$

2. Procedures are similar for all sedation machines. Each typically delivers an absolute minimum of 20%–30% oxygen, has a "fail-safe" system that prevents N_2O delivery if O_2 administration is interrupted, and employs a "pin-indexing safety system" or "diameter-indexing safety system" to ensure correct cylinder attachment. The procedure for operating and testing N_2O–O_2 sedation machines is given on p. 140.

Operating and Testing N₂O–O₂ Sedation Machines

A. Turning machine on
1. Turn on N_2O-O_2 tanks.
2. Turn machine's "on-off" switch to "on."
3. Verify that N_2O flow valve is "off."
4. Turn O_2 flow valve "on" to provide O_2 delivery rate of 5 to 8 L/min.
5. Place inhaler assembly (nasal mask) on patient.
6. Adjust total gas flow to patient's tidal volume by establishing that reservoir bag neither overinflates nor underinflates.
7. Allow patient to breathe 100% O_2 for 1 min.
8. Introduce N_2O at a rate of 1 L/min by adjusting N_2O flow value (be sure to decrease O_2 flow at an equivalent rate so total flow remains constant); pause 35–45 sec between increments; increase N_2O flow rate until baseline sedation is reached.

B. Turning machine off
1. Using N_2O flow valve, decrease N_2O flow to 0 L/min.
2. Increase O_2 flow rate so total flow remains constant (usually 5–8 L/min).
3. After patient has breathed 100% O_2 for 2 min, remove inhaler assembly.
4. Turn off N_2O at tank.
5. Turn off O_2 at tank.
6. Turn sedation machines "on-off" switch to "off."
7. Turn O_2 flow valve to 0 L/min.

C. Testing machine's "fail-safe" system
1. Turn machine on as indicated in A, steps 1–4.
2. Increase N_2O flow valve to begin flow of N_2O.
3. Turn off O_2 at tank.
4. The "fail-safe" mechanism is operational if N_2O flow drops to 0 L/min.

D. Intravenous sedation may employ psychosedatives (major and minor tranquilizers), barbiturates, narcotics, and belladonna-like agents (Table 5-3). Previously popular "fixed dosage" methods have now been supplanted by individually titrated regimens of benzodiazepines, narcotics, or barbiturates used either alone or in various combinations. Oxygen should always be available and should be routinely administered with deep sedative techniques. Patients should be informed not to drive for 24 hours after IV sedation.
1. Benzodiazepines
   a. Diazepam (Valium) remains one of the most important IV sedative agents in oral and maxillofacial surgery,

Table 5-3   AGENTS COMMONLY USED IN INTRAVENOUS SEDATION*

	Multidose vial†	Disposable syringes†	Ampules	Usual adult dose‡	Duration§
Diazepam		5 (2)	5 (2 or 10)	5–20	30–45
Fentanyl			0.05 (2)	0.05–0.1	30
Meperidine	50 (30)	50 (1,2)	50 (2)	25–100	180
Methohexital	10 (50–500)			5–250	5–7
Midazolam	5 (5, 10)		5 (2)	7–10	30
Naloxone			0.4 (1)	0.2–0.4	180–240
Nembutal	50	50 (2)		50–75	15–30

*Among manufacturers a wide variation exists in the concentration, volumes, and forms of delivery of intravenous sedative agents. Values presented here are representative and considered to be particularly suitable for oral and maxillofacial surgery, but should not be interpreted as a complete list of available products.

†Concentration in mg/ml. The number in parentheses indicates volume per vial, syringe, or ampule.

‡Expressed in mg. These are representative adult doses; all require individual titration and assessment of response.

§Duration of therapeutic effect must be assessed in patients individually. Wide variation exists. Values presented here are average effective durations of action for healthy adults expressed in minutes.

despite continuing development of numerous related compounds.

(1) Physical characteristics and composition are as follows: lipid soluble, water insoluble, available (as Valium) in a 0.5% solution (5 mg/ml).

(2) Major routes of administration are PO and IV; IM absorption is poor and erratic. Low water solubility causes diazepam to precipitate when combined with a water-based injectable. Injection into a running IV line should be made at the portal nearest the vein.

(3) Clinical effects of IV diazepam include disinhibition, drowsiness, muscle relaxation, and anticonvulsant activity. Specific circulatory, respiratory, and CNS effects have been described. Although metabolism is very slow ($t_{1/2}$ 20–40 hr), clinical effects terminate rapidly because of redistribution.

(4) Potential hazards are CNS depression, respiratory depression, cardiovascular complications (cardiac arrest, hypotension, hypertension), allergic reactions, altered mental state (coma, hysteria, hallucinations), and visual abnormalities.

   a) In the elderly patient a disproportionate sedative effect may be observed.

   b) Thrombophlebitis is a common local complication. Its incidence increases when vascular access is through the small veins of the forearm and hand. No correlation has been established between thrombophlebitis and smoking, contraceptive use, or injection by needle versus a plastic catheter. The incidence of thrombophlebitis can be decreased by slow injection through a running IV line (to increase the dilution effect) in a large vein.

   c) In general, diazepam has a high therapeutic index. The very young and the elderly are most sensitive to its effects.

(5) Recommended dosage protocols recognize the wide variability in response to diazepam and mandate administration of small incremental doses that allow its effect to be assessed before giving more of the drug. In this manner dosage is titrated to the individual patient and overdosage is avoided.

   a) The initial increment is usually 2.5 mg. Further increments of 2–3 mg are then given every 30 sec until an appropriate level of sedation is reached.

   b) A dose range of 5–20 mg is common (average total dosage is 18 mg). These dosages will be less when given in combination with other sedative medications (e.g., narcotics). The duration of an effective dose is generally about 45 min.

b. Midazolam (Versed) has many sedative properties similar to diazepam. Advantages over diazepam include its greater water solubility, lower thrombophlebitic effect, better amnestic effect, and more rapid onset. Although midazolam has a shorter half-life, actual patient recovery time is very similar to diazepam. Clinical effects and potential hazards are similar. Recommended dosage begins with an initial test dose of 1 mg, with a common total dose range of approximately 2 to 10 mg. Its increased potential for respiratory depression requires close patient monitoring.

c. Level of sedation with benzodiazepines is assessed on the basis of altered speech (most reliable index of sedation depth), ptosis (Verrill's sign), and blurred vision (least reliable index of sedation depth). Patients are carefully observed during the procedure, as described above. Afterward, they must be escorted home by a relative or friend. Reversal is available with flumazenil should adverse outcomes occur (e.g., respiratory depression) (see Reversal Agents p. 145).

d. Combination techniques involving N_2O-O_2, narcotics, and barbiturates are common, but supplementing IV benzodiazepines with either N_2O-O_2 or narcotics may be unnecessary and carries the risk of unintended passage from a state of sedation into general anesthesia. When using a combination technique, lower doses of all agents should be employed, with careful patient monitoring.

(1) For mildly or moderately apprehensive patients, a benzodiazepine alone is sufficient to allay anxiety. Complete control of pain is readily accomplished by regional anesthesia.

(2) For more fearful patients, local anesthesia and a benzodiazepine can be combined with low doses of narcotics or the barbiturate methohexital. This method may approach or intentionally produce a controlled state of general anesthesia; however, with properly trained personnel and proper facilities, the capacity for partial or total amnesia is more predictable. Pain, anxiety, and recollection of the surgical procedure are thus minimized. Methods for combining a benzodiazepine and methohexital are described in section 3.b. p. 144.

2. Narcotics (e.g., fentanyl and meperidine) are used because of their significant therapeutic value as sedatives and analgesics. They are employed alone or in combination with a

benzodiazepine, N_2O-O_2, and/or barbiturates. They must be avoided in patients taking MAO inhibitors. As in all IV sedation techniques, primary pain control still relies on effective local anesthesia. Narcotics offer the ability for reversal should adverse outcomes occur (e.g., respiratory depression) (see Reversal Agents below).

a. Fentanyl is 100 times more potent than morphine, with a typical dose of 50–100 μg (0.05–0.10 mg). Onset is almost immediate; duration is short (30 min or less); and emetic activity is low. Like all narcotics, fentanyl is a respiratory depressant; resulting alterations in respiratory rate and alveolar ventilation may persist after sedative or analgesic effects have ceased. Reports of fentanyl-induced chest wall rigidity and the potential need for treatment with narcotic antagonists and/or succinylcholine militate against the use of fentanyl by those untrained in general anesthesia or unprepared to ventilate and intubate the patient.

b. Meperidine is less potent than morphine and can be given PO, IM, or IV in doses of 25–100 mg. In addition to the intended effect of analgesia (up to 3 hr), meperidine causes sedation, respiratory depression, euphoria, bronchoconstriction, constipation, nausea, postural hypotension, diaphoresis, and xerostomia.

3. "Short-acting" (secobarbital and pentobarbital) and "ultra-short-acting" (methohexital and thiopental) barbiturates are used in oral and maxillofacial surgery. Methohexital is the most widely used barbiturate in both sedative and outpatient general anesthetic techniques.

a. Methohexital is administered as a 1% solution (10 mg/ml) given on an intermittent dosing schedule. In ambulatory general anesthesia an initial "test" dose of 20 mg (2 ml) is followed by an induction dose of 0.5–1.0 mg/kg, and then by maintenance increments of 10 to 30 mg delivered at individually determined intervals. In outpatient anesthesia, methohexital is used in conjunction with agents such as N_2O-O_2, fentanyl or meperidine, atropine or glycopyrrolate, diazepam or midazolam, and other substances.

b. Sedation and amnesia can be reliably obtained when methohexital is used to supplement IV diazepam sedation. An initial dose of diazepam (10–20 mg) is followed by small methohexital increments (5–10 mg). Local anesthesia is induced after the patient is adequately sedated. This technique offers the advantages of complete amnesia, intact reflexes (the patient remains conscious and can respond to commands), and the need for only a single operator.

    c. Light general anesthesia with diazepam and methohexital is induced with a smaller initial dose of diazepam (5-10 mg) followed by a methohexital "test dose" and an induction dose (20-50 mg). Local anesthesia is recommended; N_2O-O_2 sedation is optional. This technique affords complete amnesia and is very effective for the intractable patient. However, reflexes are obtunded and two operators trained in general anesthetic techniques are recommended.

  4. Reversal agents of various types exist, but naloxone and flumazenil are the most important.

    a. Naloxone is a synthetic agent whose configuration resembles that of oxymorphone. Naloxone reverses narcotic effects without exerting significant agonistic influences of its own. Naloxone should always be available when narcotic sedation techniques are being used.

      (1) The initial IV dose for adults is 0.2-0.4 mg and may be repeated at intervals of 2-3 min until an effect is seen.

      (2) Because the duration of narcotic-induced respiratory depression may exceed the length of time that naloxone is effective (3-4 hr), careful monitoring is needed to detect any recurrent respiratory depression.

    b. Flumazenil is a competitive antagonist of the benzodiazepine receptor, thus acting to reverse the effects of benzodiazepines. Flumazenil should always be available when benzodiazepine sedation techniques are being employed. It is available in a concentration of 0.1 mg/ml.

      (1) The initial IV dose for adults is 0.2 to 0.4 mg, and is repeated in 0.2-mg doses every minute up to a total dose of 1 mg or until an effect is observed.

      (2) Careful monitoring for re-sedation is required, since the duration of benzodiazepine-induced respiratory depression may exceed the length of time that flumazenil is effective.

III. Stress reduction protocol

  A. Several steps can be taken to help alleviate the anxiety that patients feel over the oral surgical experience.

  B. The "stress reduction protocol" outlined below acknowledges the need for managing apprehension preoperatively, intraoperatively, and postoperatively. Note that it also employs medications to enable the patient to relax before the procedure, obtain a restful sleep the night before the appointment, tolerate the procedure in comfort, and feel less discomfort postoperatively.

Stress Reduction Protocol

A. Recognize medical risk and obtain necessary consultations
B. Recognize patient's anxiety about oral surgical treatment
C. Schedule patient appointment
 1. Usually in AM
 2. Minimize waiting
 3. Shorter treatment time
D. Control anxiety during therapy
 1. Suggestion
 2. Hypnosis
 3. Local anesthetics
 4. Oral sedation
 5. N_2O-O_2 sedation
 6. Intramuscular sedation
 7. Intravenous sedation
E. Control pain during therapy
 1. Local anesthetics
 2. Systemic analgesics
F. Control pain and anxiety postoperatively

GENERAL REFERENCES

Boakes AJ, Laurence DR, Teoh PC, et al: Interaction between sympathomimetic amines and antidepressant agents in man, *Br Med J* 1:311, 1973.

Goulet J, Perusse R, et al: Contradictions to vasoconstrictors in dentistry: part III, *Oral Surg Oral Med Oral Path* 74:692, 1992.

Gustainis JF, Peterson LJ: An alternative method of mandibular nerve block, *J Am Dent Assoc* 103:33, 1981.

Holroyd SV, Wynn RL, Clark RC: *Clinical pharmacology in dental practice*, St. Louis, 1988, Mosby.

Ichinohe T, Igarashi O, Kaneko Y: The influence of propranolol on the cardiovascular effects and plasma clearance of epinephrine, *Anesth Prog* 38:217, 1991.

Jastak JT, Yagiela JA: Vasoconstrictors and local anesthesia: a review and rationale for use, *J Am Dent Assoc* 107:623, 1983.

Malamed SF: *Handbook of local anesthesia*, ed 3, St Louis, 1990, Mosby.

Spiro SR: *Pain and anxiety control in dentistry*, Englewood, NJ, 1981, Jack K. Burgess.

Trieger N: *Pain control*, Chicago, 1974, Quintessence Books.

Yagiela JA, Duffin SR, Hunt LM: Drug interaction and vasoconstrictors used in local anesthetic solutions, *Oral Surg Oral Med Oral Path* 59:565, 1985.

Postoperative Care

6

MEREDITH AUGUST

BLOOD PRESSURE CONTROL

I. All blood pressure measurements should be interpreted relative to the patient's baseline values. If a preoperative value indicates an elevated (>140/90 mm Hg) or lowered (<90/60 mm Hg) blood pressure, several measurements should be performed.

II. It is important to realize that there are no absolute values. A wide spectrum of pressure readings exists—reflecting age, systemic conditions, medications, emotional status, and other factors. All readings should be interpreted along with other vital signs.

Hypertension

Hypertension, usually defined as blood pressure >140/90, is a significant finding in a patient.

I. Etiology

A. In the older patient, previously uncontrolled borderline or frank hypertension is a leading cause of postoperative hypertension. A review of the patient's old hospital chart will be helpful, especially the anesthesia record and immediate postoperative vital signs.

1. If a patient is taking an antihypertensive medication, one should carefully question him or her with regard to compliance. Withdrawal of antihypertensive medication often contributes to the development of postoperative hypertension. Rebound hypertension is most commonly seen with cessation of beta-blocking agents.

2. A review of the medication chart will be helpful in assessing current medications for proper dosage and timing. (One must not assume that all orders are interpreted correctly.)

B. In the previously healthy younger patient, and for all persons, pain (with its catecholamine release) in the postoperative period is a significant factor in elevated blood pressure. Often, assessment of other vital signs may be helpful. The patient must be asked about his or her pain status and appropriate measures taken to ensure adequate dosage and timing of medications.

The patient may appear quite sedated but actually be very uncomfortable.

C. Drugs may cause hypertension. Positive inotropes (e.g., ephedrine and phenylephrine) may have been administered intraoperatively. Pseudoephedrine is commonly used postoperatively for maxillary procedures. If the patient was paralyzed with pancuronium or gallamine and relaxation was not adequately reversed, hypertension may result.

D. Fluid gains and losses, including blood loss, transfusions, and urine output, may cause hypertension. The patient in significant positive fluid balance may appear uncomfortable and anxious and experience respiratory distress. One should assess pulmonary status, venous distention, and the extremities for edema.

E. Poor oxygenation and/or increased P_{CO_2} may result from postoperative atelectasis or preexisting pulmonary disease and may lead to an increase in blood pressure. Narcotics may have caused the patient to retain CO_2. Unreplaced significant blood loss may lead to poor tissue oxygenation. Arterial blood gas determinations are required for properly assessing any increase or decrease in P_{O_2} and P_{CO_2}. (See section on Blood Gas Determination.)

1. The P_{O_2}, P_{CO_2}, and pH comprise the arterial blood gas determination, which may be a critical part of the preoperative workup and also the intraoperative and postoperative management of a patient.

   a. Preoperatively it is needed for:
      (1) Evaluation of the respiratory status (e.g., in a patient with chronic lung disease, marginal oxygenation, or hypercapnia)
      (2) Assessing the adequacy of ventilation (e.g., via an endotracheal tube in a severe trauma patient with intracranial or thoracic injury)

   b. Intraoperatively it is used in:
      (1) Assessing the ventilatory status
      (2) Measuring the acid-base balance

   c. Postoperatively it has multiple indications:
      (1) Acute respiratory distress
      (2) Cardiac emergencies
      (3) Prolonged wakefulness or acute agitation
      (4) Intubation or assisted ventilation
      (5) Poorly controlled diabetes

2. Technique

   a. Equipment—5–6-ml glass syringe, 19–20-gauge needle, rubber stopper or cork (or metal cap), ice-filled container, alcohol swabs for preparing skin, sponges for applying pressure after puncture

   b. Method—1 ml of heparin (1000 U/ml) is aspirated into a syringe and expelled with all the air after the barrel is

Table 6-1   SITES FOR OBTAINING ABG SAMPLES

Site	Location	Comments
Brachial artery	Accessible as it crosses medial-epicondyle of humerus proximal to antecubital space; median nerve is on medial side of vessel	Median nerve potential hazard
Radial artery	Crosses radial styloid; easily accessible with wrist and thumb extended	Allen test to confirm collateral circulation; use local infiltration to reduce spasm and provide patient comfort
Femoral artery	Largest; with patient in supine position and hip externally rotated, vessel is palpable distal to inguinal ligament; place one finger lateral to pulse, second medial to pulse; hold syringe perpendicular to pulse and puncture lateral to pulse	Puncture made lateral to pulse to avoid venous contamination

     coated; the syringe will then fill spontaneously by arterial pressure (plastic syringes do not offer this advantage)

  3. Sites—the brachial, radial, and femoral arteries are available sites for arterial blood sampling. Each has advantages and disadvantages (Table 6-1), but proficiency at each should be learned. A good pulse must be palpable at the site.

  4. Interpretation

    a. Nomograms (Fig. 6-1) are available for bedside evaluation of results. The following axioms are also helpful:

      (1) The Po_2 is meaningless without knowledge of the inspired oxygen concentration at the time of sampling.

      (2) Assume a normal pH (7.40) and normal Pco_2 (40 mm Hg).

      (3) Each 10 mm Hg shift in the Pco_2 accounts for a pH shift of 0.08.

      (4) Changes in pH from metabolic causes or compensation occur slowly unless iatrogenically produced (e.g., bicarbonate infusion). Changes produced by respiratory function occur quickly.

    b. Oxygenation varies inversely with age. Thus, the Po_2 is normally 80–100 mm Hg in room air containing 21% oxy-

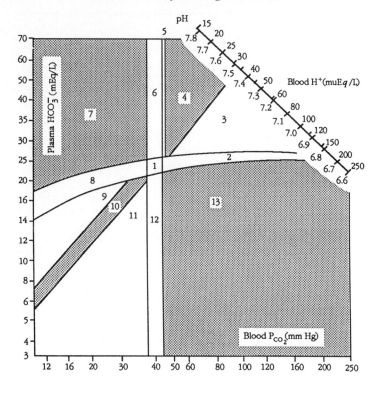

1. Normal
2. Respiratory acidosis
3. Respiratory acidosis (compensated)
4. Respiratory acidosis, metabolic alkalosis (mixed)
5. Metabolic alkalosis (compensated)
6. Metabolic alkalosis
7. Respiratory alkalosis, metabolic alkalosis (mixed)
8. Respiratory alkalosis
9. Respiratory alkalosis (compensated)
10. Metabolic acidosis, respiratory alkalosis (mixed)
11. Metabolic acidosis (compensated)
12. Metabolic acidosis
13. Metabolic acidosis, respiratory acidosis (mixed)

Fig. 6-1 Interpretation of arterial blood studies.

       gen. A Po_2 of 80 mm Hg may be normal for an elderly pa-
       tient, but not for a young one.
   c. Acidosis and alkalosis may have respiratory or metabolic
      causes. Multiple permutations are possible, since in most
      situations the observed pH is the end result of a primary
      derangement of either respiratory or metabolic function
      plus a secondary compensation. Bedside interpretation is
      possible using the axioms below. (see Fig. 6-1).

pH	Pco$_2$ (mm Hg)	Clinical status
<7.40	>40	Respiratory acidosis
<7.40	≤40	Metabolic acidosis
>7.40	<40	Respiratory alkalosis
>7.40	≥40	Metabolic alkalosis

(1) If the pH is <7.40, acidosis occurs; if >7.40, alkalosis occurs.

(2) If the Pco$_2$ is >40 mm Hg, respiratory acidosis occurs; if ≤40 mm Hg, the primary derangement is metabolic acidosis.

(3) For assessing the contribution of combined respiratory and metabolic factors to pH alteration: a Pco$_2$ of 60 mm Hg would be expected to lower the pH by 0.16 (0.08 for each 10 mm Hg difference from the normal of 40 mm Hg) to 7.24; if the actual pH is found to be 7.32, then partial metabolic compensation for the respiratory acidosis can be assumed (remember: metabolic compensation does not occur acutely); similarly, if the Pco$_2$ is 60 mm Hg and the pH is 7.20, then a combined metabolic and respiratory acidosis exists, since the Pco$_2$ alone (respiratory component) would be insufficient to account for the observed acidosis.

(4) Above all, knowledge of and experience with the actual clinical setting are most important.

F. Urinary retention may cause hypertension. A noncatheterized patient with a full bladder that has not voided within a reasonable time (8–10 hr) after a surgical procedure will often display hypertension and tachycardia.

G. Rarer causes include renovascular hypertension, Cushing's disease, hyperaldosteronism, hyperthyroidism, coarctation of the aorta, pheochromocytoma, toxemia of pregnancy, and increased intracranial pressure.

II. Diagnosis

A. Blood pressure must be measured in both arms (or legs); several readings are necessary.

B. All other vital signs must be assessed and interpreted.

C. Additional indicators may be a visibly anxious patient, flushed skin, respiratory distress, epistaxis, retinal changes, proteinuria, and a full bladder (tender to palpation, dull to percussion).

D. Symptoms may include pain at the operative site, headache, nausea and vomiting, chest pain, and respiratory distress. Visual changes (e.g., scotomas) may appear. Disorientation secondary to stroke should be noted.

E. If chest pain or respiratory distress is present, cardiac enzymes, a chest radiograph, and an ECG must be obtained.

III. Treatment

A. Elevated pressure can be tolerated by a previously healthy patient over a short time. One whose cardiovascular status is compromised may be stepping into dangerous waters with higher than normal readings. It is important to treat the cause, not the numbers!

   1. The previously poorly controlled patient needs to begin an antihypertensive regimen. A medical consultation is appropriate.
   2. Control of postoperative pain is discussed on p. 159.
   3. If the renal status is deemed adequate and the patient is urinating, pressure will often return to baseline within 12–24 hr.
   4. Drugs are a possible cause. One must check for type, dosage, and adequate reversal.
   5. Urinary retention is discussed on p. 158.
   6. Rarer causes and those associated with cardiovascular-pulmonary complications should have an appropriate medical consultation as soon as possible.

B. Hypertensive emergencies (>180/115 mm Hg) or hypertension associated with cardiovascular–pulmonary findings may be treated with the following:

   1. Labetalol HCl–20 mg IV over 2 minutes and repeat injections at 10-minute intervals based on supine blood pressure.
   2. Diazoxide—300 mg IV push or 150 mg IV followed by 50-mg increments titrated to an end point
   3. Hydralazine-propranolol—10 mg of hydralazine in 10 ml of normal saline with 1 mg of propranolol (Inderal), given in 2-ml aliquots IV
   4. Furosemide (Lasix)—initially 10 mg IV, if the patient is in positive fluid balance, or one half the oral dose
   5. Methyldopa (Aldomet)—250 mg IV q6h in 125 ml of D_5W given over 30 min
   6. Nifedipine—10 mg sublingually
   7. Morphine, if pain is the cause—begun with 5 mg IV and 2-mg increments added as needed; this will often lower blood pressure from its vasodilating effects.

   Specific antihypertensive therapy should be administered according to severity. Systemic vasodilators frequently elicit a reflex tachycardia, which may be problematic in patients with coronary artery disease. A combined alpha and beta blocker such as labetalol or a vasodilator in conjunction with a beta blocker is preferred.

Hypotension

Hypotension represents a significant lowering of blood pressure below the patient's normal values.

I. Etiology

    A. In a previously healthy patient, inadequate fluid replacement and the residual effects of anesthesia are the most common causes of hypotension. The anesthesia record must be checked for all fluid losses and gains, including significant blood loss. Nasogastric suctioning, drains, and repetitive vomiting and diarrhea may be contributing elements. Polyuria associated with diabetes mellitus or insipidus may cause volume depletion. Occult blood loss, distant from the operative site, may be a causative factor; if it is suspected, stool guaiac tests are necessary. Fluid deficits are often associated with tachycardia.

    B. Reduction of cardiac output secondary to atrial or ventricular arrhythmias, congestive heart failure, myocardial infarction, or conduction deficits may cause hypotension.

    C. Drugs (e.g., narcotic analgesics, nitrates, droperidol, hydralazine, propranolol, or curare) may lower the blood pressure.

    D. Rarer causes include septic shock, adrenal insufficiency, large pneumothorax, and positive end-expiratory pressure treatment.

II. Diagnosis

    A. Hypotension in the otherwise healthy patient is usually tolerated well.

    B. One must be very careful in the patient with existing coronary artery disease, because the heart receives its major blood supply during diastole, and reflex tachycardia is often seen in hypotensive patients. Also, patients with compromised renal function are at risk, because significant or prolonged hypotension can lead to renal failure. Patients with carotid artery occlusion cannot tolerate hypertension. Treatment of these patient groups is more aggressive.

    C. Diagnostic symptoms include:

        1. Orthostatic vital signs (supine, then sitting or standing) taken within 30 sec to 1 min of assuming each position—an increase in heart rate of 20 bpm or a decrease in systolic pressure of 20 mm Hg indicates significant volume depletion.

        2. Syncope, tachycardia, arrhythmias, or other cardiovascular findings.

        3. Laboratory values (hematocrit, osmolality, electrolytes, tests for occult bleeding)—can give clues as to the reason for an acute volume change.

III. Treatment

    A. In an emergency, 300 ml of normal saline or Ringer's lactate solution is given IV over 10 min while observing response. Fluid deficits are best replaced by giving one half volume over 12 hr and one half over the remaining 24 hr (unless cardiopulmonary status is impaired).

    B. The patient is put in the Trendelenburg position.

    C. If drugs are the cause, ephedrine, 10 mg IV, or a phenylephrine drip (1 amp in 500 ml of D_5W with a "pedi" pump chamber) is given and titrated to response.

    D. Other causes demand prompt medical consultation and coordinated treatment.

URINARY RETENTION

  I. A patient should normally void under voluntary effort within 8–12 hr postoperatively. Failure to do so is not uncommon.

 II. Etiology

    A. The usual cause is retention secondary to anesthesia, drugs, and recumbency. Heavily sedated postoperative patients are often unaware of acute bladder distention.

    B. The causes can be roughly categorized as:

      1. Prerenal—secondary to decreased cardiac output (congestive heart failure, arrhythmias, etc.) or volume depletion

      2. Renal (acute renal failure)—many underlying causes, but acute tubular necrosis is the most common

      3. Postrenal—obstructive uropathies, bladder atony secondary to medications (vagolytics, narcotics, etc.)

      4. Urinary tract infection

 III. Diagnosis

    A. Physical examination is important. The patient should be asked if he or she desires to urinate. The bladder may be palpated and percussed for tenderness and dullness. Orthostatic vital signs can indicate hypovolemia.

    B. Laboratory tests may be useful—serum hematocrit, osmolality, electrolytes, BUN, creatinine. If a urine sample can be obtained, specific gravity, occult blood, myoglobin (if transfusions were given or with crush injuries), casts, and sodium are checked.

 IV. Treatment

    A. Treatment is directed toward the cause. The most common situation is a sleepy postanesthetic patient who has received one or two narcotic injections. If physical examination indicates a full bladder, suprapubic hot packs and assisted ambulation will usually suffice.

    B. If after 10–12 hr no urine production is evident, a "straight catheter" may be inserted, with care to remove no more than 500–700 ml, because bladder spasm or syncope could result. After catheterizing a patient, it is wise to send a urine sample for analysis along with culture and sensitivity tests.

    C. Administration of parasympathomimetic agents (pilocarpine or bethanecol) can increase detrusor muscle tone in selective cases and promote micturition. However, these agents must be avoided in cases of obstruction (e.g., prostatic hypertrophy).

    D. The following box will serve as a guide for assessing urinary tests. Prolonged urinary retention demands medical evaluation to rule out renal failure.

RENAL CONSERVATION
Specific gravity high (1.040)
Osmolality high (300 or greater)
Sodium low (<10 mEq/L)

POSSIBLE RENAL FAILURE
Specific gravity isothenic or less (<1.010)
Osmolality low (<275)
Sodium high (>50 mEq/L)

   E. For treatment of volume depletion, see the section on hypovolemia.
   F. Cardiac or renal causes demand thorough and prompt evaluation and treatment coordinated with the proper medical specialty.

PAIN CONTROL

  I. Patients may exhibit a wide variety of reactions to painful stimuli. After a major oral and maxillofacial surgical procedure, most patients will require narcotic analgesics for varying lengths of time.
 II. Etiology—the source of pain is important. Besides the obvious surgical site, pain can arise from swelling, muscle spasm (secondary to intermaxillary fixation), and local factors (e.g., irritation of the gingivae from arch bars).
III. Diagnosis—a visibly anxious patient with guarding of the affected area usually is a good indicator. Associated tachycardia and hypertension can often result from pain.
IV. Treatment
   A. Systemic measures include:
     1. Meperidine (Demerol)—50-100 mg IM q3-4h
     2. Morphine—5-10 mg IM q3-4h
     3. For less painful stimuli:
       a. Codeine—30-60 mg q3-4h
       b. Acetaminophen—650 mg q3-4h
     4. If these narcotic regimens do not sustain the patient, 50 mg of hydroxyzine (Vistaril) IM along with the narcotic for increased efficacy
   B. Local measures are also important:
     1. Ice to the area for 24 hr, followed by warm, moist heat may decrease swelling and reduce muscle spasm.
     2. A rib graft donor site can be very painful. Local blockade of the afferent nerve fibers above, below, and proximal to the operative site is helpful. Bupivacaine (Marcaine), 5-10 ml, of a 2% solution with epinephrine will often obviate the need for a heavier narcotic schedule.
     3. Wax (applied to arch bars) and lip creams are helpful.

C. The patient should begin taking oral pain medications at least 24 hr before expected discharge so the efficacy of such a regimen can be ascertained. It may prevent an unexpected "emergency" call.

D. The surgeon must always weigh the side effects and psychosocial implications of pain medications and try to weigh true patient need against possible drug abuse.

WOUND CARE

I. Wound care should be part of daily patient care. It includes direct observation, indirect observation (vital signs, laboratory values), and good surgical judgment.

A. All wounds should be observed for bleeding, discharge, suture breakdowns, erythema, and necrosis.

B. Experience is needed to distinguish between the expected amount of edema and tissue discoloration from surgical procedures versus that from wound breakdown.

II. Etiology

A. Wound dehiscence or infection may occur from poor surgical technique. Prevention is best achieved by proper debridement of all necrotic or compromised tissue, sterile technique, irrigation, hemostasis, elimination of dead spaces, proper closure, and antibiotics.

B. Infection may result from intraoral or extraoral sources. Cultures are absolutely necessary for determining the cause and selecting the proper antibiotic.

C. Systemically compromised patients may be prone to infection by reduced host defenses.

III. Treatment

A. Routine care of intraoral wounds includes:

1. Daily observation.

2. A clear liquid diet for 24 hr; if the patient can be advanced to a full blenderized diet, clear liquid rinses should follow.

3. Normal saline rinses starting 24 hr after the procedure; some clinicians claim that hydrogen peroxide dissolves existing clots, leading to fresh bleeding.

4. A Water-Pik started 5–7 da after the procedure, with light pressure.

5. Wax applied to arch bars to minimize gingival swelling.

6. 0.5% Hydrocortisone cream to lips preoperatively and postoperatively to reduce swelling and discomfort.

B. Extraoral wounds require:

1. Daily observation.

2. Antibacterial ointment to sutures at each nursing shift.

3. Removal of sutures in 5–7 da, with Steri-Strips across the wound (perpendicularly) to reduce tension; collodion may be applied instead of Steri-Strips.

C. Drains should be assessed daily and removed as soon as their purpose is finished. After 24–48 hr, entrance of microorganisms into the wound via the drain becomes more likely. Antibiotics are continued for at least 24 hr after removal of drains.

D. Compressive dressings may aid in the reduction of postsurgical swelling. Gauze "fluffs" with Elastoplast and/or a neurosurgical head roll may effectively compress an extraoral surgical wound. Elastoplast placed across the chin for 3–4 da after anterior mandibular procedures is helpful for reduction of edema.

E. External pin fixation devices should be observed for loosening and discharge around pin sites. Daily application of antibacterial ointment to pin sites should be routine. Iodoform gauze between the skin and the acrylic bar of this device will help minimize irritation.

V. Complications
   A. Early wound breakdown generally results from excessive tension. If all other factors are healthy, the small wound will usually granulate without complication. Wet dressings applied to the area help prevent dehydration.
   B. Late wound breakdown (5 da) usually results from necrotic tissue or infection. More aggressive treatment is necessary—cultures, antibiotics, and thorough determination of cause.

POSTOPERATIVE FEVER

I. A fever may be defined as any body temperature that exceeds 1° above normal.
   A. In assessing a patient's fever, it is important to remember the diurnal variation of 0.5–1.0° seen when AM and PM readings are compared. It is also important in sequential temperature readings to make certain that the mode of measurement (e.g., oral vs. rectal vs. axillary) is the same.
   B. The temperature should be checked as part of every postoperative patient visit.
      1. A low-grade fever (<100° F) is not an unexpected finding during the first 2–3 da postoperatively. Fevers of this magnitude may be attributed to operative trauma or to tissue and protein absorption, and a cause need not be sought if no clinical suspicion of another source is evident.
      2. If such a low-grade fever persists beyond 3 da postoperatively, it is imperative that a fever workup be carried out and a cause sought.
      3. Fevers worthy of immediate workup may be defined as:
         a. Any that exceed 101.6° F after a single dose of acetaminophen (Tylenol) (1.2 g PO or PR) on the first postoperative night
         b. Any above 101.6° F thereafter (without antipyretic administration)

II. Etiology
   A. In the search for a cause of postoperative fever, both the timing of its appearance and its magnitude (e.g., low grade vs. hyperpyrexia) should be considered, as well as the pattern of tem-

perature troughs and peaks and any associated systemic signs
that give valuable clues as to etiology.

B. The timing of fever may be divided into three intervals:

1. Fevers that develop during surgery

   a. These are seen most often in patients who have had sepsis preoperatively. For example, in a patient with a nonreduced mobile mandibular fracture who has fever, swelling, and pain around the fracture site, manipulation of such a contaminated area will result in a bacteremia, and temperature spikes may well be noted intraoperatively.

   b. A precipitous rise in body temperature after induction with general anesthesia (with temperature rise as high as 108° F) may herald malignant hyperthermia. This is an anesthetic emergency. The procedure should be terminated and anesthesia stopped immediately.

   c. Intraoperative hyperthermia may occur in an anesthetized patient secondary to the thermal insulation provided by the drapes and by the loss of normal thermoregulatory mechanisms through the use of anticholingergic drugs and inhalation anesthetics.

2. Fevers that develop immediately postoperatively (0–6 hr)

   a. Fevers within this time interval are commonly caused by either endocrine or metabolic abnormalities. Postoperative thyroid crises are now seen less frequently than in earlier days, before the use of medications that made it easier to attain a euthyroid condition preoperatively. The actual mechanism of thyroid crises remains obscure, but altered metabolism and sensitivity appear to play a role.

   b. Blood transfusions may result in fever. This can be due to a full-blown transfusion reaction caused by administration of incompatible blood or to minor incompatibilities between donor and recipient. Signs and symptoms are noted almost immediately after the transfusion is begun and may present as any of the following: hives, chills, palpitations, chest or flank pain, and shortness of breath, in addition to fever, headache, and flushing. When any of these signs are observed, the transfusion must be stopped immediately.

   c. Dehydration secondary to inadequate fluid replacement intraoperatively and minimal oral intake postoperatively may result in fever. This is especially common in children and the elderly. Treating the underlying imbalance should normalize the temperature and help ensure adequate tissue perfusion.

3. Fevers that develop later

   a. Postoperative atelectasis is produced by inadequate ventilation or by some obstruction of the tracheobronchial tree (e.g., a mucous plug). In addition to fever, the physical findings of tachypnea, tachycardia, and moist rales upon auscultation (especially at the lung bases) are found. Atelectasis is most commonly confined to the lower lobes, is rarely lobar and is commonly seen bilaterally. A fuller discussion of atelectasis and postoperative pulmonary complications is found on pp.174. Fever secondary to pulmonary complications is most commonly found after the first 6 hr and any time thereafter and should always be high on the differential list of postoperative hyperpyrexia.

b. Another common source of fever spikes after the first 6 hr and as late as 4–5 days postoperatively is urinary tract infection (UTI). This complication is more likely to be found in patients experiencing voiding difficulties (urinary stasis) or who have had an indwelling urethral catheter placed.

  (1) Upon questioning, the patient will complain of dysuria, frequency, and pain overlying the involved part of the genitourinary tract (e.g., suprapubic, flank).

  (2) A clean voided specimen (midstream) should be examined microscopically for the presence of WBCs and bacteria.

  (3) Culture and sensitivity tests should also be ordered to ensure that antibiotic coverage is specific. The organisms most frequently isolated from patients with UTIs are gram-negative enteric bacteria, enterococci, *Pseudomonas* species, and yeasts.

  (4) The most feared complication of UTIs is gram-negative sepsis. However, other worrisome sequelae of a chronic UTI are suppurative events (e.g., periurethral, prostatic, or perinephric abscess formation and acute suppurating epididymitis). Septicemia is accompanied by shaking chills and sudden temperature spikes, along with hypotension, vascular collapse, and the release of bacterial toxins.

c. The postoperative examination of a patient should always include observation and palpation of the skin overlying the site and IV catheter placement. Nonsterile phlebitis is caused by the introduction of microorganisms into the venous system, with resultant pain, swelling, and edema surrounding the involved site. (The most common offender is thought to be a *Staphylococcus* species.) Any intravenous line that has been in place longer than 24 hr in the face of a febrile patient with no evident source of fever is suspect and should be changed. The most common infected lines are central venous and hyperalimentation lines. More often than not, however, phlebitis is a sterile process of vessel injury that is thought to be caused by the frequent infusion of irritating solutions (antibiotics, KCl, hypertonic fluids) into small venous channels.

d. Thrombophlebitis of the lower extremities is yet another later source of postoperative fever and may be suspected when a patient complains of pain and tenderness with palpation of the popliteal space, calves, or thighs. A positive Homan's sign (pain in the calf elicited by dorsiflexion of the foot) is also commonly found with this complication, as well as an increase in calf diameter compared to the contralateral extremity. Factors that predispose to the development of thrombophlebitis include prolonged bed rest, long surgical procedures, unusual bed positions maintained postoperatively (e.g., with the pelvis the lowest point and the popliteal space being pushed upon by a flexure in the bed), a previous history of either thrombophlebitis or pulmonary embolus, heart disease (with venous stasis), obesity, polycythemia, and the use of birth control pills.

e. Postoperative wound infections are generally a later (4-5 da postoperatively) source of fever. Careful daily wound inspection will alert the surgeon to the possibility of infection. In addition to increased fever, there will often be tell-tale signs around the wound itself—increased tenderness, redness, drainage (often evidenced by dressing wetness), signs of necrosis and breakdown, and reaction around sutures.

III. Formal fever workup is a logical sequence of diagnostic tests and radiographic studies that address and focus on the common sources of postoperative fever. Results of the fever workup, coupled with a thorough physical examination, should lead the surgeon not only to source identification but to prompt and appropriate treatment choices (e.g., proper antimicrobial preparation).

A. Fevers worthy of immediate workup are:

1. Any <101.6° F after a single dose of acetaminophen on the first postoperative night

2. Any <101.6° F thereafter (without antipyretic administration)

B. Fever workup should include:

1. Inspection—wound sites, drain and catheter sites, IV catheters or other lines, general cutaneous inspection for signs of urticarial drug rash or vasculitis

2. Physical examination—pulmonary and cardiac, abdominal, palpation of extremities, measurement of calf diameter

3. Cultures—blood from at least two sites, clean voided urine, any drainage from wound or IV sites (aerobic, anaerobic, and, if indicated, fungal); blood cultures must be obtained after careful preparation of the puncture site with antiseptic solutions (povidone-iodine and alcohol)

    4. Chest radiograph—which may reveal atelectasis or pneumonitis; if the patient is unable to travel, a portable flat chest film should be obtained

IV. Treatment

  A. General treatment of hyperpyrexia

    1. The primary treatment of postoperative fever is to identify its source and treat the underlying problem. In addition, measures should be taken to control hyperpyrexia, especially in patients at greater risk (children, the elderly and infirm, the cardiovascularly impaired).

    2. Local measures include cooling mattresses and baths (which do little to affect temperature).

    3. The salicylates act to reset the hypothalamic "thermostat" for normal body temperature. Heat production is not affected, but dissipation is enhanced by the increased peripheral blood flow and sweating.

    4. Acetaminophen (Tylenol), a para-aminophenol derivative, is an effective antipyretic mechanistically analogous to the salicylates and preferable for hospital use because of its decreased GI irritation. A typical (albeit somewhat arbitrary) postoperative order for Tylenol for an adult may be written: 600 mg-1.2 g q4h when temperature exceeds 101.6° F. It is imperative that the nursing staff alert the doctor when fever of this magnitude develops in a postoperative patient.

  B. Specific treatment when the cause of fever is known

    1. For fever of malignant hyperthermia the patient's body is immersed in ice water. The stomach and body are lavaged with ice, and the body surface is cooled with ice packs. Pulmonary hyperventilation is instituted and sodium bicarbonate is given. Arterial blood gases and acid-base status are carefully monitored and abnormalities treated. A diuretic is given to avert development of acute tubular necrosis of the kidney.

      a. Cardiac arrhythmias may sometimes be the initial sign of malignant hyperthermia. Procainamide is usually the drug of choice in treating these. Hyperkalemia is treated with glucose and insulin infusion, and maintenance of fluid volume prevents circulatory collapse. Dantrolene, 1-10 mg/kg, is given as soon as possible.

      b. All of the above measures are continued postoperatively in an ICU in case episodes may recur.

    2. Treatment of a thyroid crisis as it develops consists of IV hydrocortisone, sedation, oxygen therapy, cooling of the febrile patient, and IV sodium iodide. Reserpine is given q4-6h IM to reduce agitation and tachycardia (respiratory depression must be avoided). Similarly, guanethidine is used to block the release of endogenous catecholamines, and IV propranolol is useful in the control of tachycardia. Hyperthermia is prevented by use of a cooling blanket.

3. Febrile reactions may occur with blood transfusions.

   a. Severe reactions secondary to bacterial contamination of blood (generally gram-negative anaerobes) (with temperature usually $>103°$ F) necessitate immediate cessation of the transfusion. The resultant septicemia is treated with IV fluid support, antibiotics, and steroids.

   b. Minor reactions to transfusions are occasionally seen and thought to be caused by leukoagglutinins or platelet agglutinins present in the recipient. They generally require more than one half unit of infusion before symptoms (flushing, headaches, chills) are noted, and the fever is usually responsive to oral antipyretics.

4. Treatment of UTIs in a patient who is not acutely ill should consist initially of hydration while the result of urine cultures is pending. If sepsis is likely, broad-spectrum antibiotics may be started after all cultures are obtained (both blood and urine).

5. In the case of noninfective phlebitis, treatment involves removal of the cannula, elevation of the extremities, and heat to the area. If septicemia is present, appropriate antibiotic treatment is begun (often requiring massive doses). If deep venous channels are involved, it is often necessary to remove the entire vein from the catheter entrance point to where it enters the next large venous tributary. Consultation with a vascular surgeon is imperative.

6. The risks and benefits of giving postoperative prophylactic anticoagulation therapy to those at high risk of thrombophlebitis must be weighed against the possibility of postoperative hemorrhage. If thrombophlebitis does develop, treatment includes bed rest, removal of all popliteal pressure, and anticoagulation as follows:

   a. Heparin is given by intermittent IV injection or by continuous infusion.

      (1) Intermittent: 10,000–15,000 U of sodium heparin initially and then 5000–10,000 U q4h.

      (2) Continuous: 5000-U bolus and 1000 U/hr thereafter.

      (3) Treatment should be monitored by the PTT, which is maintained at 1–1½ times normal (37–60 sec).

      (4) Heparin is usually continued for 8–19 da or until symptoms have subsided and the patient is ambulatory.

   b. Warfarin (Coumadin) is not effective for 5–7 da, so it is not the agent of choice in treating an acute condition. Therapy is begun several days after heparin treatment is started and continued after the heparin is stopped.

      (1) The efficacy of warfarin anticoagulation is monitored by serial PT (obtained daily during the first week, twice weekly during the second week, and twice monthly while the patient is receiving war-

farin). The PT should be maintained at 1-1½ times normal.

(2) The maintenance dose of warfarin varies between 2.5 and 12.5 mg/da, pending the results of the PT.

(3) If prompt reversal of anticoagulation is needed, vitamin K (5-25 mg IV) may be administered. (The complication of pulmonary embolism is discussed on pp. 176.)

POSTOPERATIVE NAUSEA AND VOMITING

I. The subjective complaint of nausea and the objective and measurable phenomenon of emesis are not infrequent problems in the immediate postoperative period (generally from postintubation to 24 hr).

II. Vomiting may be an especially dangerous complication for a patient who has been placed in intermaxillary fixation (IMF). It is imperative that both scissors (or a wire cutter if IMF is done through wiring rather than elastics) and a suction source be placed at the patient's bedside if extensive emesis that the patient cannot clear ensues and the jaws must be released. Generally, when the patient is fully awake and responding to verbal commands, the clearing of emesis will rarely require the release of IMF. Nasal suctioning and suctioning in the buccal vestibules will usually aid the patient in removal of emesis from the mouth. The patient should be placed on his or her side and the head of the bed lowered (Trendelenburg position) to enable gravity to abet clearing.

III. Aspiration of gastric contents secondary to vomiting may be a disastrous event and greatly increases the morbidity of a patient's postoperative course. The mortality from massive aspiration is reported to be as high as 90%. (A complete discussion of aspiration is found later in this chapter.)

IV. Etiology

A. The cause may be one or a combination of the following:

1. Use of morphine (or other opiates), which tend to increase gastric motor activity and dampen protective reflexes.

2. Inhalation general anesthesia (especially during induction and emergence), when a vomiting center is thought to be stimulated and protective reflexes have been lost.

3. Swallowing of blood and air intraoperatively and especially postoperatively (in which case nausea and vomiting are related to the site of surgery and its extent); this is perhaps the most common cause of postoperative nausea in the oral surgical patient, especially when intraoral incisions continue to weep and blood-tinged saliva is repeatedly swallowed.

4. Gastric inflation during mask ventillation

B. It must also be kept in mind that nausea and vomiting may be due to an acute condition not directly related to the surgery or the anesthetic (e.g., acute appendicitis, stress ulcer, small bowel obstruction).

V. Prophylaxis
   A. The use of nasogastric suction in oral and maxillofacial surgery has become an important part of prophylaxis for nausea, vomiting, and the potentially fatal complications of resultant airway obstruction or aspiration pneumonitis.
   B. The use of a Salem sump nasogastric tube is indicated if the patient is to be placed in IMF postoperatively, if the operation is expected to last longer than 3–4 hr, and if hemorrhage >100 ml from the operative sites or from the nose during or after surgery is expected. The nasogastric tube ensures that the stomach can be kept clear of any blood that leaks and, hopefully, removes this trigger for vomiting. The Salem sump is inserted after the patient is anesthetized. Auscultation while air is being forced through will help ensure proper placement in the stomach. The patency of the nasogastric tube should be checked each hour (irrigate with 30–50 ml of H_2O). Thorough suctioning before extubation is the rule, so the tube is left in place in the recovery room, and thereafter if it continues to drain when connected to wall suction. Before the tube is removed, the stomach should again be irrigated with normal saline and suctioned to remove any debris. The tube must be detached from the suction source before it is pulled.
   C. Nasogastric suction, if prolonged, can remove large amounts of fluid from the upper GI tract and can lead to resultant electrolyte imbalances (e.g., decreased K^+ or decreased H^+ [alkalosis]), which may require replacement therapy.
   D. The tube must be securely taped in place so as not to apply excessive pressure to the skin, mucosa, or cartilage of the nose. A half-inch piece of tape is prepared with two tails by cutting the lower portion in half. The uncut portion is applied to the nose, and the tails are wrapped around the tube to secure it.
   E. Complaints of nausea and vomiting after discontinuing nasogastric suction are most frequently addressed by the use of antiemetic pharmacologic agents (discussed next).
VI. Treatment
   A. The following list includes the more commonly used antiemetic preparations and recommended dosage schedules. Most antiemetic preparations are H_1 antihistaminics, phenothiazines or butyrophenones:
      1. Promethazine (Phenergan)—this phenothiazine derivative is well tolerated by children. Usual dose: 12.5–25 mg q4-6h.
      2. Trimethobenzamide (Tigan)—this drug depresses the "chemoreceptor trigger zone" in the medulla. Usual dose: 250 mg tid or qid. It is not recommended for use in children because it is associated with Reye's syndrome. Extrapyramidal symptoms may be found.
      3. Prochlorperazine maleate (Compazine)—this drug and other hepatotoxins are contraindicated in children and adolescents whose signs and symptoms suggest Reye's syn-

drome. Usual dose: 5-10 mg PO q6h; rectal dose: 25 mg bid; deep IM dose: 5-10 mg PO q6h. There may be side effects of extrapyramidal tract involvement with severe opisthotonos and risus sardonicus, which are dose related; in such cases, <40 mg should be used every 24 hr.

    4. Droperidol (Inapsine), a butyrophenone neuroleptic, experimentally antagonizes the emetic effect of apomorphine in dogs. Usual dose for prophylaxis: for a person <60 kg, 0.25 ml (0.7 mg); for a person >60 kg, 0.5 ml (1.4 mg). These are not sedating doses, and they have a good effect on nausea and vomiting.

    5. Chlorpromazine (Thorazine)—this phenothiazine derivative is contraindicated in children. Usual dose: 10-25 mg q5-6h PO. If no hypotension occurs, the dose may be increased to 25-50 mg q3-4h as needed, until vomiting is controlled.

B. Our institution has empirically found the following combination of medications particularly effective in the treatment of nausea caused by antineoplastic drugs:

    1. Droperidol (Inapsine)—5 mg IM at 3 PM and 7 PM

    2. Diphenhydramine (Benadryl)—50 mg IM or PO at 2 PM and 8 PM

    3. Dexamethasone (Decadron)—12 mg IM or PO in AM.

C. All postoperative patient examinations should include both palpation and auscultation of the abdomen. If an acute process is responsible for the postoperative emesis, suspicion will be raised by rebound or pointing tenderness, loss of bowel sounds, or abdominal distention. Adynamic ileus is not infrequently encountered in patients who have had ileac bone harvested.

POSTOPERATIVE CARDIAC PROBLEMS

  I. A routine portion of the postoperative examination is careful cardiac auscultation for regularity, normal heart sounds, and no acute changes from the preoperative workup (e.g., no onset of cardiac murmur or development of S_3 gallop).

 II. Etiology

    A. The more common causes of cardiac arrhythmias in a postoperative patient include:

      1. Ischemia—which may be secondary to inadequate respiration with resultant hypoxia or to severe volume depletion and hypoperfusion

      2. Ectopy—which may be due to excessive release of endogenous catecholamines secondary to pain

      3. Acid-base imbalance—especially acidosis and hypokalemia

      4. Drugs administered intraoperatively and postoperatively

      5. Preexisting cardiac problems—e.g., atherosclerosis, left ventricular hypertrophy

      6. Hypercapnia—often contributes to the development of arrhythmias

B. Each of these should be considered individually whenever one thinks about etiology. Many cardiac arrhythmias are very serious and can lead to a precipitously downhill course.

III. Recognition and treatment

A. This review is aimed at specific recognition of such problems so that prompt cardiac consultation can be sought. Treatment is aimed at identification and, if possible, reversal of the cause.

B. Sinus bradycardia

1. Normal sinus rhythm exists; rate <60 bpm.

2. Causes include increased vagal tone, elevated intracranial pressure, and general anesthesia (cyclopropane, halothane). It is also found in trained athletes.

3. Treatment includes vagolytic agents (atropine, 1 mg IV, repeated in 3-5 min) with or without inotropes (isoproterenol, IV infusion [1 mg per 250 ml D_5W], with a pediatric drip set at 10-20 mg/min).

4. This relatively benign condition must be differentiated from complete heart block. An ECG is diagnostic, although IV atropine will also allow differentiation.

C. Sinus tachycardia

1. Normal sinus rhythm exists; rate 100-180 bpm.

2. Causes include stress (e.g., postoperative pain), fever, hypoxia, hypovolemia (with reflex tachycardia), congestive heart failure, anemia, and hyperthyroidism (thyroid storm).

3. Treatment of the underlying cause is sufficient. Beta blockage with propranolol, 1.5 mg IV (with increments up to 2 mg over 10-15 min), or propranolol, 10-40 mg PO qid, may be instituted.

D. Premature atrial contractions (PACs)

1. Irregularity of the pulse is noted. The ECG will show a nonsinus tachycardia with occasional premature P waves of varying configurations that are conducted through to the ventricle, producing a normal QRS complex. There is an incomplete compensatory pause after the PAC complex. PACs are ordinarily benign but may anticipate other atrial arrhythmias that are more worrisome.

2. If treatment is necessary, quinidine sulfate and procainamide (Pronestyl) are generally the drugs of choice. Dosage schedules and development of therapeutic levels are worked out with cardiac consultation.

E. Paroxysmal atrial tachycardia (PAT)

1. With PAT there is atrial tachyarrhythmia with a 1:1 ventricular response. Heart rates may be between 140 and 240 bpm, and the QRS complexes may be distorted at these rapid rates.

2. The cause is usually a reentry mechanism (part of the Wolff-Parkinson-White syndrome). It is often seen in patients with no cardiac history and may follow general anesthesia.

3. Initial treatment is by vagal stimulation (e.g., carotid sinus massage). If this fails, pharmacologic intervention may in-

clude edrophonium (Tensilon), a synthetic anticholinesterase, or use of digitalis, quinidine, or procainamide. Cardioversion may be necessary if these measures fail.

F. Atrial flutter and fibrillation

1. The atrial rate with flutter is 250–350 bpm; with fibrillation, it is 375–600 bpm. The pulse is often described as "irregularly irregular."

2. Frequent causes are rheumatic or coronary artery disease, thoracotomy, pericarditis, hyperthyroidism, and pulmonary embolization.

3. Treatment (always done with cardiac consultation) includes:

   a. For acute atrial fibrillation, rapid digitalization (1.5–2.0 mg q24h), to increase the AV block, and then IV propranolol in 0.5-mg increments. If no conversion occurs, quinidine sulfate or procainamide may be used.

   b. For chronic atrial fibrillation, digoxin for rate control. If cardioversion is contemplated, one must anticoagulate beforehand.

G. Nodal rhythm

1. On the ECG this is characterized by a loss of P waves (no atrial depolarization) with a normal-appearing QRS. The rate may be slowed when impulses arise from the AV node. Hemodynamic consequences follow the loss of atrial systole and decreased filling of the left ventricle. This is of little consequence in healthy patients, but is more worrisome in a person with already compromised function.

2. Causes include sinoatrial node inhibition by vagal reflex, digitalis toxicity, and acute myocardial infarction (most often noted with the use of general inhalation anesthesia, especially halothane).

3. Treatment is of the underlying cause.

H. Ventricular extrasystoles, (premature ventricular contractions [PVCs])

1. These consist of a premature QRS complex with widened abnormal configurations.

2. They are most commonly associated with ischemia, digitalis toxicity, hypokalemia, acid-base imbalance, stress, and mitral valve prolapse.

3. Treatment is indicated if there are more than six PVCs per min, if the complexes are multifocal, if they occur on or near T waves, or if there are bursts of 2 or 3 PVCs (or more) in a row.

4. Lidocaine, 100 mg IV bolus, is given, followed by an infusion (lidocaine drip) of 2 g per 500 ml of D_5W at 4 mg/min or 1 ml/min. A second bolus of lidocaine may be given in 30–40 min. If not effective, 500 mg procainamide IV or PO q4h is administered. (Because of the risk of developing a lupus syndrome with long-term procainamide use, the patient may be maintained on quinidine, 200–400 mg q6h.)

I. Ventricular tachycardia
1. On the ECG this is seen as abnormal QRS complexes at a rapid rate (150–250 bpm).
2. Ventricular tachycardia is an ominous finding, often heralding the development of ventricular fibrillation.
3. Treatment is lidocaine via bolus and infusion (as above) for immediate correction of hypoxia and the acid-base and electrolyte abnormalities. Pharmacologic intervention may include procainamide, quinidine, disopyramide, or propranolol.
4. Immediate countershock is needed if the hemodynamic state deteriorates.
J. Ventricular fibrillation
1. On the ECG this is an unmistakable, chaotic, and rapid sine wave pattern.
2. Treatment includes immediate cardioversion followed by lidocaine given as a bolus and infusion. Acidosis is corrected with bicarbonate (acidosis lowers the fibrillation threshold).

POSTOPERATIVE PULMONARY COMPLICATIONS

I. Despite many advances in the care of the postoperative patient, pulmonary complications remain frequent. To avoid dramatic increases in morbidity and even mortality of oral surgical patients, they must be addressed promptly and efficaciously.
II. Thorough postoperative examination will raise the strong suspicion of pulmonary distress, and early intervention is thus likely.
III. Many factors (both surgical and anesthetic) play a role in the development of the following entities:

Airway obstruction (acute or chronic)
Atelectasis
Bacterial pneumonitis
Aspiration pneumonitis
Pulmonary emboli and pneumothorax
Preexisting asthmatic and obstructive pulmonary disease

Airway obstruction

I. Acute obstruction is heralded by the development of increasingly stridorous inspiratory sounds, dyspnea, tachypnea, cyanosis, and pronounced use of the accessory muscles of respiration (suprasternal skin retraction during inspiration). Additional discussion of airway management is found in Chapter 12.
II. The causes of postoperative obstruction are as follows:
A. Significant laryngeal edema secondary to traumatic intubation—which can occur in oral surgical patients receiving blind nasotracheal intubation. It may have an insidious onset, with increased restlessness and irritability, yet drowsiness due to the worsening hypoxia, as early signs. It has been observed in pa-

tients with a history of recent respiratory tract infection or previous irradiation to the region of the cords.

B. Tracheal narrowing secondary to neck surgery with a significant amount of postoperative swelling or hematoma formation—this can occur with vallecula epiglottica and piriform sinus excisions, base of tongue resections, composite resections with flap procedures for head and neck cancer patients, and bilateral neck dissections. It may also result from a Ludwig-type infection or cellulitis secondary to a badly infected tooth. Other causes of tracheal narrowing are soft-tissue masses (mediastinal, oropharyngeal, and nasopharyngeal tumors) of appreciable magnitude, accumulation of viscous secretions in enough quantity to block the tracheobronchial tree, and the restrictive action of dressings placed overzealously about the neck and chest.

C. Position of the head in the unconscious patient—this may cause the tongue and epiglottis to be posteriorly displaced so they block the glottic opening and prevent exchange of air. It is noteworthy that children have significantly smaller laryngeal openings than adults, and thus even small quantities of secretions or slight compression may be sufficient to cause complete obstruction. Children also lack the forceful clearing power (e.g., cough) of adults. Lacerations of the tongue musculature or surgery of the tongue may result in massive edema.

III. Treatment of airway obstruction includes the following:

A. Early recognition of respiratory distress—this is the first step.

B. Alteration of head position if the patient is supine and unconscious—pushing forward at the angles of the mandible may permit air exchange.

C. Prompt application of a mechanical airway—if oropharyngeal and nasopharyngeal airways do not alleviate the distress, the patient must be reintubated without delay.

D. Emergency tracheotomy—with significant laryngeal edema, extensive swelling, and hematoma formation postoperatively, prompt and effective intubation is often not possible; in this case, tracheotomy will be lifesaving and should proceed without delay under local anesthesia (in the operating room only if time permits).

E. Frequent suctioning and removal of secretions, blood, and vomitus from the pharynx—use of nasogastric suction will decrease the likelihood of aspiration of gastric contents.

F. Oxygen therapy—this should be initiated immediately after the airway is cleared and modified pending the results of arterial blood gas analysis. There should be frequent postoperative inspection of dressings and bandages, as well as routine catheter aspiration through the nose and mouth.

G. In patients undergoing extensive resection of head and neck tumors, in which dramatic postoperative swelling is anticipated, elective tracheostomy may be performed to obviate the need for emergency tracheotomy (a procedure with increased risk to the patient). In these patients airway maintenance is often a critical problem for the first 48 hr and a serious one for the first 7–10 da after surgery.

Atelectasis

I. Atelectasis often presents as tachypnea, tachycardia, fever, and moist inspiratory rales (especially at the lung bases).
II. Several factors predispose to this problem:
   A. Narcotics, often given as postoperative analgesics, depress both the respiratory center and the cough reflex (deep breathing and periodic coughing tend to ameliorate atelectasis).
   B. Prolonged bed rest postoperatively hampers lung ventilation.
   C. Postoperative pain and splinting often make deep breathing difficult.
   D. Acute pulmonary obstruction will prevent large portions of the lung from being adequately aerated.

Bacterial pneumonitis

I. If atelectasis persists untreated, secondary bacterial colonization (bacterial pneumonitis) may result. This significantly complicates the patient's postoperative course and requires the use of antibiotics.
II. As part of standard postoperative orders, the nursing staff is instructed to help the patient go through the exercises of deep breathing, coughing, and rolling from side to side every 2 hr while awake and before he or she is able to ambulate. Postoperative pulmonary complications can be reduced by various lung inflation maneuvers. In addition to the above, mechanical devices such as incentive spirometers, intermittent positive pressure ventilation and continuous positive airway pressure have been employed. These conservative measures significantly decrease the occurrence of extensive atelectasis.
III. In patients with a previous history of significant smoking or chronic obstructive pulmonary disease, a postoperative order for formal chest pulmonary therapy is indicated. If atelectasis does not respond to these conservative measures, tracheobronchial suctioning or transtracheal cough stimulation should be tried. If mucous plugging of a smaller airway is thought to be responsible for an atelectatic patch, removal by means of bronchoscopy is feasible.

Aspiration pneumonitis

I. Depending on its extent, aspiration pneumonitis may be a disastrous postoperative complication with significant mortality secondary to respiratory failure. It is usually caused by gastric contents that enter the tracheobronchial tree either during anesthesia (e.g., passive aspiration with induction) or after extubation before the patient has regained protective reflexes.

II. There are factors, in addition to general anesthesia, that tend to obtund the reflexes. These include trauma, alcohol intoxication, drug overdose with resultant CNS depression, seizure disorders, a previous history of cerebrovascular accidents (CVA), and tracheostomy. Similarly, esophageal motility disorders (e.g., achalasia, spasm, hiatal hernia with reflux) place the patient at increased risk of aspiration. Bowel obstruction, either paralytic or mechanical, may also predispose to aspiration secondary to emesis.

III. Aspiration of particulate matter may lead to occlusion of airways, hypoventilation of a lung segment, and subsequent collapse.

IV. The pH of the aspirate has also been implicated in the extent of damage. If the pH of gastric fluid is over 2.5, minimal lung damage ensues. However, with a pH $<$2.5 and the amount of aspirate $>$50 ml, pulmonary parenchyma and blood vessels are severely damaged and significant bronchospasm (secondary to chemical irritation) ensues.

V. Several findings are diagnostic of aspiration pneumonitis.
   A. Physical evidence—dyspnea, cough, wheezing (rhonchi and rales), fever, tachycardia, hypotension, shock, and cyanosis
   B. Radiographic evidence—unilateral radiodense infiltrates, most commonly seen in the right upper lung if the patient is supine at aspiration, or possibly bilateral diffuse infiltrates
   C. Laboratory evidence—leukocytosis (12,000–15,000 WBCs), arterial blood gases with hypoxia, and normal or decreased P_{CO_2}. (Approximately 30% of these patients will have negative bacterial cultures. When cultures are positive, the most common etiologic flora is an oropharyngeal species, with anaerobes outnumbering aerobes by 10:1.)

VI. As soon as aspiration pneumonitis is noted or suspected (with active vomiting or passive refluxing), the patient should be placed in the Trendelenburg position. Pharyngeal and endotracheal suction should be started immediately and, if necessary, bronchoscopy for the removal of particulate matter from the airway.
   A. If the patient's level of consciousness is significantly deteriorating secondary to hypoxia (Pa_{O_2} is a worrisome value) and he or she is laboring to breathe, mechanical ventilation with positive pressure should be instituted (to maximize oxygenation).
   B. If wheezing is present, bronchodilators (aminophylline) should be used. IV steroids are of value only if administered within 5 min of aspiration.
   C. Antibiotic therapy should be started only in response to a strong suspicion of a bacterial component of the aspirant (e.g., organisms on Gram stain or, preferably, positive culture results) and should be specific for the major offending organisms isolated.
   D. The use of corticosteroids to decrease acute imflammation and stabilize membranes remains controversial. Most studies showing efficacy have been anecdotal and uncontrolled. Prolonged use of steroids may also mask the presence of secondary infection.

E. The most effective treatment of aspiration pneumonitis remains prevention. This includes identification and appreciation of patients who are at risk. They may be treated prophylactically with cimetidine or an antacid (e.g., Maalox) in an effort to decrease the acidity and amount of gastric secretions. Rapid-sequence intubation is recommended in these patients, and they should be extubated in an alert and fully awake condition. A suction source should be readily available at the bedside at all times.

Pulmonary emboli

I. The origin of pulmonary emboli (PE) is most commonly thrombi in the venous circulation, especially of the lower extremities, which affix themselves to the intima of the host vessel.

II. Factors predisposing to the development of PE include:

Prolonged postoperative bed rest
Bed positions favoring the stagnation of venous bleeding
Previous history of thrombophlebitis or pulmonary emboli
Heart disease
Obesity
Polycythemia
Use of polychlorinated biphenyls (PCB)

III. Signs and symptoms of pulmonary emboli are:

A. Positive leg signs (e.g., pain, tenderness) may occur in 10% of patients. However, frequently there will be no presenting symptoms.

B. The classic triad of acute onset of chest pain, dyspnea, and hemoptysis is seen in only a small percentage of cases.

C. The classic auscultatory sign of a friction rub may be present.

D. If emboli obstruct over 60% of the pulmonary artery tree, physical examination will show signs of acute cor pulmonale—loud P_2 sounds, distention of neck veins, hepatomegaly, tachypnea, tachycardia, cyanosis, and hypotension.

E. In such cases ECG signs will include definite evidence of right ventricular strain—right ventricular hypertrophy and right axis deviation, ST segment depression in leads II, III, aVF, V_2, and V_3, and inversion of T waves in leads V_1 through V_3. These findings usually precede the development of shock and vascular collapse.

F. The chest radiograph will occasionally show decreased lung markings (Westmark's sign) and evidence of right ventricular enlargement. The classic wedge-shaped density is frequently seen. However, the most common plain film finding is that of a normal chest radiograph.

G. In less than one third of the cases of PEs, pulmonary infarction ensues. The patient may then have dyspnea, pleuritic pain, hemoptysis, cough, fever, tachycardia, and tachypnea.

H. Noteworthy laboratory results include an increased WBC count and an increased lactate dehydrogenase level on chest radiography.

I. Pulmonary emboli should be suspected in any postoperative patient who presents with the above symptoms and laboratory and radiologic findings (especially one who is at greater risk). Small emboli are considerably more difficult to diagnose because they are often asymptomatic and show no characteristic ECG or chest radiographic signs.

J. The role of the radionuclide ventilation/perfusion ($\dot{V}/\dot{Q}$) lung scan for the diagnosis of pulmonary embolism is well known. The scan is most valuable when the findings are either normal or considered to be of high probability (>85% $\dot{V}/\dot{Q}$ mismatch).

K. The most reliable diagnostic technique is pulmonary angiography. Because of the inherent risks of invasive arteriography, alternative methods of diagnosis are being sought. Dynamic contrast-enhanced CT and MRI are currently able to identify larger PE.

IV. Treatment is as follows:

A. Oxygen therapy is begun and, depending on the patient's Pao_2, may be accompanied by intubation. Ventilatory assistance is begun if needed. Central venous pressure is routinely monitored.

B. If hypotension and heart failure develop, they must be promptly treated.

C. Either morphine or meperidine (Demerol) is given to decrease pain and anxiety.

D. Anticoagulation with heparin is begun right away. It may be given by either IV intermittent injection or continuous IV infusion after the diagnosis has been made or the index of suspicion significantly increased.

1. Intermittent injection—initial dose 10,000 U IV, then 7500-10,000 U q4h for 24 hr; thereafter, the dose is decreased and warfarin treatment is started concurrently.

2. Continuous infusion—initial dose 5000 U IV, followed by 100 U/kg; heparin therapy monitored by the PTT, which is maintained at 1 to 1½ times the normal value (37-60 sec); this is usually continued for 8-10 da, by which time the venous thrombi have presumably become firmly adherent to the vessel wall.

E. Warfarin therapy is begun 2-3 da after heparin, and the drugs are given concurrently until heparin is discontinued.

1. Usual dose of warfarin—10-15 mg/da (the PT is drawn daily during the first week of therapy, twice weekly during the second week, and weekly or less frequently thereafter); levels 2-3 times normal are found to be therapeutic, and dosage may be adjusted to achieve this.

2. Duration—anticoagulation maintained for a minimum of 6 mo after PE in an effort to prevent recurrence.

F. The use of fibrinolytic agents (to speed dissolution of the clot) has been advocated, especially in the case of massive PE. Two plasminogen activators, streptokinase and urokinase, have been extensively studied for this purpose.

1. Streptokinase is not suitable because of an increased incidence of allergic reactions.

2. Urokinase (a natural fibrinolysin obtained from human urine) is more suitable, although its use has been associated with a high incidence of bleeding and its prohibitive cost makes it a less than ideal agent; unequivocal demonstration of its efficacy in decreasing the mortality and morbidity of PE remains to be shown.

G. Surgical interruption of the inferior vena cava (IVC) is done in an effort to safeguard against recurrent and possibly fatal PE. Surgery is indicated in patients who are unable to receive anticoagulation treatment (e.g., trauma patients with major visceral, brain, or spinal cord injuries; patients with other bleeding lesions; patients with blood dyscrasias or clotting disorders secondary to liver disease) or in those in whom anticoagulation has previously been unsuccessful. IVC interruption is also advocated in patients with a history of recurrent PE and documented septic phlebitis. IVC ligation results in total impedance of blood flow through the vessel. Partial occlusion of the vessel may be obtained by use of a slotlike clip, grid, or IVC "umbrella." The principle of partial occlusion is that emboli will be trapped, although some blood flow may continue. In actuality, it is likely that the small openings quickly become occluded with either newly formed thrombi or recurrent emboli. To date, no significant differences in results obtained from either technique have been demonstrated. Anticoagulation therapy should be reinstituted several days after IVC interruption.

H. Pulmonary embolectomy is the mechanical removal of a clot from the pulmonary artery. This highly invasive and risky procedure is indicated only in patients with progressive circulatory collapse, chronic pulmonary hypertension, or documented occlusion of the right or left main pulmonary artery. At best, embolectomy under direct vision through pulmonary arteriotomy carries a 33% mortality risk.

Pneumothorax

I. Pneumothorax is defined as air entering the pleural cavity, which thereby reduces the normal negative intrapleural pressure and results in partial lung collapse.

A. The index of suspicion of postoperative pneumothorax is raised when the surgical procedure itself involves an area close to the lungs (e.g., the harvesting of autogenous rib grafts for mandibular reconstruction). Supraclavicular approaches to the brachial plexus (for regional anesthesia) and the insertion of subclavian central venous lines, likewise, carry a finite risk (usually <1%) of producing a pneumothorax.

   B. Pneumothorax develops occasionally as a result of injury to the apex of the pleural reflection at the inferior limit of the neck during neck dissections. Care must be taken when approaching this area to avoid entering the pleura.

II. Signs of pneumothorax include tachypnea, tachycardia, and cyanosis.

   A. On physical examination there is hyperresonance over the involved area, absent breath sounds, and loss of normal diaphragmatic movement on the affected side.

   B. On chest radiography the margin of the collapsed lung is seen outlined by air.

   C. Decreased Pao_2 (secondary to a functional shunt) may be found.

III. Treatment consists of intermittent needle aspiration or prophylactic chest tube insertion. Treatment of all traumatic pneumothoraces is chest tube emplacement (with underwater seal) checked by sequential chest radiographs.

IV. After chest trauma or placement of a central venous line, signs and symptoms of a tension pneumothorax may develop. Patients demonstrate tachypnea, tracheal deviation away from the side of injury, distention of neck veins, decreased breath sounds, and signs of shock. Frequently, diagnosis must be made emergently without the help of a radiograph. Placement of a long, 14-gauge angiocatheter in the second intercostal space, midclavicular line, results in a gush of air under pressure and the patient should respond. A formal chest tube is then placed.

GENERAL REFERENCES

American College of Surgeons: *Manual of preoperative and postoperative care*, Philadelphia, 1983, WB Saunders.

Condon RE, Nyhus LM: *Manual of surgical therapeutics*, ed 9, Boston, 1996, Little, Brown.

SECTION III

Specific Care of the Oral Surgical Patient

7

Dentoalveolar Surgery

RAY ENGLISH, JR.

Exodontia

GENERAL CONSIDERATIONS

I. A major goal of contemporary dental medicine is the preservation of the natural dentition. However, extraction of teeth is often indicated and remains an important part of oral and maxillofacial surgery.

II. The application of proper surgical technique and compassionate patient management will permit removal of teeth in a painless and atraumatic fashion. Managing a patient's fears and apprehensions is every bit as important as the execution of proper technique.

PREOPERATIVE MANAGEMENT

I. Patient treatment starts with the initial assessment. A concise history is obtained to determine whether preexisting medical or dental problems might affect the planned procedures.

II. A physical examination should precede any surgical intervention. The entire oral cavity is examined for other abnormal conditions that may exist, in addition to the problem for which the patient was referred.

III. Radiographs are taken so the problem at hand can be evaluated, as well as the teeth, alveolar bone, sinuses, etc. The relationship of the teeth to structures such as the inferior alveolar canal and maxillary sinuses should be ascertained.

IV. After a complete history, physical examination, and radiographic examination, a surgical plan is developed. This plan includes a determination of the patient's general management, surgical management, and anesthetic needs.

V. Several surgical principles must be considered.

A. The surgeon must have good access to the surgical field. The patient is positioned to allow maximal exposure. Good lighting is essential. The assistant should also be able to suction the field as necessary.

1. Bleeding in the field must be controlled and attention given to maintaining good surgical anesthesia.
2. Whenever necessary, a flap should be developed to afford maximal access to the field. A flap will heal much better and faster than a torn, traumatized area of tissue.

B. The forces used to remove teeth must be under control at all times. The force used with rotary drills must also be carefully controlled. The surgeon has to develop a feel for the amount of bone removed by the drill with light pressure and must be careful to protect the adjacent tissues.

C. The path for removal of a tooth must be unimpeded. An adjacent tooth may block the extraction path of a malpositioned tooth, in which case the tooth to be removed may need to be sectioned before removal.

1. A multirooted tooth may need to be sectioned because the curves in the roots may be blocked by bone, or the distance between the roots may be too wide for removal through the tooth socket.
2. Sectioning of teeth, when indicated, reduces trauma and prevents complications related to the use of excessive force, as in extensive bone removal, maxillary tuberosity fracture, or sinus exposure.

D. When access to the surgical field is compromised by soft tissue or when bone removal is necessary, a soft-tissue flap should be raised to provide access to the field. The flap should be large enough for access to the entire field of surgery.

1. To ensure adequate blood supply, the base of the flap should be wider than the crestal margin.
2. The flap should be designed so that, when repositioned, the marginal incision rests on bone.
3. Papillae of adjacent teeth should be protected.

VI. The following are some of the common indications for removing teeth:

A. Carious destruction that cannot be restored
B. Extensive and advanced periodontal disease that cannot be treated
C. Malpositioning that jeopardizes adjacent structures or teeth
D. Orthodontic therapy
E. Caries and/or periodontal disease, along with impacted teeth in a patient undergoing radiation therapy. (These teeth should be removed at least 7–10 da before therapy.)
F. Tooth infection that is considered to be a potential source of systemic bacteremia in a patient with cardiac valvular and septal disease or with prosthetic valves. (Teeth with extensive caries and periapical or periodontal disease are the potential problem. Coronary artery bypass graft surgery is not an indication for extraction. [A complete discussion of this important topic is found in Chapter 4.])

G. When they interfere with the placement of prostheses

TREATMENT PROCEDURE
Elevator and forceps extraction

I. Elevators are very useful in the removal of teeth. They should, however, be used with care because serious complications can occur when they are used improperly. Most problems with elevators stem from misjudging of the amount of force delivered or from improper positioning.

   A. Trauma can result in fracture of the mandible, tuberosity, or alveolar bone and tooth segments or in loosening of teeth.

   B. Bone, not an adjacent tooth, should be used as a fulcrum when positioning the elevator.

II. Elevators are used in the following ways:

   A. Straight elevator (no. 40 or 301). This is the most versatile type.

      1. It is used to luxate an erupted tooth. Placed perpendicular to the long axis of the alveolar ridge on the mesial aspect of the tooth, with the rounded side of its tip resting on bone, it is rotated away from the tooth, creating a "scooping" action to elevate the tooth. The elevator may also be rotated toward the tooth to luxate and move it posteriorly. Once the tooth has some mobility, the elevator can be worked in an apical direction on the labial side. The labial bone plate is used as a fulcrum for further elevation.

      2. The straight elevator is also useful for sectioning a tooth. After a slot is made with a rotary drill at the point where the tooth is to be split, the elevator is placed in the slot and rotated to separate the halves.

   B. Bayonette elevator. This offset-shaped instrument is designed for removing maxillary and mandibular third molars.

   C. Potts and Miller elevators. These are useful for removing deeply impacted maxillary third molars. Their curved shape allows them to be seated at the cervical area to prevent the tooth from being inadvertently pushed superiorly into the maxillary sinus.

   D. Cryers, or east-west, elevator. This type is useful for removing fractured roots of molars.

III. Extraction forceps are designed to fit the anatomic shape of the crown and root of specific teeth and for the application of specific forces on individual teeth in different anatomic positions. Generally speaking, straight-handled forceps are used for anterior teeth, and curved-handled or bayonette-handled forceps are used for posterior teeth.

IV. Proper use of forceps and elevators promotes the efficient removal of teeth with minimal discomfort and tissue damage. There are many types of forceps available, all variations of a few basic designs. It is important to select the proper forceps for the specific tooth to be removed.

V. The basic techniques for removing teeth are:

A. Maxillary incisors and canines—the upper straight forceps (no. 99-C) is used to remove maxillary central and lateral incisors and canines. It is placed on the crown, and apical force is applied to seat the beaks at the neck of the tooth. The tooth is removed with alternating labial and palatal pressure, followed by mesial rotation.

B. Maxillary premolars—the upper universal forceps (no. 159) is used to remove these teeth. The first premolar frequently has two roots and is removed by buccopalatal pendulum movements until loose. Slight rotation may be used to deliver the tooth, preserving the buccal plate. The second premolar has a more conical root and is removed in a similar fashion, except that more rotation may be employed.

C. Maxillary molars—the upper universal (no. 150) forceps is used for most maxillary molars. More difficult or extensively decayed molars may be removed with the upper molar cowhorn forceps (no. 88-R or 88-L). Great care is needed with the latter, because the risk of bone fracture is increased by the large forces that these forceps can deliver. Buccal movement is used to remove the maxillary first and second molars. A firmly anchored molar may occasionally need to be sectioned with a rotary drill so it can be removed without damage to surrounding structures. The two buccal roots are sectioned from the crown, and the forceps is used to remove the crown and palatal root. The buccal roots are then removed individually.

D. Mandibular incisors—these are most efficiently removed with the Ashe forceps, but the lower universal forceps (no. 151) may also be used. The roots of the incisor teeth are delicate and relatively flat on their mesial and distal surfaces, with thin labial and lingual plates. To prevent labial bone destruction, short buccolingual movements are best for removing these teeth.

E. Mandibular canines and premolars—the Ashe forceps is the most efficient for removal of mandibular canines and premolars. The lower universal (no. 151) forceps may also be used. Short buccolingual forces followed by a rotary motion are used to remove the canines, preserving the buccal plate.

F. Mandibular molars—the lower universal forceps (no. 151) is used for most mandibular molars. The lower molar cowhorn forceps (no. 23) is useful for difficult molars with divergent roots. The cowhorn forceps has sharp buccal and lingual beaks that seat between the mesial and distal roots. As the forceps is firmly seated between the roots, a vertical force is placed on the tooth and the tooth is delivered with buccal movement. If the crown fractures in the process of removal, the roots will usually be separated, and this makes their removal relatively simple. It is occasionally necessary to section a molar between the roots with a rotary drill and remove the roots individually.

Postoperative complications

I. Most of the complications of exodontia can be avoided with proper presurgical planning. These problems are usually the result of poor access and visualization, poor surgical technique (most often the use of excessive force), or incorrect use of instruments.

II. Surgical complications should be approached with a specific plan and not as a haphazard addition to the procedure. Poorly handled complications often lead to more extensive problems. It is important that the patient be informed when problems occur.

A. Fractured roots (mandible)—when a portion of a root is fractured, the operator should stop and take a few moments to analyze the situation and plan an approach to the problem.

1. The following should be reevaluated before proceeding:

   a. Patient position should promote optimum visualization.

   b. Light should be adequate and positioned to give maximum visibility.

   c. Suction, along with adequate irrigation, is essential for keeping a clear field.

   d. Assistants should be positioned to retract the soft tissues effectively and suction without obstructing the surgeon's field of vision.

   e. Surgical access—the field should be well suctioned and flaps retracted if necessary for optimal visualization. (A radiograph may occasionally be useful in locating the root fragment.)

2. The root segment should be gently manipulated with the appropriate elevators to luxate it superiorly. Excessive force in the posterior region can cause displacement of a tip mesially through the thin lingual bone plate into the submandibular space or inferiorly into the inferior alveolar canal.

3. When a root is displaced mesially, it can be palpated with a finger in an attempt to manipulate the tip back through the lingual plate defect into the extraction site, permitting removal through the socket. If this is unsuccessful, a mucoperiosteal flap is elevated and the tip is visualized and removed. It is important that the lingual tissues be well protected with retractors.

4. If a root tip is displaced into the inferior alveolar canal, it is almost impossible to remove bone through the socket to retrieve the root. Excessive bleeding from the socket may make visualization difficult, increasing the risk of damage to the neurovascular bundle. These root tips may sometimes be left if there are no symptoms. If removal becomes neces-

sary, it is best done in the operating room by an experienced surgeon.

B. Fractured roots (maxilla)—the same principles of access discussed for recovery of mandibular root tips are true for the maxillary teeth. Every attempt is made to remove the root with minimal damage to adjacent structures and minimal resection of bone.

1. Fractured premolar roots are easily removed by elevating a conservative mucoperiosteal flap for access and removing a portion of the buccal plate. The root tip can then be elevated or extracted with a root tip elevator or forceps.

2. Molar root tips may be removed in a fashion similar to that used for premolars. It is important that the force applied with the elevator does not push the tip apically. If this happens, the tip may be displaced into the maxillary sinus. Such a root may then be:

   a. Displaced apically but still within the bony socket

   b. Displaced through the buccal bone plate and into the lateral soft tissues

   c. Lodged between the socket apex and the bony sinus floor

   d. Lodged against the sinus membrane at the socket apex, within the sinus, having penetrated the sinus membrane

3. A minimally displaced root may be removed using a small suction tip placed in the socket. If the root penetrates the membrane, it can usually be removed with small instruments through the socket. If the root has penetrated the membrane, it is often best to close the socket and recover the root tip via a Caldwell-Luc operation.

C. Postoperative bleeding—in patients without a defective coagulation mechanism, this can usually be avoided with good surgical technique and appropriate postoperative care by the surgeon and patient.

1. Attention to the following points will significantly reduce the incidence of postoperative bleeding problems:

   a. History—a patient with a history of postoperative bleeding, easy bruising, etc., should be evaluated in the appropriate manner to rule out a bleeding disorder before surgery.

   b. Patient instructions—these should be clearly explained to the patient or to the person responsible for the patient, as well as given to the patient in written form. The patient should be instructed to bite on a compact gauze sponge placed directly over the socket for at least 30 min after surgery without checking to see whether the bleeding has stopped. He or she should be instructed how to place the sponge properly in case it becomes dislodged.

   c. Foreign bodies—fragments of tooth, bone, calculus, etc., should be removed from the socket, because these may become a focus for bleeding or infection. If the buccal or lingual bone plates have been expanded, they should be compressed before suturing the socket.

d. Active bleeders—any active bleeding sites in soft-tissue or bone must be controlled. Soft-tissue bleeding can usually be stopped with pressure; however, it may be necessary to ligate a large vessel or compress the bone around a nutrient vessel.

e. Sutures—adequate sutures should be placed to close the soft tissues and approximate the papillae to bone, because most postoperative bleeding is from unsutured papillae.

2. If bleeding occurs after the patient has left the office, he or she should be told how to replace the gauze sponge directly over the socket and bite firmly for 20–30 min. A tea bag over the socket may also prove helpful. If bleeding persists, the patient must be seen so the problem can be evaluated. The following steps should be used in managing these cases:

a. Anesthesia—the surgical area should be obtunded with a local anesthetic agent containing a vasoconstrictor. This will allow the patient to be thoroughly examined without pain and will help reduce bleeding.

b. Access—patients with postoperative bleeding will usually be apprehensive and need reassurance. It may occasionally be necessary to administer a sedative to comfort them. A calm patient, as well as good light and suction, is essential for a thorough examination and treatment.

c. Surgical site—the old clot should be cleared from the socket so the operator can examine the socket and surrounding tissues. A large clot protruding from the socket is easily disturbed by the tongue and teeth, causing continuous and prolonged bleeding.

d. Pressure—a gauze pack is placed over the site and firm pressure maintained until bleeding is controlled. The socket should be coapted with sutures through the papillae to put pressure on soft tissues.

e. Direct hemostasis—any soft-tissue bleeding sites not controlled by pressure over the socket may be clamped and sutured or cauterized. Bone bleeders may be compressed around the site. If bleeding is over a large area or persistent, it may occasionally be necessary to place bone wax or a hemostatic agent (e.g., Gelfoam, Surgicel, Avitene, or topical thrombin).

f. Assurance—the patient should not be discharged until it is clear that the bleeding has been controlled. He or she should then be reassured that the problem is under control and will remain so if instructions are followed precisely.

D. Tuberosity fracture—this is usually the result of excessive force during removal of maxillary second and third molars.

1. When removing teeth, the surgeon should keep the tooth and surrounding soft tissues visible at all times and should palpate as pressure is applied. Particular attention should be given to teeth that stand alone in the arch and to those that have a low extension of the maxillary sinus viewed radiographically.

2. When a fracture occurs, the segment should be retained, if possible. If the segment is relatively large and well attached to the periosteum, it should be replaced and the mucosa closed. If the segment is excessively mobile, it may be necessary to splint it until it heals. If it is small or detached from the periosteum, it should be removed and a flap rotated to close the defect.

3. It is important to recognize the fracture immediately, while it is occurring, so the soft tissue over the defect can be retained. If a tooth is being removed blindly, bone and attached mucosa may be removed with it, leaving a large sinus communication that may be difficult to close.

E. Postoperative pain—pain following oxodontia is usually well controlled with mild to moderate analgesic agents.

1. When the pain persists, it is usually a sign of an underlying problem. The patient should be examined clinically and radiographically.

2. The following are some of the common causes of persistent pain after tooth extraction:

a. Postoperative infection—this should be treated as soon as possible with antibiotics (and drainage when indicated). Localized osteitis ("dry socket") can occur in teeth other than third molars and is caused when the blood clot in the socket is lost prematurely, exposing the bare walls of the socket. The patient has delayed increasing pain not controlled by mild analgesics. Appropriate antibiotics, analgesics, and a topical analgesic dressing are used. The dressing is placed in the socket and changed daily until the symptoms have resolved.

b. Retained root, bone, or foreign body—the extraction site should be examined clinically and radiographically for any extraneous fragments. They may appear within the socket or between the alveolar plate and the mucosa.

c. Alveolar plate fracture—the socket should be examined for evidence of alveolar plate fracture. Small fragments of bone may need to be removed, but larger ones with periosteal attachment can be left and supportive care given until the symptoms resolve.

d. Maxillary sinus problems—persistent pain in maxillary teeth after surgery may be the result of odontogenic infection or a coincidental sinusitis (nonodontogenic pain). The sinus should be evaluated clinically and radiographically and treated with appropriate antibiotics and surgical intervention when necessary.

e. Adjacent teeth—the teeth adjacent to an extraction site should be examined to determine whether the pain is arising from another tooth or associated tissues.

f. Muscle spasm—postoperative pain may be caused by prolonged mouth opening during a procedure, aggravation of a chronic or subclinical problem, or trismus from an anesthetic injection.

g. Nondental origin—facial pain may persist after an extraction and may have no obvious dental source. Various problems should be considered when a patient reports this. The oral surgeon must always look carefully before performing further extractions. It is not at all uncommon to see a patient with a history of multiple extractions done before the diagnosis of trigeminal neuralgia.

h. Prevarication—finally, one must be mindful that there will be the occasional patient who complains of pain falsely in an attempt to secure narcotic medications.

Preparation of the Mouth for Dentures

GENERAL CONSIDERATIONS

I. The removal of teeth and preparation of the mouth for dentures require attention to numerous details so the alveolar bases will be suitable for long-term function and comfort.

A. To prevent root fracture and destruction of the labial plates, teeth are removed as atraumatically as possible.

B. Flaps should be kept to a minimum because excessive flap elevation may compromise the labial vestibule. This can be particularly damaging in the anterior mandible area, where the vestibule may be lost when the flap is sutured.

C. Alveoloplasty is kept to a minimum. If the width of the ridge is to be reduced, the buccal plate should not be removed, if possible. To reduce the amount of resorption, the interradicular bone is removed and the plates compressed (or osteotomized and then compressed) to narrow the ridge over time.

II. Providing a patient with an immediate "surgical" denture is a very satisfying experience for the surgeon and a service for which patients are extremely grateful.

A. It has several advantages over the conventional denture.

1. The patient is never without teeth.

2. The immediate denture acts as a surgical bandage to reduce postoperative bleeding.

3. Postoperative edema and discomfort are reduced.

4. The patient is able to eat with relative comfort, thus assuring

adequate nutrition. This may be of particular importance for patients such as diabetics in whom the nutritional status is critical.

5. Speech is not significantly impaired.
6. The denture acts as a stent to preserve the vestibules.

B. Although the immediate denture is only a "temporary" prosthesis and often has to be replaced by a "permanent" denture 6–12 mo after surgery, this is not always the case. The immediate denture patient is followed closely by the prosthodontist, and the denture is adjusted or relined as indicated.

C. The disadvantages of immediate dentures include:
1. Possible unsatisfactory healing
2. Need for a second regular prosthesis
3. Discomfort if not done optimally

SURGICAL TECHNIQUE

I. There are two techniques for placement of immediate dentures—a two-step and a one-step technique.

A. The two-step technique is used when the patient has a full complement or a significant number of posterior teeth. This method requires two surgical procedures. The posterior teeth are removed at the first procedure, and the ridge is allowed to heal. The anterior teeth are removed at a second procedure, and the denture is placed.

B. With the one-step technique, all remaining teeth are removed and the immediate denture is placed at the same time. To preserve alveolar bone and the vestibule, the teeth are removed as atraumatically as possible.

II. A clear acrylic tray and a duplicate of the trimmed cast are used during surgery to reveal where the prosthodontist has anticipated bone removal when making the denture. The tray may be used to fine-tune any necessary alveoloplasty. Small high spots that prevent the denture from seating may sometimes be corrected by selective trimming or thinning of hyperplastic gingival mucosa and fibrous papillae rather than removal of bone. Minimizing surgery is the best rule in immediate denture patients.

III. The immediate denture placed during surgery should be checked by the dentist within 2–3 da. If the patient is relatively comfortable the denture should not be removed prematurely, because it will not likely be possible to replace it until all the swelling has resolved.

IV. A soft denture reline material may be necessary in some patients for adequate denture retention immediately postoperatively.

Impacted Teeth

GENERAL CONSIDERATIONS

I. Third molars are the largest group of impacted teeth and the most frequently removed.

II. The indications for removal are:
  A. Infection—pericoronitis is a common infection associated with impacted third molar teeth. It occurs when food and debris collect under the mucosal covering or operculum of the impacted tooth. The infection should be controlled before the tooth is removed. Treatment consists of appropriate antibiotic therapy, irrigation to remove debris, and incision and drainage if necessary. Any source of irritation (e.g., an opposing erupted maxillary tooth) should be removed. Uncontrolled pericoronal infection can lead to more serious infections.
  B. Pathologic conditions—clinical or radiographic evidence of disease associated with a third molar is indication for removal.
  C. Pain—caries, inflammation, and infection may all cause pain, which is an indication for removal.
  D. Effect on adjacent teeth—third molars that contribute to infection of adjacent teeth (e.g., caries and periodontal disease) should be removed.
  E. Orthodontic considerations—third molars may need to be removed to facilitate orthodontic therapy.

PREOPERATIVE PREPARATION
  I. Patient preparation
  A. Explanation of the radiographic and clinical findings and of the surgical procedure removes the mystery from the experience and also helps correct any false preconceptions that a patient may have regarding the surgery. The anesthesia to be used should also be discussed before surgery.
  B. Potential complications should be explained and discussed without unduly frightening the patient. These should include, when applicable:
    1. Possible lingual and labial paresthesias
    2. Possible mandibular fracture with deep mandibular impactions
    3. Anesthetic complications
    4. Damage to adjacent teeth
    5. Possible sinus involvement with high maxillary impactions
  C. Finally, the postoperative course should be discussed. The patient should know what to expect after emerging from anesthesia and should have some general idea of how long he or she may need to recuperate, how much pain to expect, and how long he or she can expect to be swollen.
  II. Radiographs
  A. Appropriate radiographs are important in planning for third molar surgery. Classification of the teeth according to their anatomic position (mesioangular, distoangular, horizontal, vertical) aids in determining the surgical approach.
  B. The relationship of impacted teeth to important structures (e.g., the mandibular canal, adjacent teeth, the maxillary sinus, the infratemporal space) should be assessed.

III. Clinical examination
   A. It is essential in every case that a thorough examination be done before surgery. One needs to be sure that any pericoronal or other infection is resolved.
   B. Restorations in adjacent teeth are noted and their effect on the surgical plan considered.

SURGICAL TECHNIQUE

   I. General considerations
      A. Use of the surgical drill rather than the hammer and chisel is suggested for the following reasons:
         1. Modern technology has produced high-speed turbine drills that allow fast, efficient, low-temperature bone removal.
         2. The drill is much more comfortable for the awake patient.
         3. It is technically easier to use and is safer.
         4. Bone can be removed in a more controlled fashion, reducing the amount of osteotomy.
         5. It places less strain on the temporomandibular joints.
      B. The importance of good access can hardly be overemphasized. Before bone surgery is begun, a flap should be raised for clear and unobstructed access to the surgical area. It must be retracted to prevent damage to it by the rotary drill. An envelope flap raised to the first molar area is adequate for removal of most impactions.
   II. Mesioangular impactions
      A. The rotary drill with a fissure bur is used to remove labial bone from around the crown. It then makes a slot in the buccal groove following the long axis of the tooth into the pulp chamber.
      B. A thin straight elevator is used to section the tooth and remove the distal root and crown. The mesial section is then elevated and removed. To avoid rotating the tip of the root onto the roof of the mandibular canal, the surgeon should be careful to elevate the mesial section in the direction of its long axis rather than vertically.
      C. The socket is generously irrigated to remove bone and tooth fragments, and any remnants of the dental sac are removed.
   III. Vertical and distoangular impactions
      A. The drill removes labial bone and bone covering the crown. This creates a groove extending to the cemento-enamel junction (CEJ). A horizontal slot is made in the tooth at the CEJ extending into the pulp chamber.
      B. A straight elevator placed in the slot is rotated to separate the crown from the tooth. The labial groove is deepened with the drill, and a purchase point is made just below the horizontal cut.
      C. A Crane pick is used to elevate the tooth.
      D. If the roots are curved or widely separated, they may have to be separated and removed in sections.

IV. Horizontal impactions

   A. The crowns of horizontally impacted teeth are frequently covered with bone. The drill removes the bone, exposing the crown to a point below the CEJ. Then a vertical slot is made at the CEJ and the crown is separated.

   B. The crown often cannot be delivered intact and must be divided horizontally and removed in sections.

   C. Superior and labial bone is removed from the roots, and a labial purchase made.

   D. The Crane pick is used to elevate the roots anteriorly. The roots may have to be separated and removed in sections.

Surgical Endodontics

   I. Conventional endodontic therapy should always be the treatment of choice in treating irreversible pulpal and periapical disease. There are, however, indications for surgical management of endodontic problems.

   A. A periapical lesion that does not resolve after conventional endodontic therapy should be surgically treated.

   B. Periapical lesions other than granulomas should be treated surgically, and the lesions examined histologically.

   C. Endodontically treated teeth in which the canal has not been completely filled can be treated surgically.

   D. Teeth in which endodontic instruments have been broken can be treated surgically.

   E. Teeth with a wide or "blunderbuss" apex that cannot be filled by conventional therapy may be treated surgically.

   F. Overfilled canals that are symptomatic can be treated surgically.

   G. Teeth that continue to be symptomatic after conventional therapy often respond to surgical management.

   H. Teeth with fractures in the apical one third to one half can often be treated successfully by surgical means.

   I. Teeth into which access is impossible because of the presence of canal calcification, crowns, or posts can be treated surgically.

   II. Apicoectomy

   A. Two types of incisions may be used to approach the apical region for apical surgery.

   1. A linear or semilunar incision should be used at the midportion of the root if the tooth is crowned. This prevents disruption of the papillae and gingival margin. This may also be the best incision if only a thin margin of crestal bone remains.

   2. A mucoperiosteal flap elevated from the neck of the teeth with a relaxing incision should be used in the posterior mandible because this allows for best visualization of the mental foramen without injury to the nerve.

   B. If the periapical lesion has not perforated the labial plate, a drill is used to remove bone for access to the apex of the tooth. It is important that adequate bone be removed to allow complete extirpation of the lesion and resection of a full one third of the tooth apex.

C. The apex of the resected tooth must be sealed. Failure is more likely by performing apicoectomy alone without paying particular attention to the apical seal. The best seal is achieved with dental amalgam. If the tooth is filled with gutta-percha, the gutta-percha may be heated to seal the apex.

D. The apical defect is thoroughly irrigated and the flap carefully closed with 3–0 or 4–0 gut sutures.

Replantation and Transplantation of Teeth

I. The oral surgeon is frequently required to replace teeth that have been partially or completely avulsed. The success of these procedures depends in large part on the timing of treatment.

II. Partially avulsed teeth should be returned to the proper position and stabilized. To avoid unnecessary tissue damage, surgical intervention is kept to a minimum. Gingival lacerations are sutured, and the alveolar bone is remodeled around the tooth with digital pressure. Intruded teeth are brought back to their proper position, as are teeth that have been extruded. If partially avulsed teeth are stable, they may not require any splinting. When stabilization is required, rigid fixation should be avoided; periodontal packing or orthodontic-type splinting is recommended.

III. The prognosis for avulsed teeth is indirectly proportional to the time that the tooth is out of the socket. Teeth replaced within 30 min have the best prognosis for long-term success without root resorption.

IV. Avulsed teeth are managed as follows:

A. Storage—the best recommendation is for the lost tooth to be immediately replaced in its socket. When this is not possible, the tooth should be retained in the buccal sulcus while the patient is transported to the office. Because it may not be a good idea for a young child to hold an avulsed tooth in his or her mouth, in these cases the tooth should be transported in milk or tap water.

B. Root cleaning—the tooth should be handled by the crown, not the root. The root should not be touched before replantation, unless there is dirt or debris on it, in which case it may be gently rinsed with saline and the debris removed with cotton pliers. The root should not be scraped, brushed, or cleaned with medicines or chemicals of any kind.

C. The socket—the socket should be left alone unless it contains dirt, debris, or a blood clot, in which case it should be gently irrigated and suctioned. The tooth is replanted in the socket, and the socket manually compressed.

D. Splinting—the tooth is splinted with orthodontic brackets and wire. In some cases it can be stabilized with sutures over the occlusal surface. It should remain splinted for at least 7–10 da, with the patient on a soft diet.

E. Endodontic therapy—a tooth with an open apex will usually reestablish its blood flow and remain vital. A replanted tooth should be followed closely and, if signs of pulpal disease develop, the pulp should be extirpated and the canals filled with calcium hydroxide. A tooth whose apex is closed will usually not remain vital, and its pulp should be extirpated within the first 2 wk after replantation. The canals are filled with calcium hydroxide, which should be removed and replaced every 3–4 mo; after 1–2 yr a permanent root filling (e.g., gutta-percha) can be inserted. However, such therapy should never be started while the tooth is out of the mouth and socket, for this wastes time during which the tooth could be returned to the mouth.

F. Antibiotics—a patient should be given antibiotics for 1 wk after treatment and tetanus toxoid as necessary according to the patient's history.

TRANSPLANTATION

I. The third molar is the most commonly transplanted tooth. The usual situation is for an unerupted or partially erupted third molar to be transplanted in the site of a first or second molar that has been lost prematurely.

A. The prognosis is best when cases are selected in which the roots of the tooth to be transplanted are approximately one third to one half formed, with wide-open apices, and the labial plates of the recipient site are intact. The space available at the recipient site must be assessed for adequacy. When the crown of a first molar is decayed, the second molar may drift forward, reducing the mesiodistal space.

B. The surgical technique is as follows:

1. The first or second molar to be replaced is removed as atraumatically as possible to preserve the labial plate of bone. It may be necessary to section the tooth to prevent damage to the plate. The interseptal bone is removed to make room for the transplant, and the socket is curetted to remove any periapical disease, bone fragments, or soft tissue. The socket is then irrigated.

2. An envelope flap is reflected to expose the impacted third molar, which is removed atraumatically to prevent damage to its root structure.

3. The tooth is placed in the recipient socket and positioned slightly out of occlusion. It should not be wedged into the socket. If it does not fit, bone should be removed from the socket to allow the tooth to fit without being wedged.

4. A transplanted mandibular tooth can frequently be secured with a suture or small-gauge wire placed over its occlusal surface. It may also be stabilized by placing acid-etched

resin at the contact points.

5. The patient is given appropriate antibiotic coverage for 7–10 da postoperatively and advised to maintain a soft diet and avoid masticating on the transplanted side for 2 wk.

II. Canines are the next most frequently transplanted tooth. Transplantation is not a substitute for orthodontic positioning and should be performed only when the tooth cannot be positioned by conventional means.

A. The surgical technique is similar to that for third molar transplantation, except that the socket usually must be better developed. The socket should be large enough that the transplant does not require wedging into position and is slightly out of occlusion. Splinting can be accomplished with periodontal packing, cold-cure acrylic, or acid-etched acrylic placed at the contacts.

B. As is true with a transplanted molar, it is important that a canine not be in a functional position during the healing period.

C. All transplanted teeth should be followed radiographically for signs of possible pulp necrosis, periapical pathology, or infection.

Alveolar Ridge Retention

I. Once the teeth are removed, the alveolar ridges undergo progressive bone resorption. As resorption progresses, denture function is increasingly compromised. Many of the factors that cause resorption are difficult to control. It has been observed, however, that as long as a tooth is present, the alveolar bone is preserved.

II. The following procedures are designed to preserve bone by retaining or replacing the tooth roots.

A. Supramucosal root retention
1. Teeth are amputated above the mucosa and copings are placed on the root stumps. A complete denture prosthesis, referred to as an *overdenture,* is constructed to fit over and be partially supported by the prepared root stumps.
2. The patient must be observed closely so that any periodontal or periapical problems can be intercepted early.

B. Submucosal root retention
1. Teeth that have sound root structure may be amputated at the level of the alveolar bone and covered primarily with alveolar mucosa. The roots may be vital or may have undergone root canal therapy before being buried.
2. The success of this procedure depends on keeping the roots covered with mucosa. The mucosa is permitted to heal before denture construction so the risk of dehiscence over the roots will be minimized.

C. Hydroxyapatite root cones
1. Hydroxyapatite root form cones usually lead to mucosal dehiscence and are therefore no longer used.

Canine Exposure to Assist Orthodontics

I. Impacted canines can often be moved into position orthodonti-
cally. To do this, the canine tooth must be exposed so that an orthodontic appliance can be placed on its crown.

II. The position of the canine tooth must be evaluated before surgery
by periapical radiographs taken at different angles to determine
whether the cuspid is buccal or lingual to the adjacent tooth roots.
   A. If the tooth is buccal, an apically repositioned flap should be
   utilized to preserve the attached gingival tissue.
   B. If the cuspid is impacted palatally in the maxilla, electrocautery
   can be used to remove overlying tissue and locate the crown.

III. If bone overlies the impacted crown, this must be removed very
carefully with curettes rather than a drill to prevent injury to the
crown enamel. The adjacent dental sac should also be removed
with curettes.

IV. Care should be taken not to expose the cementum or tooth root.

V. After achieving hemostasis, an orthodontic bracket or button
should then be placed. The tooth is then activated using a light
wire or elastic thread from the tooth to the existing arch wire.

VI. The same technique can be used in managing other impacted
teeth for orthodontic exposure.

IMMEDIATE IMPLANT PLACEMENT

The reader is referred to Chapter 8 for a discussion of this subject.

GENERAL REFERENCES

Guernsey LH: Preprosthetic surgery. In Kruger GO, ed: *Textbook of oral and maxillofacial surgery*, ed 6, St. Louis, 1984, Mosby.

Kruger GO: Impacted teeth. In Kruger, GO, ed: *Textbook of oral and maxillofacial
surgery*, ed 6, St. Louis, 1984, Mosby.

Obwegeser HL: Surgical preparation of the maxilla for prosthesis, *J Oral Surg*
22:127, 1964.

Peterson LJ, et al: *Contemporary oral and maxillofacial surgery*, ed 2, St. Louis,
1990, Mosby.

Starshak TJ: *Preprosthetic oral and maxillofacial surgery*, St. Louis, 1980, Mosby.

Preprosthetic Oral and
Maxillofacial Surgery

8

WILLIE L. STEPHENS

GENERAL CONSIDERATIONS

I. Preprosthetic surgery is that part of oral and maxillofacial surgery designed to establish the best hard- and soft-tissue bases for prosthetic appliances. Its scope spans the spectrum, from simple extraction technique and preparation of the mouth for dentures to bone grafts and alloplastic implants.

II. The development of new biomaterials and improved prosthetic techniques, along with a better understanding of oral physiology, has contributed to great strides in the success of prosthetic appliances for edentulous patients.

PREOPERATIVE MANAGEMENT

I. A thorough evaluation of the patient is most important in determining whether he or she is a candidate for surgery and which procedure would be the appropriate treatment.

II. The patient's physical and psychological ability to tolerate a conventional prosthesis must be determined early in the evaluation process. Some patients will not be able to adapt to a conventional denture regardless of how well made and well fitting it is. A clue in this regard may be the patient's intolerance of multiple apparently well-made dentures. Such a person may be a candidate for an implant rather than a ridge extension procedure (e.g., a mandibular bone staple or an osseointegrated device).

III. Consultation with the prosthodontist is most important in determining the appropriate procedure to address each individual patient's prosthetic requirements.

IV. Other considerations—the patient's age, physical, and mental health status, and financial constraints, as well as the condition of the hard and soft tissues of the alveolar ridges—must be taken into account.

SIMPLE TREATMENT PROCEDURES

I. A poorly fitting denture can be a significant contributor to alveolar ridge resorption and soft-tissue problems (i.e., hypertrophy).

II. Minor osseous and soft-tissue defects can prevent proper denture fit and contribute to the need for later major reconstructive preprosthetic surgery. A number of limited surgical procedures can be performed under local anesthesia to improve denture fit.

Alveolar and mylohyoid ridge reduction
Alveoloplasty

I. Conservation of alveolar bone is of paramount importance; therefore, any hard-tissue corrective procedures should be conservative. Minimal flap deflection is recommended for preservation of the vestibule.

II. When isolated prominences of the alveolar ridge must be removed, an incision is made directly over the prominence and a minimal flap is elevated for exposure. Rongeurs and bone files are used to reduce and smooth the area, and the incision is closed with resorbable sutures.

III. A knife-edged ridge is reduced by making an incision along its crest. A mucoperiosteal flap is elevated, exposing the ridge, and the sharp portion of the ridge is appropriately recontoured and smoothed with a bone file. A rotating bur or rongeur and file may be used as indicated.

Mylohyoid ridge reduction

I. A prominent mylohyoid ridge may prevent proper lingual flange extension and cause pain from impingement by the denture.

II. To remove this prominence, an incision is made along the crest of the ridge adjacent to the area. A mucoperiosteal flap is elevated over the mylohyoid ridge and a wide periosteal elevator is placed to retract and protect the lingual tissues. The ridge is removed or reduced with a chisel that is approximately 1 cm in width. A bone bur is used to smooth the area further. The operative site is irrigated and closed with resorbable sutures.

Tuberosity reduction

I. Enlargement of the maxillary tuberosity may result from excessive fibrous tissue or bony enlargement.

II. Fibrous tissue reduction is accomplished by means of a wedge resection over the crest of the ridge, followed by submucosal resection of fibrous tissue under the buccal and palatal flaps. If bony enlargement is present, it may be reduced with rongeurs and smoothed with a bone file. The operative site is irrigated and closed with interrupted or continuous resorbable sutures.

Removal of maxillary and mandibular tori and exostoses
Maxillary tori

I. These may interfere with denture placement and cause discomfort by irritation of the thin overlying mucosa.

II. A maxillary occlusal radiograph is taken before removal to determine whether the torus is pneumatized, since removal of such a torus could create an oronasal communication. An exploratory bur hole can be used to test for pneumatization.

III. A midpalatal incision is made over the torus, with a Y-shaped extension at one or both ends of the incision if necessary for access. A fissure bur is used to section the lesion, and each section is carefully removed with a curved osteotome to prevent accidental creation of an oronasal communication. The site is smoothed with a bone file or bur, and the incision is closed with interrupted sutures.

Mandibular tori

I. These usually occur on the lingual aspect of the mandible adjacent to the premolar area.

II. The incision for removal is made over the crest of the ridge and should extend beyond the immediate area of the lesion to allow for retraction of the mucoperiosteum without tension and to prevent lingual flap tears. A large periosteal elevator is used to retract and protect the lingual anatomy. Large broad-based tori are sectioned with a bone bur and removed with a chisel and mallet. Those with a narrow-pedicled base may often be removed with just a mallet and osteotome. After removal, the site is irrigated and the incision is closed with interrupted sutures.

Exostoses

I. Lateral exostoses occur most frequently in the posterior maxillary areas. They should be removed when they interfere with proper extension of the buccal denture flange.

II. An incision is made over the crest of the ridge, and a mucoperiosteal flap is elevated to expose the lesion. A retractor is placed to protect the mucoperiosteum, and the exostosis is removed or recontoured to produce a smooth ridge. The incision is closed with interrupted sutures.

Submucosal vestibuloplasty

I. Submucosal vestibuloplasty may be used to restore maxillary vestibular depth when the bone height is adequate but the mucosa and muscles are attached on or near the crest of the ridge. Additionally, the overlying mucosa must be free of pathologic changes.

II. A vertical incision is made through the mucosa in the midline of the maxillary labial vestibule. Dissecting scissors are inserted into the incision, and a submucosal tunnel is extended from the midline to the tuberosities bilaterally. In wide, broad arches, additional vertical incisions may be required to gain access to the tuberosity regions. The vertical incision is then extended to the periosteum, and the scissors are again used to make a corresponding supraperiosteal dissection. Any abnormal muscle attachments are released from the crest of the ridge and displaced superiorly. If these tissues are redundant, they are simply excised. The incision is then closed with interrupted sutures, and a stent or denture is used to take a compound impression with the flanges extended to the depth of the newly created sulcus. The denture is secured with perialveolar wires for approximately 10 da. A palatal screw (in the middle of the hard palate) may also be used.

III. When redundant soft tissue is present, it is resected as necessary, and the submucosal extension is performed through the open incision. In the open incision procedure, sutures may be placed to secure the mucosa in the depth of the sulcus to periosteum. The incision is then closed along the crest of the ridge. A stent is also used in this procedure and is placed as described previously.

Secondary epithelialization procedures

I. Over the years, numerous secondary epithelialization procedures have been described to provide ridge extension in limited areas when adequate bone height is available. Such procedures are virtually limited to the mandible, however, because in the maxilla they have proved to be poor with respect to relapse.

II. Two of the more commonly used secondary epithelialization techniques are the Kazanjian and the lip-switch.

A. In the Kazanjian procedure, a horizontal incision is made in the mucosa of the lip. A mucosal flap is reflected to the crest of the ridge, and a supraperiosteal dissection is extended to the depth of the labial sulcus. The success of this procedure depends on maintaining a thin mucosal flap and a periosteal base free of muscle and submucosal fatty tissue. The mucosal flap is sutured to the periosteum in the depth of the sulcus, and the raw lip surface is left to granulate. A compound impression is taken with a stent or denture, and the denture is left in place for 10 da.

B. The lip-switch procedure is similar to the Kazanjian except that the raw surface of the lip is covered with periosteum. After the mucosal flap has been developed, an incision is made through the periosteum along the crest of the ridge, and the periosteum is dissected from the labial side of the alveolar ridge and turned onto the raw surface of the lip. The periosteal flap is sutured to the lip mucosal incision. The remainder of the procedure is the same as described earlier.

COMPLEX TREATMENT PROCEDURES
Vestibuloplasty with grafts

I. Vestibuloplasty with split-thickness skin or mucosal grafts has been widely used in the United States since the 1960s for increasing the relative alveolar bone height and improving the soft-tissue base for construction of a denture prosthesis. Suitable cases exhibit a relative loss of vestibular depth from a combination of alveolar bone loss and high soft-tissue attachments; however, there should be adequate bone available if exposed.

II. The indications for vestibuloplasty with grafts include the following:

    A. Severe atrophy of the alveolar ridge leading to poor retention. A minimum of 9–10 mm of residual bone is needed in most cases for an acceptable result. This is not the procedure of choice when severe resorption of basal bone has created a pencil-thin mandible requiring additional bulk for strength.

    B. High soft-tissue attachments that prevent adequate flange extension for denture stabilization. This includes high mucosal, muscle, and frenum attachments that cause displacement of the denture base.

    C. High mylohyoid muscle attachments. A prominent mylohyoid ridge muscle attachment prevents adequate lingual flange extension and may also become painful from flange impingement.

    D. Redundant soft tissue on the ridge and in the vestibulum. Soft-tissue accumulations (e.g., epulis fissurata) cause obliteration of the sulcus and also create a mobile soft-tissue base that compromises denture stability.

III. Preoperative planning includes the following:

    A. Thorough history and physical evaluation. The patient must be in generally good health and able to undergo general anesthesia lasting at least 3 hr. There should be no uncontrolled medical problems. Underlying disease of the mandible is eliminated before surgery.

    B. Thorough oral examination. The alveolar ridge should be rounded rather than sharp or knife-edged. If it is sharp, this may require correction before surgery. The width of the ridge is equally as important as ridge height for denture retention and is therefore a presurgical consideration. The mylohyoid ridge also is examined so it can be determined whether revision will be necessary at the time of surgery.

    C. Radiographic examination of the mandible. This should consist of at least panoramic and lateral cephalometric studies, which are used in making determinations of the size and shape of the alveolar bases, the position of the mental nerves, and whether residual disease exists. The lateral cephalometric radiograph can be used to assess the angle at which the mandible flares as it extends toward the inferior border and will help in determining how much flare to give the extended flange of the denture or stent placed at the time of surgery.

    D. Impression of the mandible. This is taken for stent preparation. A tray that is overextended with dental compound is used to fabricate a stone model. The labial vestibule of the model is further extended to the depth that is to be achieved surgically. The angle at which the vestibulum is to be extended inferolaterally is determined from the cephalometric radiograph. The flanges of the patient's denture or an acrylic tray is extended to the new vestibular depth and is used to maintain the graft during healing.

Mandibular split-thickness skin graft vestibuloplasty

I. Skin graft harvesting and donor site

   A. The donor site must be as free as possible of hair growth. The lateral thigh is a site commonly selected. The area is prepared and draped and the skin to be harvested is lubricated with mineral oil.

   B. The Brown or Padgett dermatome is set to take a graft approximately 0.012–0.015 in. thick. A strip of skin 4–8 ×10–15 cm is usually required for vestibuloplasty. The harvested graft is stored on saline-moistened gauze until it is placed on the recipient site.

   C. The donor site is covered with a thrombin-soaked gauze pad, and a temporary pressure dressing is placed until the intraoral procedure is completed. It is then covered with an Opsite dressing, which remains in place until spontaneously exfoliated. Compress gauze or scarlet red-impregnated gauze may also be used as a dressing.

II. Surgical technique

   A. The labial mucosa is infiltrated with 2% lidocaine and 1:200,000 epinephrine.

   B. A no. 15 blade is used to make an incision just labial to the crest of the ridge, extending for a second molar region to the midline bilaterally. Posteriorly the incisions are extended distolabially one half to three fourths in a 45° angle to the ridge.

   C. Dissecting scissors and a periosteal elevator are used to perform a careful supraperiosteal dissection exposing the labial and anterior aspects of the alveolar ridge. The dissection should not extend below the external oblique ridge or a blind pocket that will trap food may be created.

   D. If the mentalis muscle is attached superiorly, only about one half of it should be detached; otherwise, there may be a prolapse of the soft-tissue structure of the chin (the so-called witch's chin).

   E. The mental nerves are protected during surgery.

   F. If the neurovascular bundle exits from the crest of the ridge or if there is a lateral bony prominence, it may be desirable to dissect the structure gently and create a new channel into which the bundle can be placed. However, even minimal manipulation of the mental nerve tissue will be attended by sensory disturbances at least temporarily and perhaps over a much longer time.

   G. Any fat or muscle remnants are removed from the periosteal base to allow firm healing of the skin graft to the periosteum.

   H. The small Obwegeser awls, designed for vestibuloplasty, are used to pass nine circummandibular (2–0 chromic) sutures around the inferior border of the mandible. These attach the lingual mucosa and muscle and the labial mucoperiosteal flap to the lower portion of the mandible. After all nine sutures are placed, they are tied into the labial sulcus to secure the repositioned lingual and buccolabial tissues. The inferior placement of the flaps creates a new, deeper labial vestibule and a lower floor of the mouth. If the floor of the mouth does not require revision, these sutures may be placed through the floor adjacent to the lingual alveolus. The buccolabial flap can be further secured by suturing it to the periosteum in the depth of the vestibule.

I. An impression of the newly exposed alveolar ridge is made with impression compound and the previously prepared stent. The compound should extend to the depth of the new vestibule. The inner aspect of the stent is painted with benzoin or another adhesive agent to secure the graft, which is then placed in the stent epithelial side down. When the adhesive has dried and the graft is securely attached to the stent, it is ready for placement. The graft and stent are carefully placed on the ridge and secured with two or three circummandibular wire or nylon sutures. The stent is held in place for 10 da and then removed for trimming of necrotic skin edges and removal of any debris from the sulcus. The stent is also trimmed slightly, if necessary, for comfort and is worn until a new denture is fabricated.

J. Antibiotics should be given prophylactically at the time of circummandibular suture removal. Penicillin V or erythromycin in a dose of 2 g is given 2 hr before the procedure and 250 mg is given every 6 hr for 1 da after the procedure.

III. Factors contributing to success

A. When the basic principles of patient selection, technique, and skin grafting are followed, a consistently good to excellent result can be expected.

B. The principles essential to success of the vestibuloplasty procedure include:

1. Selecting a donor site that is free of hair follicles. Harvesting from a hairless area, as well as taking a very thin graft (0.012–0.015 in.), reduces the possibility of having hair grow from the grafted site.

2. Preparing the alveolar recipient site by supraperiosteal dissection. This will create a clean periosteal bed. The periosteum should be free of fat and muscle tissue remnants so there can be firm attachment of the graft to the periosteum.

3. Good hemostasis at the recipient site. Bleeding and subsequent hematoma will prevent complete attachment of the graft to the periosteum.

4. Graft coverage of the entire recipient site. This will prevent granulation tissue formation and wound contracture and relapse.

5. Immobilization for 7-10 da. To ensure complete healing, a stent should hold the graft.
6. Leaving at least 9-10 mm of residual bone. The ridge should have a relatively broad and rounded shape, not a sharp crest.
7. Avoidance of extending the vestibular dissection into three critical regions:
   a. Posterior buccal area—the dissection should in most cases not extend beyond the external oblique ridge, because this will create a blind pocket that can trap food.
   b. Mentalis muscle—when the dissection must involve the mentalis, one third to one half of the muscle fibers should remain attached to prevent the patient from having a "witch's chin."
   c. Genioglossus muscle—when the genial tubercles and attached muscle fibers are involved, approximately one half of the genioglossus should remain attached to prevent postoperative tongue control problems.

Floor of mouth procedure

I. A floor of the mouth procedure is frequently necessary before labial vestibuloplasty because bleeding problems, although infrequent, are more likely to occur in this location than in the labial vestibule.
II. The surgical technique is as follows:
   A. Lidocaine and 1:200,000 epinephrine are injected along the lingual aspect of the mandible bilaterally for vasoconstriction.
   B. A no. 15 blade is used to make an incision just medial to the crest of the ridge extending anteriorly from the second molar area to the midline bilaterally.
   C. Using blunt dissection and finger pressure, the surgeon exposes the mylohyoid muscle and resects it at its attachment to the mylohyoid ridge. Extra care is taken to tie or coagulate any bleeding vessels immediately to prevent them from retracting and bleeding later.
   D. When the genial tubercles are superiorly positioned and would appear to interfere with future denture placement, they may be selectively reduced.
   E. The genioglossus muscles may also be resected at the bone attachment, but one third to one half of the muscle should remain attached to avoid postoperative tongue control problems that might result in airway obstruction or difficulties with swallowing or speech. Nine 2-0 chromic sutures are symmetrically spaced through the mucosa-muscle flap to be attached later to the labial flap.

Mandibular mucosal graft vestibuloplasty

I. Buccal mucosa and palatal mucosa have been used as an alternative to skin in the vestibuloplasty procedure. They have the advantage of eliminating an external donor site and may therefore be an excellent alternative when a skin graft is contraindicated, as in the patient with a history of keloid formation or other dermatologic disorder.

II. Buccal mucosa may be used for full-thickness as well as split-thickness grafts. The full-thickness graft is taken freehand with a scalpel and dissecting scissors. After the graft is resected, it is carefully "defatted" before placement on the alveolar ridge. If fat is left on, the graft may not attach firmly to the periosteal base, leading to a mobile soft-tissue base. The ridge extension procedure is performed as described for the split-thickness skin graft vestibuloplasty. The graft is secured with absorbable sutures, and a compound-lined stent or denture is placed.

III. Palatal mucosa may also be used as graft tissue for ridge extension procedures.

   A. However, its use is limited by the amount that can be harvested. Removing the entire palatal mucosa leaves a wound that heals slowly and results in prolonged discomfort. A horseshoe-shaped graft is taken freehand. Excess fat and salivary gland tissue are removed to prevent mobility of the graft after healing. The graft can be enlarged by means of a graft expander when necessary for complete coverage. The graft is sutured in place, and a stent is placed to secure it.

IV. A disadvantage of mucosal grafting is that the amount of mucosa available for harvesting may not be sufficient to cover the entire ridge. In such instances use of a graft expander will both increase the size of the graft and allow excellent adaptation to the ridge, thereby lessening the risk of hematoma under the graft because of the fenestrations present.

Alveolar ridge augmentation for conventional dentures
Alloplastic augmentation

I. Hydroxyapatite implants

   A. Hydroxyapatite (HA) is a biocompatible, nonresorbable calcium phosphate substance with physical and chemical characteristics similar to those of dental enamel and bone. Clinical and laboratory studies have produced no evidence of local or systemic inflammation or foreign body response to its use. Apparently it can become strongly adherent to bone. It provides a nonresorbable supporting matrix for deposition of bone by chemically bonding without an intervening fibrous capsule. Radiographic evaluation is easy because its high calcium content renders it radiopaque.

   B. Hydroxyapatite implants alone can restore a variety of types of alveolar ridge defect. They may be used to restore the width of the ridge, ridge height, undercut areas, and mandibular height and width when moderate to severe loss exists as a result of resorption, prior surgery, or trauma. When extensive resorption has occurred with loss of basilar bone and when the mandible is pencil-thin, it is suggested that HA be combined with autogenous bone.

C. The material is supplied in prepackaged 1–2-ml plastic syringes or in vials with syringes that are filled by the surgeon at the time of surgery. The HA-filled syringes use either saline or blood as a cohesive agent to aid in the control of the particles during placement and to minimize postoperative migration. Approximately four syringes are required to augment the posterior ridge bilaterally or to augment the anterior ridge, and approximately eight syringes are needed for a total ridge augmentation. The surgical procedure may be done under general anesthesia or in many cases under local anesthesia in the operating room.

II. Maxillary augmentation

A. The single vertical midline incision technique is sufficient for most maxillary augmentations.

B. The procedure may be done with or without submucosal vestibuloplasty, depending on whether a ridge extension is necessary.

1. If the augmentation is done without submucosal vestibuloplasty, the vertical incision is carried through the periosteum immediately. A small periosteal elevator is used to develop a subperiosteal tunnel along with the portion of the ridge to be augmented. It is sometimes necessary to elevate the mucosa on the palatal side of the ridge to develop an adequate tunnel size.

2. When a submucosal vestibuloplasty is necessary, the initial vertical incision is carried through the mucosa to the periosteum. The submucosal dissection is then performed, with the vertical incision extended through the periosteum and a subperiosteal tunnel is formed. The periosteum is incised if a larger tunnel size is needed.

C. Traction sutures are placed on each side of the incision to aid in keeping the incisions open for insertion of the syringes that will be used to deliver the implant material.

1. The implant syringe is placed in the tunnel, and the pockets are filled from the posterior aspect to the midline bilaterally.

2. To prevent the inclusion of implant particles in the incision during closure, the traction sutures may be used to lift the tissue edges away from the implant while the incision is being sutured.

D. The incision is closed with interrupted horizontal mattress sutures. Soft stents or dentures prepared on a preoperative model may help retain ridge form in maxillary cases but can cause tissue breakdown.

III. Mandibular augmentation

A. Bilateral vertical incisions approximately 1 in. long placed over the lateral aspect of the alveolar ridge in the canine area are used for most mandibular procedures. Occasionally a single midline vertical incision is used for augmentation of the anterior mandible only.

B. The mental nerve is carefully visualized and protected during surgery.

C. A small periosteal elevator is used to develop a limited subperiosteal tunnel along the crest of the ridge from the vertical incision posteriorly to the third molar area bilaterally. If augmentation of the anterior ridge is necessary, the tunnels are extended anteriorly as necessary.

D. Care should be taken not to extend the dissection beyond the external oblique ridge, for this could allow excessive lateral migration of the implant particles.

E. Traction sutures are placed on each side of the incision to aid in keeping the incision open for insertion of the implant syringes.

F. In total mandibular augmentation the posterior pockets are filled with the implant first. The syringe is inserted to the posterior extent of the tunnel, and the pockets are filled from the posterior area to the canine area bilaterally. As the implant is injected, it is guided into position and molded to form with finger pressure as needed. The anterior pockets are then filled from the midline back to the canine incision.

G. When the implant is packed around the mental nerve, various alterations in nerve function have been noticed. Omitting the implant in this area does not compromise the prosthetic result.

H. Traction sutures are useful for lifting the tissue edges from the implant, and the incision is closed with interrupted horizontal mattress sutures.

I. Splints are not used as frequently in the mandible as in the maxilla but are helpful for undercut cases.

J. Antibiotics are started preoperatively and continued for 1 wk postoperatively.

K. Clinical judgment is the best indicator of when new dentures can be constructed. Most ridges are well healed and firm enough for denture construction approximately 6 wk after surgery.

L. When inadequate vestibular depth remains after augmentation, a secondary vestibuloplasty with a graft may be performed over the implant after sufficient healing has occurred. Approximately 3–4 mo healing time should be allowed before vestibuloplasty is performed. The standard vestibuloplasty procedure is used.

M. Hydroxyapatite has several uses in mandibular augmentation:
   1. It can be applied in conjunction with the mandibular staple implant.
   2. It can also be mixed with cancellous bone. Augmentation of a very atrophic mandible is a suitable indication.

3. In solid blocks it offers the clinician greater control over placement and it reduces migration. The basic methods are similar, although in the mandible more extensive lingual tissue dissection will permit tunnel development with less loss of buccal vestibular depth. Wound dehiscence is a common and major problem.

Autogenous bone grafts

I. Autogenous bone grafts are the treatment of choice when maxillary or mandibular augmentation is deemed necessary. Despite graft resorption after the procedure, sufficient bulk for adequate function remains after the resorption has been stabilized.

II. Bone graft augmentation is recommended in the following circumstances:

A. When there is inadequate bone height and width for vestibuloplasty

B. When additional bulk is required to strengthen the mandible with extensive resorption

C. When the bulk of an implant substance (e.g., HA) would be too large to restore a functional denture base and strengthen the mandible

III. Superior border rib grafts

A. Superior augmentation of the mandible with a graft from the ribs, placed by means of a transoral approach, has been well described. Resorption is one half to two thirds within the first 18–24 mo, and vestibuloplasty procedures are often necessary following the graft. Thus the patient must be able to tolerate three procedures: harvest of the rib graft, placement of the graft, and vestibuloplasty.

1. Two rib segments 6–8 cm long are used. The first is contoured by vertical scoring on its internal surface to allow it to be bent and adapted to the curvature of the mandible. The second is cut into small pieces to be packed around the first after it is placed.

2. The buccal vestibule is infiltrated with lidocaine and 1:200,000 epinephrine.

3. An incision is made at the crest of the ridge from the retromolar region to the midline bilaterally.

4. The mucoperiosteal flap is elevated labially and lingually to expose the alveolar ridge, and a periosteal releasing incision is made to provide adequate tissue to cover the graft if necessary.

5. When the anterior mandible is higher than the posterior mandible, a groove of sufficient width to accept the rib is made in the anterior region to compensate for the difference in bone height.

6. The rib strut is placed toward the lingual over the mylohyoid ridge. Three wire sutures are used to secure it.

7. A continuous horizontal mattress suture is recommended for closure. Eversion of the tissue edges is stressed to encourage early closure and prevent wound dehiscence. A periosteal releasing incision can be used to reduce flap tension. Closure is started posteriorly. As the closure proceeds anteriorly, a pocket develops between the graft and the mucoperiosteum; this is filled with the bone chips from the sectioned rib. Bone chips are placed primarily on the buccal aspect of the rib to form a well-contoured ridge.

8. After closure with the mattress suture is completed, a running spiral suture is recommended for added security of closure.

9. The patient is started on a regimen of antibiotics preoperatively, and this is continued for 1 wk postoperatively.

10. Approximately 4–6 wk are allowed for healing if a vestibuloplasty procedure is anticipated.

B. Augmentation of the maxilla

1. Ribs have also been used for maxillary ridge augmentation. Resorption is usually in the form of decreased ridge circumference, with more vertical bone loss anteriorly than posteriorly. The graft is therefore placed lateral to the atrophic ridge to compensate for the resorption and restore optimal alignment with the mandibular ridge.

2. The graft may be placed through an open incision extending from the tuberosity to the midline bilaterally. Lateral periosteal relaxing incisions are usually necessary to allow closure of the incisions with minimal tension. The graft is secured with four wire sutures. Anteriorly the strut is usually not in contact with the basal bone; posteriorly it is in direct contact. Two figure-8 wires are placed to secure the graft without basal contact. This area between the graft and basal bone is later filled in with bone chips. Two wires are placed posteriorly to further secure the graft.

IV. Inferior border rib grafts

A. Inferior border grafting for mandibular augmentation is designed to eliminate some of the problems associated with transoral graft procedures. Resorption is less with inferior border grafts because the graft does not bear the pressure of the denture, and secondary vestibuloplasty is often not necessary. This is also an excellent procedure for the repair of fractures or malunions of the severely atrophic mandible. It does require an extensive extraoral approach, but with only slight added risk to the mandibular branch of the facial nerve.

B. Surgical technique

1. Two ribs are harvested, and each is scored on its inner surface with cuts approximately 1 in. apart.

2. Rongeurs or osteotomes are used to remove alternating notched sections of bone to allow the ribs to bend easily. The bone sections removed are stored for later use.

3. The inferior border of the mandible is exposed from angle to angle through a submandibular incision.

4. One rib is adapted to the lingual aspect of the mandible, and the second is adapted to the buccal side. The bone segments previously removed are used to fill the space between the two rib struts.

5. Intraosseous or submandibular wires are placed as necessary to secure the grafts. Bone plates and screws may be used for more rigid fixation.

6. The surgical incision is closed in layers.

7. A temporary denture can be placed as soon as the patient is comfortable because it does not put pressure directly on the graft. If a vestibuloplasty is necessary, 2–6 mo of healing time should be allowed.

V. Superior border iliac block grafts

A. Augmentation of the superior border of the mandible with iliac crest block grafts has been performed successfully for years.

1. Treatment of atrophic mandibles with iliac crest bone placed transorally gives better results than treatment using cartilage. Iliac crest onlay grafts may be placed through an extraoral approach as well. The advantages of an extraoral approach are elimination of oral contamination, reduced risk of oral mucosal dehiscence, ease of closure of the surgical site, and reduced incidence of the need for secondary vestibuloplasty.

2. The risks of an extraoral approach have already been discussed.

B. Surgical technique

1. The graft is placed through a submandibular incision adequate to expose the mandible from the second molar region to the midline bilaterally.

2. The superior crest of the mandible may need to have any sharp areas reduced to allow good adaptation of the graft blocks.

3. After the bone blocks are placed along the entire crest, the spaces between and around the blocks are filled with cancellous bone taken at the time the bone blocks are harvested. The bone blocks are secured by intraosseous wire sutures, and the incision is closed in layers.

4. Three to six months of healing should be allowed before a functioning denture is placed or a vestibuloplasty performed.

VI. Ridge augmentation with pedicled bone grafts

A. Mandibular augmentation procedures using pedicled bone grafts are designed to take advantage of lingual muscle attachments, which provide a rich blood supply to the bone flap. Continuity of the blood supply may limit resorption associated with onlay graft procedures. Two types of osteotomy have been used for mandibular augmentation—the horizontal with an interpositional bone graft and the vertical or visor.

B. Horizontal/interpositional osteotomy

1. The horizontal osteotomy is generally indicated for patients in whom resorption has been more extensive in the buccolingual dimension, producing a narrow mandible. This allows the osteotomy cut to be made above the mental nerve. A corticocancellous bone graft is taken before the procedure is started.

2. A mucoperiosteal incision placed just lateral to the crest is extended from the retromolar area to the midline bilaterally.

3. A buccolabial mucoperiosteal flap is reflected, and the mental nerves are exposed and dissected free of soft tissue so they can be protected.

4. A fissure bur is used to make vertical bone cuts through the posterior aspect of the alveolar ridge bilaterally. These cuts go through the buccal and lingual bone and extend from the crest of the ridge to just above the mandibular canal.

5. The lateral wall of the canal should be partially or completely uncovered so the level of the nerve will be revealed and the nerve protected against damage during surgery.

6. The horizontal bone cuts can be made with either a thin fissure bur or a reciprocal saw. The blade must be angled slightly inferiorly so it does not enter the canal.

7. Small osteotomes may be used to complete the lingual cortical cuts. The bone flap is reflected upward in preparation for placing the interpositional graft.

8. The corticocancellous graft is cut to the thickness corresponding to the desired increase in bone height.

9. The graft blocks are placed as necessary to fill the interpositional space, and the remaining gaps are filled with cancellous bone and marrow.

10. Three wires or nylon sutures are usually adequate to secure the bone segment. The incision is closed with a continuous horizontal mattress suture followed by a continuous spiral suture.

C. Vertical or visor osteotomy

1. The visor osteotomy was first described by Harle in 1975. Other workers modified the procedure by raising the pedicled graft along the entire length of the arch, grafting the buccal aspect of the superior segment with cancellous bone, and performing a simultaneous vestibuloplasty.

2. Surgical technique
   a. An incision is made just labial to the crest of the ridge and extended from the retromolar area to the midline bilaterally.
   b. A vertical mucoperiosteal tunnel extending from the crest of the ridge to the inferior border is developed on the lingual side of the mandible in the third molar area.
   c. A fissure bur is used to make a vertical bone cut from the crest to the inferior border in this tunnel on each side. An air-driven reciprocating saw is used to make the sagittal cut between the buccal and lingual cortical bone.
   d. In the posterior mandible the saw blade must be angled laterally so the cut will extend through the inferior border.
   e. The mobilized segment is elevated to its new position and secured with wire or nylon sutures. When alignment of bone segments is adequate, bone screws may be used.
   f. Mucosal closure is started posteriorly with horizontal mattress sutures, and the labial tunnel created lateral to the raised bone segment is filled with cancellous bone. A new denture is usually constructed 4–6 mo after surgery.

VII. Maxillary interpositional bone graft
   A. An interpositional bone graft for maxillary ridge augmentation has been suggested as an alternative to conventional onlay bone grafts. Less graft resorption is anticipated. A simultaneous interpositional bone graft with vestibuloplasty to restore the atrophic maxilla has also been described.
   B. A Le Forte I osteotomy is performed in preparation for bone graft insertion. After the maxilla has been inferiorly positioned, iliac crest bone struts or a solid horseshoe-shaped graft is inserted to provide the preoperatively determined amount of augmentation. The segments are stabilized with intraosseous wires or preferably with bone plates and screws to attain rigid fixation and increased stability. The incision is then closed with sutures.

Autogenous bone graft sites for endosseous implant reconstruction

I. The increasingly routine use of endosseous implant reconstruction in preprosthetic surgery has led to its use in patients with less than adequate residual bone volume. When implants are to be placed in sites with inadequate bone for their support, it is then necessary to bone graft the site before implants are placed. This section outlines some of the techniques that can be used for site preparation, but will not specifically discuss when to place the bone and implants simultaneously and when to place the bone and implants in separate procedures, because many times this will depend on the surgeon and his or her experience and personal philosophy. Some general factors that may be used in this decision will be made along the way, however.

II. There are many factors and principles that affect the success or failure of bone grafts. The following are some that are important to any graft procedure. Some of these are particularly important when grafting small areas of the alveolar ridges. Soft-tissue limitations are often crucial to the success of bone grafts as well to the size and shape of the grafts.

   A. Absolute rigid fixation is essential to the early and late success of bone grafts. This may be more important as the size of the graft decreases. A mobile graft is likely to become infected or cause a wound dehiscence. If the graft does not become infected, the mobility causes disturbance of early vascularization, leading to resorption and fibrous tissue formation. Bones, screws, and plates are much better than wires or sutures for absolute rigidity. Multiple screws should be placed at divergent angles from each other to prevent graft mobility during the resorptive phase of bone healing. Rigid fixation of the graft becomes paramount if a soft-tissue dehiscence occurs. A dehiscence is more likely to heal if the graft is absolutely rigid than if there is the slightest amount of mobility. If the soft tissue does not heal over the exposed area, the amount of bone loss is likely to be limited to the exposed region.

   B. The size, shape, and contour of the graft has to be accurate and fit the area to be grafted with precision. If the graft is overcontoured, has sharp edges, or does not fit the ridge precisely, the graft is not likely to be successful or may not be useful even if it heals.

   C. Soft-tissue management is extremely important, and flap design must be carefully thought out before any incisions are made. There is usually a minimum of excess soft tissue; therefore, one usually has one chance to get the design right. Whenever possible, the flap should be thick enough for a two-layer closure. In most cases, the incision is either on the crest of the ridge or on the lip or cheek side of the buccal sulcus. An incision on the crest should not extend more than approximately 4 mm palatal to the crest, or the risk of necrosis at the incision is increased. This incision should be made in two layers. The initial incision is made transversely through the mucosa. The flap is then elevated 3–4 mm to the ridge crest at the submucosal/supraperiosteal level. The blade is now used to incise the periosteum on the crest of the ridge. The flap is elevated with a periosteal elevator exposing the defect. The exposure to the site should be adequate to restore the defect without excessive tension on the flap during retraction. Vertical incisions into the sulcus are usually required for site preparation, graft placement, and rigid fixation. The vertical incisions should be clean and precise, extending obliquely in a direction that produces a flap base wider than the crestal incision. Because the graft increases ridge width and/or height, the flap will likely not close without tension. To allow tension-free closure, a new no. 15 blade is used to make a horizontal incision through the periosteum only, superior to the flap base. This will allow extension of the flap for a tension-free, layered closure. If the periosteal incision is too close to the apex of the flap, necrosis at the incision line may occur. The flap is closed in layers using 4-0 or 5-0 resorbable suture for the periosteal/submucosal layer and 4-0 or 5-0 nonresorbable, interrupted or vertical mattress sutures for the mucosa. Removal of these sutures usually requires loop magnification. If the incision is made in the lip or buccal region, it is made of sufficient thickness to allow a two-layer closure. If there is any question about coverage or incision closure, the buccal incision will be safer than a crestal incision in most cases. It does, however, often cause more compromise of sulcus depth after healing. Because of the elasticity of the sulcus and buccal mucosa, one must be careful not to get the apex of the flap wider than its base at the ridge crest. This tends to be more of a problem with smaller defects. This incision is also closed in layers using 4-0 or 5-0 resorbable sutures for the deep layer and 4-0 or 5-0 nonresorbable, vertical mattress sutures for the mucosa.

It is impossible to overemphasize the importance of soft-tissue management in these patients. The use of nonresorbable sutures for mucosal closure, with their careful removal under magnification, is critical. After the suture knot is resorbed, the suture tract remains open for an unpredictable length of time, potentially leaving an inflammatory tract that may communicate with the graft.

The position of the incision may be influenced by its relationship to the graft. It is best to keep the incision away from the graft, if possible, to prevent having the closure directly over the graft. The incision for a sinus floor augmentation may be ideally made over the alveolar crest, whereas the incision for an onlay to the anterior ridge may be better placed on the lip side of the sulcus.

D. Bone graft donor sites. Localized site preparation for implants has created the need for smaller, locally accessible autogenous donor sites from which bone can be harvested without using a distant site such as the ilium. There are a number of potential donor sites available. The following are some of the common sites available, many of which can be used under local anesthesia or local anesthesia with sedation on an outpatient basis setting as well as in the operating room.

1. Implant sites. A commonly overlooked donor site during implant surgery is the implant site itself. The bone that fills the twist drill flutes is an excellent source of bone for small sites such as for a fenestration defect. A large amount of bone can be harvested by using a trephine rather than a twist drill to make the largest hole before the tap is used, then additional bone from the tap flutes can be carefully harvested. If the assistant removes bone from each rotary instrument, one is often surprised at the amount of bone collected. The trephined bone plug is cut into fine chips with a sharp bone cutter or ronguers.

2. Tori. Maxillary and mandibular tori, as well as lateral exostoses, may be resected and used as particulate grafts. A large torus could be contoured to fill in an alveolar defect.

3. Tuberosity and retromolar region. The tuberosity region is an easily accessible donor site, particularly if the third molars have been removed. The retromolar region of the mandible may also be used.

4. Anterior mandible (chin). The region of the mandible between the mental foramen is an excellent source of bone for small block grafts and is easily accessible for the use of a trephine to harvest bone plugs that can be cut into small particles. It is obviously important to use a small anterior incision to avoid the mental nerves completely. If a larger exposure is required for a larger harvest site, the nerves should be identified, exposed, and protected during the procedure. When harvesting a larger graft with a bone cut near the mental foramen, the anterior loop of the canal should be carefully assessed to avoid inadvertent injury. A clear panorex or preferably a CT scan or tomograms should be used to assess the position of the loop anterior to the foramen, and an explorer or other small instrument should be used clinically to determine the anterior extent of the canal before the bone cut is made. When possible, minioscillating and reciprocating saws, rather than a rotary drill, are used for bone removal. The movement of the saw blades in each direction is only a few millimeters, and, as a result, potential damage to soft tissues against the saw blade is minimal. The use of a rotary osteotomy or drill requires more exposure and retraction, and if soft tissue is caught by the bur, serious tissue damage can be done. This could be particularly damaging to a nerve. In addition, with a saw, less bone is lost from the bone cuts and there is less thermal damage. If a bur is used, an inline bone filter can be used to harvest fine bone chips from the irrigation. The patient should have the procedure, potential risks, and expected

postoperative course carefully explained preoperatively. The fact that the chin is the donor site does not mean that this is a benign procedure. Harvesting a large chin graft can be associated with morbidity similar that of a small iliac graft. The patient should be made aware of:

a. Potential permanent nerve damage
b. If nerve exposure, the likelihood of some level of temporary sensory change due to retraction and swelling
c. Likely a feeling of sensory loss in the mucosa around lower anterior teeth and possibly alteration of sensation to anterior teeth
d. Possible significant postoperative discomfort due to swelling, sensory changes, and bone pain
e. Possible small change in chin contour, particularly if a large graft has been harvested

To prevent possible changes in the lip and chin postoperatively, the following factors should be considered:

a. It may be reasonable to leave a vertical bone strut in the midline to prevent soft-tissue collapse into the defect.
b. Large defects may need to be filled with HA or other bone substitutes.
c. Placing the incision on the lip side of sulcus should minimize scar formation and contracture.
d. It is absolutely essential that the mentalis muscles be carefully and securely reapproximated to prevent soft-tissue chin droop and other aesthetic changes. Placing a tape or Elastoplast chin dressing can be useful to reduce tension on the incision line and may also reduce discomfort.

5. Other maxillary and mandibular sites. The cortical borders of the pyriform rim, nasal floor, zygomaticomaxillary buttress, and external oblique ridges are all sites from which small grafts can be easily harvested. Bone can be harvested from any of these sites with trephines, small osteotomes, small rotary drills, or saws. When harvesting from the external oblique ridges of a patient with atrophy, one should be careful because the inferior alveolar neurovascular bundle may not be very deep to the bony cortex.

6. Harvesting by iliac marrow aspiration and percutaneous iliac trephine. A bone marrow aspiration needle can be used to harvest bone marrow on an outpatient or inpatient basis. The harvest from this procedure is usually mixed with a bone substitute or filter for grafting. Instrumentation is available for the use of a trephine to harvest bone from the ilium percutaneously or through a minimally open incision. The trephine bone cores are cut

into small bone chips to be used alone or in combination with other graft material. The procedure can be done on an outpatient or inpatient basis.

7. Iliac harvest. The harvest of bone from the ilium is done under general anesthesia. It can, however, be done as an outpatient, surgical day care procedure for a small to medium harvest. The surgical procedure has to be very clean, with a secure closure. There must be complete hemostasis around the surgical site before closure to avoid the need for a drain. The anterior approach is most commonly used for the harvest.

Technique. The iliac crest and anterior superior iliac spine are marked. The incision is marked approximately 6 cm below the crest. The skin is pulled superiorly so that the incision mark is directly over the iliac crest and an incision 4–6 cm in length is made parallel to the crest. The incision is extended through the fascia lata and periosteum to bone. The periosteum and iliac muscles are elevated to expose the medial table. Retractors are placed to protect the medial or lateral soft tissues. After the crest is exposed, bone can be harvested from the lateral table, medial table, or crest of the ilium. The crest can also be split when cancellous bone only is needed. When a corticocancellous graft is needed, the patient may be more comfortable postoperatively if the muscle and periosteum are left intact on the lateral table and the graft is harvested from the medial table. Minioscillating and reciprocating saws are routinely used for bone harvest. They allow more precise, less traumatic graft removal than the use of osteotomes alone. After the bone cuts are made, osteotomes may be used to divide the graft from the donor site. When a bicortical graft is needed, the lateral as well as the medial tables are exposed and the soft tissues are protected with retractors. The saws are then used to resect the graft, leaving the entire crest completely intact.

Careful surgical closure is very important to minimize postoperative discomfort. Bone wax is used to completely control bone bleeding and a soft-tissue hemostatic agent is used, if necessary, to prevent soft-tissue bleeding. The periosteal layer and fascia lata layers are carefully closed, followed by closure of Scarpa's fascia, the subcutaneous layer, and skin. A pressure dressing is then placed.

8. Other donor sites available include:
   a. Cranium
   b. Fibula
   c. Tibia and tibial plateau
   d. Rib

E. Equipment and instruments. Whether bone graft procedures are done in the office, outpatient surgical day care unit, or operating room, the proper equipment, lighting, and instruments are essential to the efficient, safe, and effective surgical procedure. The following are some of the essentials that should always be available.

   1. Good overhead lighting is adequate for most procedures. Procedures such as the sinus elevation/graft procedure may require a headlight for adequate illumination of this and other small, tight areas.

   2. Saws and rotary osteotomes (drills). Minioscillating and reciprocating saws are excellent and may provide a margin of safety over the drill when working in tight areas such as bone harvest from the chin. They are also less traumatic for all harvest/donor sites.

   3. Saw blades, drills, and trephines. An adequate stock of reciprocating and oscillating saw blades of various sizes and shapes should be available, as should a good stock of side-cutting, round, and hole-drilling burs for placing bone screws. New, sharp burs are very important and should be used whenever cutting bone, including the careful shaping of the graft on the table with copious irrigation to prevent overheating of the bone. A generous supply of 2.5–3.5-mm diamond round burs are helpful for use in creating the bone window in cases of sinus augmentation. Trephines of various diameters should be available for bone harvest.

   4. Mini bone screws. A set of small bone screws 1.5 mm and 2.0 mm diameter should be available to stabilize solid block bone grafts. Bone screws are also useful to stabilize barrier membranes.

   5. Sinus graft instruments. A set of instruments designed for sinus membrane elevation is needed for consistent atraumatic sinus mucosa elevation and retraction. Instruments are commercially available.

   6. Osteotomes. A set of small sharp osteotomes is essential. The need for having a sharp instrument cannot be overemphasized. A sharp osteotome allows one to make a sharp, accurate cut with consistent mallet strokes. A dull osteotome requires an unpredictable amount of force, thus decreasing control of the instrument. A set of osteotomes of varying thicknesses should be available for ridge-splitting procedures.

   7. Retractors. A lip retractor and a few right-angle retractors of various lengths should be available.

   8. Graft templates. Paired bone-graft templates are commercially available. They provide one set of horseshoe-shaped templates in several sizes to measure the intraoral

mandibular or maxillary defect. A matched sterile set is used to measure and shape the graft in situ at the donor site. These templates are very helpful in accurately shaping the graft.

9. Loop magnification can be invaluable when working in close spaces such as the posterior maxilla and sinus region and when working around vital structures such as the mandibular neurovascular structures. There are times when the relatively fragile oral mucosa is best closed with sutures smaller than the 3-0 or 4-0, which is more customarily used. Loops are helpful in placing the sutures and are essential in the atraumatic and complete removal of nonresorbable suture. A single suture left in place may compromise a complex graft procedure.

10. Bone cutters. Some type of sharp bone cutter with which the operator is familiar should be at hand. A standard rongeur used for removing alveolar bone spicules is not adequate. An instrument that can be used to cut bone into small, fine particles without completely crushing the bone is best.

11. Mini bone mill. Although not absolutely essential, a mini bone mill can be very helpful in converting solid bone into particulate graft. One has to be careful with a very small bone plug or chip because some bone will be lost in the mechanisms, and therefore very small bone pieces may be better cut into particles by hand.

12. Bone filter. Small, inline bone filters are available and can be used to filter bone chips from the suction tubing. This can be helpful when harvesting bone with a drill or can be used to recover bone from irrigation during implant procedures. The filters are disposable and the remainder of the system is autoclavable.

13. Bone stabilizing clamps. Bone clamps to stabilize a large graft for total maxillary or mandibular reconstruction are commercially available. They can be invaluable in temporarily stabilizing the graft while placing the first few implants or bone screws. An assortment of smaller clamps should also be available for smaller grafts or for added stability of larger grafts. These are also commercially available but can be easily made by bending and modifying available instruments such as Allis clamps.

F. Barrier membranes have been developed to allow guide tissue regeneration. They allow bone regeneration by the principle of osteopromotion. This is the principle of creating secluded space protection with a barrier membrane, which allows only bone-forming cells to populate the space, to the exclusion of competing, more rapidly migrating connective tissue-forming cells. Expanded polytetrafluoroethylene (e-PTFE) is the more widely used membrane material. The material is chemically and biologically inert. Because membranes are nonresorbable, they must be removed during a subsequent procedure. Resorbable membranes are also commercially available; however, the nonresorbable e-PTFE (Gore-Tex, W.L. Gore, Flagstaff, AZ) remains the most widely used membrane.

It is essential that the space under the membrane is maintained and that the membrane does not collapse. If this happens, the volume of bone regenerated may not be adequate. Membranes are available in several sizes of oval and rectangular shapes for bone graft reconstruction. They are also available with titanium reinforcement trips to help prevent membrane collapse. Small defects may be treated with a membrane alone, without a bone graft or bone substitute. Miniscrews may be used to "tent" the membrane and to secure the membrane in place. For larger defects, bone chips or bone substitutes are used to maintain the space under the membrane and to provide a scaffold for bone formation. Very large defects should be treated with autogenous bone. Barrier membranes may be used simultaneously with implants, when indicated, or used to develop sites for future implant placement. Clinical experience and judgment are essential in determining when to place implants and bone grafts and/or membranes simultaneously.

The following are some of the important factors in the successful use of non-resorbable barrier membranes.

1. The site should be clean and free of infection.
2. The membrane should be carefully trimmed and contoured to precisely cover the defect or graft extending a few millimeters beyond the defect margin.
3. There should be no sharp edges on the membrane.
4. The membrane should be trimmed so as not to contact adjacent teeth.
5. Whenever possible, the membrane should be rigidly fixed with mini bone screws to prevent postoperative mobility. If an implant is placed simultaneously, a hole can be punched in the membrane and a cover screw used to give additional stability. Mobility is most likely a significant factor leading to infection or early membrane exposure, or both.
6. Flap closure, as in the case of bone grafts, is one of the most important aspects of the procedure. The flap must be closed, tension free with mattress sutures. Nonresorbable sutures are strongly recommended.
7. Whenever possible, the membrane should be left in place until re-entry for implant placement or an implant second-stage procedure.
8. If the membrane becomes exposed after 6–8 wk, it should be removed. If the exposure occurs before 6–8

wk, the site should be irrigated several times a day with chlorhexidine and the membrane removed after 8 wk.

G. Specific osseous defects. The following are specific examples of some of the many osseous defects that may require bone graft site preparation for immediate or delayed implant placement. Implants must be placed with far more precision than they did just a few years ago. The aesthetic and functional expectations are extremely high today. As a result, a high degree of precision placement is performed in aesthetic areas. Enhanced precision is resulting in increased numbers of implant procedures in the more functionally important posterior regions. There is often inadequate residual bone available for implant support, and when this is the case, site preparation with bone grafts is needed. This discussion is limited to use in autogenous bone, the gold standard for reconstruction. The issue of immediate versus delayed implant placement in graft sites is not specifically addressed formally because this often depends on the surgeon's experience and the degree of placement precision required for a specific site. There is, however, one absolute rule—there must be adequate residual bone to stabilize the implant. If the implant is stabilized primarily by the graft, the implant success rate is unfavorable. If there is any question about placement timing, it is probably best to wait until the graft has healed.

1. Extraction sites and small alveolar defects. Extractions that are to have implants may have them placed immediately if the socket is intact, or the sites may be developed for future implant placement. In cases in which one or two teeth are removed and the adjacent teeth are healthy with good bone and soft-tissue height, the implant should be placed or the site grafted immediately. If the socket heals normally, there is a risk that the normal resorption of the thin bone walls will cause a loss of height that will make it more difficult to get the proper ridge height and emergence profile for the prosthesis relative to the adjacent normal teeth. The options are to:

a. Place the implant immediately. If there is a crestal void between the socket and implant, a barrier membrane alone or with a graft or bone substitute should be placed. The implant should extend several millimeters beyond the tooth apex; this may provide adequate bone to fill any voids. If there is a fenestration defect, a titanium-reinforced membrane or bone filler should be used to prevent membrane collapse over the implant threads. Primary closure of the mucosa will likely require flap elevation with releasing incisions into the sulcus, with a periosteal releasing incision to allow the flap to advance palatally over the socket.

b. If implant placement is delayed, the socket may be covered with a membrane only or a membrane with bone or bone substitute. If a membrane alone is used, it may be wise to use a titanium-reinforced membrane to prevent collapse into the socket. If there is a fenestration or other osseous defect, a bone graft or bone substitute should be used to maintain the space and prevent membrane collapse. The site should be ready for implant placement in 6–8 mo.

Small alveolar defects in areas that are particularly aesthetic should be carefully assessed for bone graft site development. Many of these areas should be grafted and the implants placed after the graft has fully healed. If the ridge is of adequate height and wide enough that the buccal and lingual or palatal bone plates can be separated with a thin osteotome, the ridge may be split and the space between the bone plates grafted. When the ridge is very narrow and cannot be split, a small graft is harvested from an intraoral site such as the chin or external oblique ridge and contoured to fit the defect. If increased height is also required, the graft is contoured to an inverted L shape with the foot of the L extending over the ridge. The underlying and adjacent bone, particularly in the mandible, is perforated with a small, round bur, which allows for bleeding from the marrow space. Whenever possible, at least two mini screws are placed at angles divergent to each other to secure the graft. The screws should be placed as lag screws to ensure compression of the site. A barrier membrane is placed and secured with miniscrews. The site is reopened and the implant placed after complete healing.

2. Knife-edge ridges. Whenever the knife-edge ridge, particularly in the maxilla, is wide enough for the two bone plates to be separated with a special osteotomy described below, the ridge should be split and the space between the two bone plates grafted. If possible, the elevation of the periosteum from the bone should be minimized. If the bony base above or below the narrow ridge is wide enough and of adequate bone density to stabilize the implants, the implants may be placed simultaneously depending on the degree of placement precision needed.

a. Procedure. The ridge should be wide enough to place a few holes in the ridge crest with a 2.0-mm round bur. A very thin osteotome in thickness (millimeter) is used to make the initial incision between the bone plates with gentle mallet strokes. The depth of the cut should be increased evenly along the entire defect to prevent a fracture. The cut should extend to the depth in the base, where width is adequate for the implant. Osteotomes of increasing thickness are then used to sequentially increase the width between the plates to the width necessary for the implant to be used. If implants are to be placed immediately, the implant sites are prepared in the usual manner. Bone chips or wooden or metal wedges may be used to keep the bone plates apart. The bone at the base must be of sufficient depth and density to stabilize the implants. Once the implants have been placed, the wedges are removed, the defect between the implants is filled with bone, and a membrane is placed and secured. The implants should not be countersunk. If implants are not placed, the site is grafted by placing a few solid bone wedges or struts to prevent inward collapse of the bony walls. The space between the struts is filled with a particulate bone graft and a barrier membrane is placed.

When a ridge is too narrow or too dense, as in the mandible, it is best to maintain a narrow ridge graft, if possible, rather than resecting ridge. (Reconstructing a true vertical loss is difficult.) Whether the defect is large or small, thin veneer grafts rigidly fixed with miniscrews and covered with a barrier membrane give excellent results.

3. Anterior maxillary vertical defects are often the result of a full maxillary denture being traumatically occluded by retained mandibular anterior teeth. There is usually a step between the anterior and posterior ridge height, although the posterior ridge below the maxillary sinus is usually not thick enough for implants. There is often a "flabby" soft-tissue anterior ridge with connective tissue filling the space created when the alveolar bone is resorbed. This tissue is carefully "filleted" open to provide coverage for a bone graft and should never be resected. These defects are best reconstructed with an onlay graft buttressed against the step at the posterior ridges.

    a. Procedure. The incision is placed well into the lip side of the sulcus. The flap extends through the full thickness of mucosa. The mucosa is dissected toward the alveolar ridge 4–5 mm. The blade is then used to make an incision that extends to the alveolar ridge. This incision should be thick enough to be closed in two layers. A periosteal elevator is then used to lift the "flabby" ridge mucosa from the alveolar base, with this dissection extending past the ridge into the palate. The blade is now used to make an incision. The flabby mucosa from the periosteal side extends to within approximately 2–3 mm of the crest. Dissecting scissors and a surgical blade may be used to carefully remove the submucosal connective tissue from the underside of this flabby tissue, creating space for the bone graft without perforating the mucosa. A bone graft is then harvested and contoured to fit the defect precisely, with the graft buttressed against the step at the posterior region. The graft is rigidly fixed with bone screws. Implants may be placed simultaneously, but only if there is adequate basal bone for implant stability and if the implants can be placed with the precision required of the planned prosthesis. Soft tissues are carefully closed in two layers using resorbable 4-0 or 5-0 suture for the submucosal layer and 4-5 nonresorbable suture for the mucosa.

4. Posterior maxillary defects are often the result of alveolar resorption and inferior impingement by the maxillary sinus. Although a knife-edge ridge is much less common in the anterior region, there is often an associated loss of transverse dimension owing to the circumferential loss associated with maxillary atrophy. Onlay grafts can be done if adequate freeway space is available. The amount of height increase possible by onlay grafting may also be limited by the amount of soft tissue available for a tension-free closure. As a result, the sinus floor augmentation procedure is a commonly used procedure. This may be combined with grafting to increase alveolar width.

a. Procedure. The incision can be placed in the sulcus; however, a crestal incision may be preferable because it gives excellent access, is easier to elevate, has excellent hemostasis, and is not directly over the graft site. If a lateral ridge graft is placed, it may be safer to place the incision on the cheek side of the sulcus. The alveolar ridge and lateral wall of the maxillary sinus are exposed. A small, handheld light on a flexible stem can be placed in the nose with the room lights off to identify the anterior and inferior sinus margins. This can be helpful for the optimal placement of the bone cuts for the lateral window. A 2.5-3.0-mm round diamond bur is used to outline the dimension of the bone window over the sinus. If the bony wall is thick, a regular round bur is used to remove bone to within 1-2 mm of the sinus lining. The inferior bone cut is 2-3 mm above the sinus floor, and the anterior vertical cut is made at the anterior sinus margin. The cuts are completed with the diamond bur because it will not cut the sinus membrane as easily as a regular bur and will not catch the lip of the bone window, which can pull the bur into the membrane further, but diamond burs are easier to control, thus reducing the risk of membrane perforation. The membrane is then elevated with special instruments designed for this purpose. Freer periosteal elevators of various sizes can also be modified for this purpose. The membrane elevation starts with the sinus floor and is then extended anteriorly, medially, and posteriorly. The bone window is elevated with membrane attached and becomes the new sinus floor. Retraction can be difficult but can sometime be facilitated by using a 10-ml syringe with a 25-gauge needle passed through the membrane, using the syringe to evaluate air from the sinus. This creates a vacuum effect, which elevates the lining and bone window. A particulate bone graft is then densely compacted and used to graft the sinus floor to the desired height. If there is 4–5 mm of residual bone thickness, implants may be placed simultaneously. However, if there is any question about bone quality or implant position, it is best to wait until the graft has healed. Placement of bone block with immediate implant placement has been recommended; however, considering the normal pattern of resorption of bone grafts in the ideal environment, one would expect unpredictable bone resorption in a graft that is difficult to fill to the sinus floor and wall contours and that is unprotected at the superior surface (the sinus membrane provides little vascular supply for revascularization). The most predictable procedure is to place a densely packed particulate-cell-rich autogenous graft with a barrier membrane with implants placed after the graft heals. This provides a graft and an environment conducive to rapid vascularization of the graft. If the ridge requires widening, this can be done by placing a veneer graft simultaneously. Mucosal closure should be in two layers with nonresorbable suture to close the mucosa.

5. Severe resorption of the total maxilla. The severely atrophic maxilla presents a number of problems that make osseous and implant reconstruction particularly challenging.
   a. There is bone loss in all dimensions.
   b. Severe resorption often affects the relationship of the maxilla to the mandible creating a relative mandibular prognathism. Surgical correction may be indicated to achieve appropriate implant functional placement.
   c. Atrophy after tooth loss is often followed by significant anatomic changes in the relationship to adjacent structures, specifically the maxillary sinuses, the nasal floor, and the zygomaticomaxillary buttress.
   d. The bone quality of the maxilla is normally less dense than that of the mandible. When the maxilla becomes atrophic, it is often even more spongy, with thin cortical places, further complicating reconstruction.

III. The following are three procedures that can be used for total reconstruction of the atrophic maxilla. This does not represent all possible procedures, but is a representative example of procedures that address most of the potential reconstructive problems.

A. The onlay bone graft procedure is best utilized when there is adequate freeway space to accommodate the increased height and the anteroposterior (A-P) discrepancy is not excessive. If there is not adequate freeway space, the patient may not have enough space for the prosthesis. This procedure is also especially good for those patients with extensive anterior atrophy where the posterior ridge is more normal in height. The disadvantage of the procedure is that the patient must leave his or her denture out for a few weeks to a few months. There is also the potential for problems with the incision because of its extent.

1. Procedure. The procedure is done in the operating room under general anesthesia. Virtually every step of this procedure is or can be critical to success. The position of the incision is critical to successful tension free mucosal closure. The incision really cannot be made too far laterally for all practical purposes. It is placed well into the lip and cheek side of the buccal vestibule. It is a circumvestibular incision extending posteriorly to at least the zygomaticomaxillary buttress. The incision should be stepped and thick enough to be closed in two layers. The mucosal incision extends through the mucosa, then extends submucosally toward the ridge approximately 5 mm or more. The surgical blade is then used to make the step incision, which then extends to the alveolar ridge. The periosteal elevator is used to completely expose the alveolar ridge and to raise the palatal side of the graft. The incisive nerve can be resected and the foramen packed with bone chips, allowing anterior implant placement if needed.

The alveolar ridge is now prepared for graft placement by removing small, sharp spicules and irregularities. It is especially important that any retained connective tissue remnant, such as that in the tooth socket or old periapical defect, be completely removed. The sinus floor can be grafted simultaneously if the ridge is thin enough. This site should also be prepared before the bone harvest so that the amount of bone needed can be determined. A template of the exposed maxilla is utilized in harvesting and shaping the graft. Matched sets of templates are commercially available; one template is matched to the ridge, and the matching template is used at the donor site. The graft is harvested from the ilium, although cranial grafts have been used. The graft is contoured to fit as precisely as possible to the ridge. It is secured with multiple bone screws if the implants are to be delayed. If the residual ridge is of adequate thickness and density, implants can be placed simultaneously. This decision may also depend on the planned prosthesis. If the prosthesis is to be fixed/removable, such as in a spart erosion design, immediate placement can be used because the position of each individual implant is not critical. If, however, a conventional fixed bridge is planned, it is best to delay implant placement until the graft has healed, and a template is used to place the implants in the optimal position as determined by the prosthesis.

After the graft has been rigidly fixed in position, it is further contoured with a large round bur to remove excessive contour or bulk to facilitate soft-tissue closure. The sinus graft is placed if needed. Barrier membrane can be carefully placed to protect the lateral surface of the graft. The incision is carefully closed in layers using 4-0 or 5-0 Vicryl or other resorbable suture to close the submucosal layer, and 3-0 and 4-0 nonresorbable suture to close the mucosa. Vertical mattress sutures are placed

B. Le Forte I osteotomy with interpositional bone graft. Combining a total maxillary osteotomy with an interpositional bone graft should be considered when:
   1. There is severe total atrophy.
   2. There is a significant increase in freeway space.
   3. There is a significant A-P discrepancy.
   4. There is a significant decrease in the transverse discrepancy.
   5. There is loss of facial vertical dimension.
   6. It is important that the temporary prosthesis be placed immediately after surgery.

When there are significant discrepancies in the relationship of the maxilla to the mandible, it is important to correct or improve the relationship if possible. A severely resorbed maxilla with an increased freeway space, an A-P discrepancy, and a decreased transverse dimension whose position to the mandible is not corrected before implants are placed, creates a situation in which there is an unfavorable crown-root ratio, a significant anterior cantilever effect, and transverse bilateral crossbite. The specific advantages of the procedure are:
   1. The maxillary vertical dimension, A-P discrepancy, and transverse dimension can be corrected simultaneously with the graft.
   2. Implants can, under many circumstances, be placed during the same procedure.
   3. The patient can wear a properly fitting denture immediately or within the first 2-3 wk after surgery.

Procedure. The standard approach for a Le Forte I osteotomy is used to expose the maxilla. The horizontal bone cut from the pterygomaxillary fissure to the lateral nasal rim is made with a reciprocating saw and is placed a few millimeters above the sinus floor. Osteotomes are used to separate the maxilla from the pterygoid plate and the lateral-nasal walls. Unlike the Le Forte I procedure in the dentate patient, the maxilla cannot be "downfractured." All of the bone cuts must be completed so that the maxilla can be mobilized with digital pressure to prevent a transverse palatal fracture. The sinus mucosa is completely removed from the sinus floor. A horseshoe-shaped graft is harvested and contoured to fit the nasal and sinus floors. Any voids between the graft and sinus and nasal floors are packed with bone chips. A bone clamp is used to stabilize the graft to the maxilla. Bone screws or implants are used to stabilize the graft to the maxilla. The bone graft–maxillary complex is repositioned and rigidly fixed with bone plates and screws and/or wire fixation. Maxillary and mandibular dentures or splints are used to establish the A-P position, and the vertical dimension is best established utilizing an extra-oral reference point such as a small bone screw at the nasal processor forehead. The mucosa is closed in two layers using 4-0 Vicryl or other resorbable suture for the submucosal layer and 4-0 nylon or other nonresorbable suture for the mucosa. Sutures should be removed with loop magnification. The patient's denture can be placed approximately 1–2 wk postoperatively depending on the level of swelling. The denture should be carefully relieved over the alveolar ridge and flange area. The area directly over the alveolar ridge and implants only is relieved with a soft liner. The entire palate is intentionally not lined with a soft material to ensure that most of the denture is displaced here and not on the alveolar ridge.

If implants are placed with the graft, they are exposed 6–8 mo later. If implants are not placed with the graft, they are placed 6–8 mo afterward. If a fixed/removable, spart erosion type prosthesis is planned, placing fixtures at the time of the graft may be an excellent idea. However, if a precision conventional fixed prosthesis is planned, it may be best to delay implant placement until the graft has healed and to place implants with a prosthetically derived template for precision placement.

C. Combination sinus floor graft and anterior onlay graft. Patients with retained lower anterior teeth may present extensive anterior vertical bone loss often extending superiorly to the level of the anterior nasal spine and nasal floor, combined with inferior displacement of the maxillary sinus and alveolar ridge. They usually have a flabby anterior soft-tissue ridge at the same level as the posterior osseous ridge, but with a significant alveolar bone step between the anterior and posterior osseous ridges.

    1. Procedure. This type of atrophic ridge is best corrected by placing an onlay graft in the anterior region extending posteriorly to the osseous step. The technique has been described earlier in this chapter. This restores the anterior alveolar ridge to the level of the posterior ridge. The posterior regions are augmented with bilateral sinus membrane elevation and particulate bone graft. The patient's denture can usually be placed relatively soon after surgery. Because the sinus graft is particulate, the implants are usually delayed and placed after the graft has healed.

IV. Severe total mandibular resorption

    A. Despite very extensive resorption, the mandible can usually be treated without bone grafting for implant reconstruction. There are, however, cases in which a bone graft is indicated. These are cases in which:

        1. The level of resorption is so extensive that the mandible is at risk of fracture from the increased biting efficiency after reconstruction.

        2. The extent of resorption is such that the mandible is at risk of fracture from the implants themselves.

        3. The atrophy is such that there simply is not enough bone for the implants.

        4. There are contour differences or differences in size from trauma, tumor surgery, infection, etc., that make prosthetic reconstruction difficult without correction.

        5. The extent of atrophy is such that the crown-root ratio compromises function, aesthetics, and long-term implant success.

    B. Procedures

        1. Onlay grafts. The most commonly used procedure for total mandibular reconstruction in the onlay graft is the most direct approach to the problem. The principal potential problem is soft-tissue closure.

           As the procedure is usually done transorally, the incision is placed well into the lip and cheek side of the buccal sulcus. The flap should be thick enough to be closed in two layers. Care must be taken not to cut the mental nerves, as they are very superficial in these cases with the mental foramen being at or near the crest of the ridge. A template is used to harvest and contour an iliac graft to fit the alveolar ridge precisely. If implants are to be used, they are placed anteriorly to the point of exit of the mental nerves and must engage the residual mandible for stabilization. The implant sites in the graft are not countersunk because the graft cortex is not thick enough. If the posterior residual mandible is thick enough for the implants, the inferior alveolar neurovascular bundle can be removed from the canal posteriorly to allow more posterior implant placement. Otherwise, a posterior implant can be placed in the graft above the canal after healing. If implants are not placed immediately, conventional bone screws are used to rigidly fix the graft and implants are placed 6–8 mo later.

2. Interpositional bone graft procedures are excellent procedures because, in effect, they provide an autogenous bone tray with a vascular pedicle. This allows placement of an autogenous graft that can be rigidly fixed between two vascularized bone flaps. The two procedures most likely to be used are the anterior horizontal osteotomy of the mandible and the visor osteotomy, which is described earlier in this chapter. The horizontal osteotomy is performed by making a critical bone cut anterior to the mental foramen or removing the neurovascular bundle to allow a more posterior vertical cut. These cuts extend to the mid-body and are connected with a mid-body horizontal cut. The superior bony segment is elevated to the desired height, and a graft is placed between the bony segment. Either implants or bone screws are placed through the superior bony segment extending through the graft into the inferior bony segment.

With the visor osteotomy, implants are placed after healing is complete. A particulate bone graft is placed in a pocket created between the lateral surface of the lingual bone plate, the superior border of the labial bone segment, and the buccal mucosal flap. The osteotomy can be modified to have a horizontal anterior component. An interpositional graft could be placed for immediate or delayed implant placement.

Maxillomandibular discrepancies

I. Severely compromised denture function may be experienced by a patient with significant maxillomandibular disharmonies. Compromised denture stability presents functional as well as aesthetic problems and contributes to accelerated alveolar bone loss.

II. When severe discrepancies compromise denture function, an orthognathic surgical procedure should be considered. A complete clinical evaluation and diagnostic survey are as essential as they would be for the dentulous patient considering orthognathic surgery. A complete physical examination, radiographic examination, and analysis of mounted diagnostic casts are essential in developing a successful treatment plan. In addition, close collaboration with the prosthodontist treating the case is essential.

III. Developmental discrepancies may be accentuated by the normal resorption patterns of the alveolar ridges. A patient who did not have discrepancies with the natural dentition may exhibit relative discrepancies caused by the pattern of ridge resorption. The surgeon and prosthodontist should be aware of differences in maxillary and mandibular resorptive tendencies.

    A. Maxillary resorption reduces the circumference of the maxilla because most of the bone loss is on the buccofacial aspect.

    B. The mandible loses bone primarily from the lingual aspect, with most of its vertical loss occurring in the posterior region.

    C. These patterns, together with overclosure from vertical bone loss, accentuate prognathic tendencies.

IV. When orthognathic surgical procedures are performed, stabilization of the osteotomized unit presents significant problems that must be considered in developing a treatment plan for the edentulous patient.

    A. Surgical splints secured to the mandible and maxilla are necessary for stability. The exact postsurgical positions must be established by use of mounted casts. When the new maxillomandibular position is determined, splints or dentures are constructed on the casts and interlocked in this position. The splints are secured to the mandible and maxilla and, when locked together, will secure the osteotomized units to the desired position.

    B. Lag screw and rigid internal fixation devices may also be useful.

Dental implants

  I. There has long been a search in the dental profession for a successful implant to stabilize or totally support tooth replacement prosthetics. Endosteal, subperiosteal, and transosteal implants are presently the principal types in clinical use.

    A. Endosteal implants have been used since the 1950s with success rates less than 50% until the introduction of the osseointegrated implant. This is the most widely used implant at this time and one of the three or four most important advances in oral and maxillofacial surgery.

    B. Subperiosteal implants are still used by some practitioners; however, the results remain less predictable than with osseointegrated or transosteal implants. This implant procedure is not discussed in detail, except to say that it is a two-step surgical procedure. The first step requires complete exposure of the atrophic mandible intraorally to take a precise bone impression. A model of the bone is used for fabrication of a precision-fitting bone framework with four transmucosal pins, which is then placed during a second open surgical procedure. A precision bone fit of the framework is essential to its success, and if the fit is not accurate, a new impression must be taken for a new framework. A computer-generated CAD/CAM alveolar bone model can be generated from a 3-D CT scan, thereby eliminating the first surgical step. This implant will not be discussed further in this chapter.

C. There are two transosteal implants currently in use—the fixed mandibular bone plate developed by Dr. Small, and the transmandibular implant developed by Dr. Bosker. Both are placed during a single surgical procedure and may be used for either fixed or removable prostheses, although both are most commonly used with a removable or fixed/removable prosthesis.

II. Osseointegrated implants

A. The concept of osseointegration is the basis for modern endosteal implants and has, in fact, been extrapolated to a greater or lesser extent to explain the biology and biotechnology of most other implant systems. The term *osseointegration* was introduced and scientifically and clinically defined by Professor P.I. Branemark of the Laboratory of Experimental Biology at Gothenburg University, Gothenburg, Sweden, in the 1960s. The Branemark implant was introduced in North America in 1980. Branemark described osseointegration as direct contact between living haversian bone and implant without any intervening fibrous tissue layers. The implants developed by Branemark are made of commercially pure titanium. This system was the first endosteal implant to be scientifically controlled in its development and in its clinical studies, with long-term follow-up to substantiate its long-term efficacy for clinical use. Before 1980, the generally accepted definition of implant success was that issued in 1978 by the Harvard Consensus Conference. Its definition of success was that "The dental implant provide functional service for five years in 75 percent of the cases." The principal problems with earlier implants were that the materials, principles, and techniques of placement did not provide a combination of biocompatibility and preservation of tissue (bone and soft tissue) viability to allow a consistent soft-tissue–free implant to bone interface.

B. The first clinical trials began in Sweden in 1965, and by 1983, 3510 osseointegrated fixtures had been placed. In 1980, the procedure was introduced in North America. The system was initially recommended for full arch reconstruction, with particular emphasis on the mandible. After success was established and documented for this indication, studies were then undertaken to establish the long-term safety and efficacy for partial jaw reconstruction and, later, for single tooth replacement.

The implant fixture is a precision manufactured screw milled from 99.75% pure titanium. The standard outer diameter is 3.75 mm and is available in lengths of 7, 8.5, 10, 13, 15, 18, and 20 mm. Fixtures are also available in 4 mm and 5 mm diameters to be used for better stability and biocortical stabilization in sites with porous bone. The standard fixtures are placed after the site has been threaded with a tap. Self-tapping fixtures are also available.

C. The procedure is well defined and designed for careful, precise preparation of the implant site to minimize bone trauma. Experimental studies in Sweden demonstrated that temperatures above 47°C at the drill–bone interface causes bone cell necrosis, the healing of which results in connective tissue at the implant–bone interface. For this reason, the drills used are special spiral drills of increasing diameter, run at a speed of approximately 1500 rpm. The tap used to tread the fixture site and the drill used to place the fixture are run at 10 to 15 rpm to reduce surgical trauma.

After implant fixture placement, the bone and fixture must be left in an unloaded state in which healing can occur, allowing bone to heal directly to the titanium fixture. The healing period for the fixture is approximately 3–6 mo in the mandible and maxilla, at which time the fixtures are uncovered and prepared for progressive loading, leading to full masticatory function. The following is a brief summary only of the procedure for full arch reconstruction.

The specific procedure for fixture placement is the same for the mandible and maxilla. A horizontal mucoperiosteal incision is made on the labial aspect of the alveolar ridge and a mucoperiosteal flap is raised to expose the bony alveolar ridge. Normally six or more fixtures are placed in the mandible between the mental foramen, and four to six can be placed in the maxilla anterior to the maxillary sinuses. Small contour irregularities or knife-edged ridges are leveled with ronquers.

The site preparation begins in the midline with the first two fixtures placed approximately 4 mm on either side of the midline. Fixtures are generally not placed directly in the midline, and they are usually approximately 7 mm apart, as the bone height, volume, and contour allow. The site is started with a 2-mm round but to define the position on the alveolar ridge. A 2-mm spiral drill is used to define the direction and depth of the fixture site as determined from preoperative tomograms or CT scans. A 3-mm pilot drill is used to increase the size of the site, and a 3-mm spiral drill is used to increase the site to 3 mm in diameter over the entire desired depth. All of the drilling procedures are done with copious irrigation to minimize surgical trauma from elevated temperatures. A special countersink drill is used to widen the opening of the site, and a drill tap of the appropriate length is used to prepare the thread in the site. When this is completed, a fixture of the appropriate length is placed, a cover screw inserted, and the mucosa closed with 3–0 or 4–0 vertical mattress sutures.

Three to six months after fixture placement, the mucosa is opened and abutment cylinders placed in preparation for prosthetic reconstruction.

III. Transosteal implants. There are two types of transosteal implants currently in use: the fixed mandibular staple bone plate and the transmandibular implant.

A. Fixed mandibular bone plate

1. The fixed mandibular staple bone plate is the present day evolution of the mandibular staple bone plate conceived by Small in 1964. Two years of laboratory research on dogs was followed by a 5-year clerical trial from 1968–1974. The original three-pin model was soon revised and manufactured in three configurations: the five-pin, seven-pin, and modified seven-pin. The five-pin was the most frequently used model and one of the models used until recently, when the design was changed to provide more stability and more resistance to vertical loading by the addition of two self-tapping compression screws. The implant is still made of corrosion-resistant titanium, aluminum, and vanadium alloy. There are now two-pin configurations available. The three-pin configuration is a five-pin implant that has four transosteal pins and may be utilized to stabilize various types of removable prostheses. It can also be used to support a fixed mandibular prosthesis. Both configurations are stabilized by a 9-mm central stabilizing pin and two compressions of varying lengths, depending on the thickness of the mandible.

2. The previous generation implant was designed as a stabilizing device that resisted lateral displacing forces. The prosthesis was entirely soft tissue supported with placing vertical loading forces on the implant. The additional stability provided by the compression screw allows the implant to resist displacement from vertical loading and, as stated above, the implant with four transosteal pins can be used to support a fixed removable or a fixed prosthesis.

3. Preoperative preparation, indications, and contraindications remain essentially unchanged, except for the fact that in some cases in which space between the mental foramen permits, one may choose the four transosteal pins and treatment plan for a fixed prosthesis. Preparation includes a careful assessment of the mandibular hard and soft tissues. Requirements for use of the implant included at least 10 mm of bone height in symphyseal region. If the patient does not have adequate residual bone height, the mandible may be augmented with bone of hydroxyapatite. Discontinuity or other osseous defects are best corrected before implant placement. Bone grafting procedures should be done at least 6–9 mo before implant placement; hydroxyapatite augmentation may be done 6–8 wk before the implant. Other bone defects or problems (bone spurs, ridges, etc.) are corrected, and re-

tained tooth roots and other foreign bodies are removed properly.

4. The patient should be in generally good health and be able to undergo general anesthesia of at least 2 hr duration. The soft tissues are assessed to determine whether adequate attached mucosa exists in the areas where the transoral pin will penetrate the oral mucosa and to determine whether there is adequate available vestibule. If there is inadequate attached mucosa, a palatal mucosal or skin graft should be done before surgery to correct this problem. Redundant tissue problems or infections are also treated before surgery. Vestibuloplasty procedures, lowering of the floor of the mouth, or other revisions should be completed 6–8 wk before the implant surgery. Numerous surgeons have reported success performing the accessory procedure (e.g., vestibuloplasty and hydroxyapatite augmentation) simultaneously with the staple.

5. The operative technique used is that described by Small (1980) with modifications for the armamentarium used to place the implant. Under satisfactory nasotracheal general anesthesia, the submental region and oral cavity are prepared and draped in the standard fashion. Small believes that maintaining isolation of the surgical site from the oral cavity is extremely important to the success of the implant system; however, other authors have been less strict in this respect and have noted no adverse effects. Preoperative antibiotics are given routinely and continued for 7 da postoperatively. After a local anesthetic is administered with a vasoconstrictor, an incision approximately 4 cm long is made in a skin crease in the submental region following the curves of the mandibular symphysis. Dissection is carried down to the inferior border of the mandible. The periosteum is reflected, care being taken to clear all soft tissue from the exposed bone. Any irregularities in the bone surface may be smoothed with a bone bur for better adaptation on the staple base if necessary. The drilling guide assembly is placed with the anchoring jaws of the drill assembly on the alveolar ridge and the leveling plane on the inferior border. A special planing rotary osteotomy is provided with the placement implant kit, which is used with a Hall drill to level the inferior border of the mandible. The drilling chamber is the place with the leveling plane guide remaining in place.

6. The drill guide has seven holes and is used for the placement of both the two and four transosteal pin implants. To place the two transosteal pin implant, the intraoral anchoring jaws are placed in the most lateral positions of the intraoral assembly. A 2-mm twist drill is used to place

a hole 9 mm in depth in the middle hole of the drill chamber, which is the hole in the no. 4 position of the chamber, and a stabilizing pin is placed. The same drill is then used to drill the two transoral holes in the no. 2 and 6 positions of the chamber, and two stabilizing pins are placed. A 2-mm reduction guide is placed in the no. 3 and 5 hole positions, and a 2-mm twist drill is used to drill holes to a depth of 9 mm in the no. 3 and 5 positions. The reduction guide is removed and the 3-mm twist drill is used to widen the 2-mm hole to 3 mm in diameter, but only to a depth of approximately 1 mm to facilitate placement of the compression screws. All of the holes are drilled with copious amounts of irrigation to minimize heat-induced bone trauma. The drill assembly is removed and the staple implant placed with finger pressure; a seating instrument is provided and may be used with one or two taps from a small mallet to finish seating the implant to the inferior border. The two 9-mm self-tapping screws are then tightened to fix the implant in place. Longer screws are available for use in mandibles with more bone height. A special cutter is used to remove the excess intraoral pin height, leaving the remaining pin approximately 5 mm above the mucosa. Special ball attachments with a highly polished sleeve that extends to the bony crest are placed at the time of surgery or at a later time by the surgeon or prosthodontist. The attachments eliminate the contact between the implant threads and mucosa, thus eliminating this potential source of irritation and inflammation.

7. Complications should be relatively uncommon and minor in nature when they do occur. The most frequent problem with the previous generation implant was gingival hyperplasia and inflammation caused by frictional irritation of mobile mucosa against the pin threads. The new ball attachment has a polished sleeve that extends to the bony crest covering all exposed threads. This has greatly reduced the problem of gingival inflammation hyperplasia. When inflammation and hyperplasia do occur, they are treated by local excision and may, on occasion, require skin or mucosal grafting. Silver nitrate sticks may also be used, but electrocautery should not be used. Loosening or extrusion used to be an occasional problem when the implants were located occlusally, but should no longer be a problem with the addition of the compression screws in the new design. Poor placement of the implant probably represents the most significant potential problem.

B. The transmandibular implant was developed by Dr. Hans Bosker. The implant is fully functional and constructed of a gold alloy for biocompatibility. The implant is indicated for reconstruction of the severely atrophied mandible for removable or fixed prosthesis. The published success rates are consistently between 96% and 97%. The implant is particularly suitable for the severely atrophied mandible (bone height <10 mm) because the prosthesis is completely implant supported. The implant's design transmits masticatory forces to the mandible via the inferior border base plate. The implant developer has reported increased bone height in the mandibular saddle area in severely atrophic cases. Because the prosthesis is completely implant borne, patient satisfaction is consistently very good.

C. Surgical procedure

Unlike the mandibular staple type implant in which the base plate, transosteal pins, and stabilizing pins are one piece, the transmandibular implant is designed with the base plate and transosteal and stabilizing pins as separate components. A special instrument set with drill guides, drills, taps, etc., are required to place the implant.

A curvilinear incision over the submental region of the mandible is used to expose the inferior symphyseal area. The base plate is used to determine the length of the incision, and a template is used to remove irregularities of the inferior border. A drill guide is placed and used as a guide to drill three holes for cortical screws. A drill guide is locked in place with three cortical screws. Two additional holes for cortical screws are drilled. An adjustable drill guide is then placed and used to determine the direction of the holes for the threaded transosteal posts. These four holes are tapped, the drill guides removed, and threaded posts placed. The base plate is attached to the threaded posts with locking screws, and the cortical screws are then placed. The intraoral superstructure is placed and attached with screws to the transosteal pins, and impressions for the prosthesis are taken. The prosthesis is usually started 4–6 wk after surgery.

GENERAL REFERENCES

Baker RD, Connole PW: Preprosthetic augmentation grafting-autogenous bone, *J Oral Surg* 35:541, 1977.

Bosker H: *The Transmandibular Implant*. Dissertation submitted to fulfill the requirements for the degree of Doctor of Medicine, May 1986.

Bosker H, Van Dijk L: The transmandibular implant: a 12-year follow-up study, *J Oral Maxillofac Surg* 47:442–492, 1991.

Branemark P-I et al: Regeneration of bone marrow, a clinical experimental study following removal of bone marrow by curettage, *Acta Anat* 59:1–46, 1964.

Branemark P-I et al: Intra-osseus anchorage of dental prosthesis. I. Experimental studies, *Scand J Plast Reconstru Surg* 4:81–100, 1969.

Branemark P-I et al: Repair of defects in mandible, *Scand J Plast Reconstr Surg* 4:100–108, 1970.

Branemark P-I et al: Osseointegrated implants in the treatment of the edentulous jaw. Experience from a ten-year period, *Scand J Plast Reconstr Surg* (suppl 16) 1-132, 1977.

Eriksson RA, Albrektsson T, Albrektsson B: Heat caused by drilling bone. Temperature measured in vivo in patients and animals, *Acta Orthop Scand* 55:629-631, 1984.

Guernsey LH: Preprosthetic surgery. In Kruger GO, ed, *Textbook of oral and maxillofacial surgery*, ed 6, St. Louis, 1984, Mosby.

Helfrick J et al: Implants used in preprosthetic reconstructive surgery. In Fonseca RJ, Davis WH: *Reconstructive preprosthetic oral and maxillofacial surgery*. Philadelphia, 1986, WB Saunders.

Kent JN et al: Alveolar ridge augmentation using nonabsorbable hydroxylapatite with or without autogenous cancellous bone, *J Oral Maxillofac Surg* 41:629, 1983.

Keller EE, et al: Prosthetic reconstruction of the severely resorbed maxilla with iliac grafting and tissue-integrated prostheses, *Int J Oral Maxillofac Implants* 2:155-163, 1987.

MacIntosh RB, Obwegeser HL: Preprosthetic surgery: a scheme for its effective employment, *J Oral Surg* 25:397, 1967.

Power PP et al: The transmandibular implant: from progressive bone loss to controlled bone growth, *J Oral Maxillofac Surg* 49:904-910, 1994.

Sailer HF: A new method of inserting endosseous implants in totally atrophic maxillae, *J Craniomaxillofac Surg* 17:299-305, 1989.

Schnitman PA, Schulman LB: Recommendations of the consensus development conference on dental implants, *J Am Dent Assoc* 98:373, 1979.

Small IA: The mandibular staple bone plate for the atrophic mandible, *Dent Clin North Am* 24:565, 1980.

Small IA: The fixed mandibular implant: its uses in reconstructive prosthetics, *J Am Dent Assoc* 121 (3):369-374, 1990.

Tatum JR, H: Maxillary and sinus implant reconstruction, *Dent Clin North Am* 30:207, 1986.

Differential Diagnosis
of Orofacial Pain
and Headache

DAVID A. KEITH

Mouth, face, and head pains are common complaints, and the etiology can be readily determined in the majority of cases. However, in some instances, the complex anatomy, vague descriptions, equivocal physical findings, and emotional overlay make diagnosis difficult. At the present time, many pains in the face and head are attributed to the temporomandibular joint (TMJ) and the muscles of mastication. Because these problems receive much attention in the media, the diagnosis is readily accepted. It is incumbent on all practitioners to make a responsible effort to determine appropriate diagnoses on the basis of scientific principles. The key components of any differential diagnosis are a thorough knowledge of anatomy and a detailed history.

HISTORY OF COMPLAINTS

A protocol for the rigorous examination of the area is presented. It is imperative that a detailed history be obtained before the patient is examined or special tests or imaging studies are ordered, because in a majority of cases the diagnosis may be made from this information alone.

I. Chief complaint. It is important to obtain the patient's description of the pain in his or her own words, as this may provide a clue to its etiology. Primary neuralgias are frequently described as sharp and lancinating, vascular headaches as throbbing, and muscle pain as a continuous deep, dull ache. The patient may not be able to give all these descriptions at the first interview, and corroborating information from relatives and friends may be needed to build up a general picture of the pain as it affects the patient. Each pain complaint should be listed in order of severity.

II. Present complaint. The intensity of the pain needs to be measured against the patient's own experience of pain, need for medication, and effect on life-style. For example, does the pain interfere with work, sleep, or social activities? The origin of the pain should be determined by asking the patient to indicate the site of the pain or its maximal intensity. Its anatomic distribution should be accurately traced in terms of local anatomy.

The patient should be encouraged to remember the events surrounding the onset of the pain, even if it was several years ago. Any other instance of similar pain should be ascertained, even though the patient may not associate these with the present problem. The time relations of the pain should be clarified in terms of duration and frequency of attack, as well as possible remissions.

Aggravating factors should be determined. Is the pain aggravated by the ingestion of specific foods or beverages, by lying down, during times of stress, or by other identifiable factors? In other instances, determine any relieving factors; for example, heat and cold are important clues.

The effect of past treatment needs to be elucidated. Which medications helped? Has surgery altered the nature of the pain? Has endodontic treatment or extraction affected the pain? Finally, the presence or absence of associated factors (e.g., swelling, flushing, tearing, nasal congestion, facial weakness) needs to be ascertained.

III. Previous medical history. The patient's current health situation needs to be ascertained by recording previous diagnoses, recent illnesses, and the results of previous physical examinations. All relevant data should be recorded.

IV. Previous treatment. All medical and surgical treatments related to the chief complaint(s) should be described in detail and listed in chronological order, including the names of the health care professionals involved. The effect of these treatments and any complications should also be noted.

V. Review of systems. A complete review of each of the various body systems should be recorded. These may indicate abnormalities or diseases that are relevant to the chief complaint (e.g., sleep disorder, previous psychiatric history, joint mobility, headache disorders, generalized arthritis).

VI. Trauma history. The patient is specifically questioned regarding trauma to the mouth, face, or head area, including previous injuries, assaults, abuse, or accidents.

VII. Family history. A previous history of related problems should be recorded, including the result of prior treatments (e.g., migraine history, cancer of the mouth or face).

VIII. Psychosocial history. Evaluate and record the patient's emotional and mental status (e.g., angry, unresponsive, evasive, confused or disoriented, distressful, tearful, tangential speech). The patient's feeling regarding his or her chief complaint needs to be documented, as well as its influence on his or her job and home responsibilities. Record the number of sick days or days lost from school related to the problem and how it interferes with social and sporting activities. The influence of the pain problem on grades should also be noted. Inquire about the reaction of family, friends, and employer to the problem and note recent changes in stress, anxiety, or depression levels. Inquire as to whether the patient is seeing a therapist, counselor, or psychiatrist.

IX. Litigation or disability history. List whether any disability claims are pending or planned and establish if litigation is pending or planned and, if so, establish the details.

X. Medication history. Review the exact types and daily dosage of any medication the patient is taking.

XI. History of surgeries and hospitalizations. Be sure that a complete list is available.

XII. Physical examination. The physical examination begins as soon as contact is made with the patient. Expressions, movements, speech, emotion, reaction to questions, posture, general appearance, etc., are all important to this evaluation. Casual movements, actions, and reactions during general questioning and history taking may be more revealing than the findings from physical examination.

The purpose of the examination is to discover any possible anatomic or physiologic basis for the pain. It is therefore important to proceed in a stepwise and consistent fashion. Pain patients should have a complete head and neck examination, not an examination directed by a presumed diagnosis.

Headaches, cranial neuralgias, and facial pain have been classified by the International Headache Society. The specific descriptions and criteria for the evaluation of temporomandibular disorders have been refined by Okeson (1996). From a clinical point of view, pain in this region can conveniently be classified as shown in the box.

Pain caused by local disease

I. Pain secondary to local disease accounts for the greatest number of diagnoses encountered in clinical practice, and, by means of a detailed history and appropriate diagnostic tests, the etiology can be detected.

II. Pain arising from the teeth, jaws, and periodontal structures is usually diagnosed with a high degree of accuracy. A detailed discussion of the various types of dental pain is beyond the scope of this article. Temporomandibular disorders are discussed in a separate section at the end of this chapter. However, several conditions can give rise to confusion and should be considered.

III. Referred pain in the jaws is occasionally encountered. The patient may complain of pain in the mandible, and a maxillary tooth may be found to be the cause, or vice versa. The complaint of an earache from a diseased mandibular tooth is also a well-recognized pattern. Experimental stimulation of various areas in the nose and paranasal sinuses can refer pain to well-

Classification of Oral and Facial Pain

PAIN CAUSED BY LOCAL DISEASE
Teeth, jaws, and periodontal structures
TMJ and muscles of mastication
Salivary glands
Nose and paranasal sinuses
Blood vessels

PAIN FROM NERVE TRUNKS AND CENTRAL PATHWAYS
No abnormal neurologic signs (primary neuralgias)
Abnormal neurologic signs (atypical neuralgias,
posttraumatic neuralgias, secondary neuralgias)

PAIN FROM OUTSIDE THE FACE
(EYES, EARS, HEART, CERVICAL SPINE, ESOPHAGUS)

ATYPICAL FACIAL PAIN
Usually chronic and often associated with psychiatric
diagnoses
Nature of the pain may change over time and sometimes has
features consistent with myofascial, vascular, or neurogenic
pain.

defined regions of the mouth and face. A tooth that is cracked and not yet separated can pose a diagnostic challenge. In the initial stages, the pain may be stimulated by applying pressure to the appropriate cusp. In the later stages, visible separation of the tooth, periodontal signs, and radiographic findings confirm the diagnosis.

IV. On occasion, patients complain of pain in a particular tooth, and, although no diagnostic abnormality is noted, a filling is placed. The pain persists, and, although no specific pathology is noted, root canal treatment is undertaken. This may be followed by retreatment and often by an apicoectomy and subsequently extraction of the tooth. The pain may persist and the patient may continue to insist on further dental or surgical interventions, all of which fail to relieve the pain. This condition is called *atypical odontalgia or phantom tooth pain* and is considered to be a deafferentation neuralgia. In experimental animals, pulpectomy can lead to functional and morphologic changes in the central trigeminal system. How this situation creates chronic pain has yet to be determined, but trivial and often forgotten trauma to the dental apparatus can produce a chronic pain in some individuals. This pain may stay localized in one quadrant of the mouth, and the extensive interventions may lead to edentulous spaces in an otherwise healthy mouth. On other occasions, the pain moves from one quadrant to another, and the patient may be rendered almost entirely edentulous. A detailed history will reveal that the dental treatment was undertaken without a significant cause for the pain being determined and that, although the pain may have been relieved for a few days or weeks, it invariably returned. The appropriate evaluation would include full neurologic evaluation, including a magnetic resonance imaging scan to rule out pathology of the trigeminal system. Treatment with clonazepam, 0.5 to 2 mg at bedtime, sometimes supplemented with a tricyclic antidepressant, is appropriate. The patient should be cautioned not to undergo any further dental treatment unless specific local disease is demonstrated.

V. Although poorly recognized, pain of vascular origin can occur in the facial area.

   A. Giant cell arteritis, usually involving the temporal vessel, presents in patients over 60 years of age. There is dull persistent pain in the temple during chewing. The temporal artery is nonpulsatile, tortuous, and tender. The erythrocyte sedimentation rate will be elevated, and a biopsy will demonstrate giant cell arteritis. If this diagnosis is suspected, even before pathologic evidence is available, the patient should be referred to an ophthalmologist to rule out central retinal artery involvement, with the possibility of permanent blindness. Corticosteroids will ameliorate the condition.

   B. Cluster headaches are most often unilateral and occur in the ocular, frontal, and temporal regions, but may also start in the infraorbital region (i.e., maxilla). These headaches predominantly affect men and usually start when the patient is between 18 and 40 years of age. Bouts may last 4–8 wk, with one to three attacks every 24 hr, with a maximum of eight attacks. The patient describes the pain as excruciating and as a constant stabbing, burning, and throbbing. Pain-free intervals lasting several months separate the bouts. Associated features include ipsilateral ptosis and myosis, tearing, rhinorrhea, and nasal congestion. Treatment is with ergot preparations, prednisone, methysergide, or calcium channel blocking agents.

   C. Chronic cluster headaches are similar to cluster headaches but occur less commonly. The diagnosis requires at least two or more attacks per week over a period of more than a year. Treatment can be the same for cluster headaches, but lithium carbonate tends to work better for chronic clusters.

   D. Chronic paroxysmal hemicrania involves the ocular, frontal, and temporal regions and occasionally the occipital, infraaural, mastoid, and nuchal areas, invariably on the same side. It occurs predominantly in females, and patients have attacks every day. Characteristically, the attacks fluctuate in frequency and severity. They may last from 5–45 min and at their maximum are excruciating. Ipsilateral conjunctival injection, lacrimination, nasal stuffiness, and rhinorrhea are seen in most patients. Attacks occur at regular intervals throughout the day and night, and the patient may be awakened by a nocturnal attack. Indomethacin provides relief.

When these vascular phenomena start in the infraorbital region, diagnostic confusion can result. In a study of patients attending a chronic facial pain group, 14% presented with pain of vascular origin. Half of those patients had vascular pain alone, and the other half had vascular pain associated with a psychiatric disorder, myofascial pain, or some other diagnosis. In these patients, the pain started in the maxilla or the maxillary teeth and involved the eye and the supraorbital and lateral orbital regions.

Primary neuralgias

I. Primary trigeminal neuralgia is a well-defined condition in which the patient experiences severe, lancinating pain when a trigger zone in the anatomic distribution of the trigeminal nerve is stimulated. Typically, the trigger zones are in the area of nasolabial fold or the upper and lower lip and may be stimulated by washing, shaving, talking, or any slight movement of the area. There is no sensory loss, and the pain lasts only for a matter of seconds. Between attacks, the patient is pain free. Because of the intense nature of the pain, the untreated patient will be extremely fearful of stimulating the area and may be unwilling to move or touch the mouth and face. Typically, remissions for months or years are anticipated. Although this description is classic, patients may have had various treatments in the past, which may have altered their pain and sensory examination. The appropriate evaluation will include a thorough neurologic examination and magnetic resonance imaging to rule out any mass impinging on the trigeminal system. It should also be pointed out that patients with multiple sclerosis may have similar neurologic pain in the face, and space-occupying lesions in the cerebellopontine angle may mimic a trigeminal neuralgia.

II. A similar condition, glossopharyngeal neuralgia, has the same characteristics, except that the trigger zone is in the tonsillar area, lateral pharyngeal wall, or base of the tongue. This condition should not be confused with Eagle's syndrome, in which an elongated styloid process is said to impinge on the soft tissues of the throat, or with Trotter's syndrome, in which a tumor of the nasopharynx gives rise to pain in the lower jaw, tongue, and side of the head. In these cases, deafness secondary to obstruction of the eustachian tube and asymmetric mobility of the soft palate secondary to tumor invasion of the levator palati should be sought.

III. Postherpetic neuralgia is also encountered in the trigeminal distribution. The first division (ophthalmic) is especially affected, and the possibility of corneal scarring should be borne in mind. Many patients are over 70 years of age, and the older the patient, the more severe the pain appears to be. The pain is described as a constant burning that may or may not be accompanied by a stabbing sensation and some hyperesthesia or hypoesthesia. The diagnosis is readily made on the basis of a painful rash in the area.

Treatment

I. Treatment of the first episode of primary neuralgias is medical, with carbamazepine or phenytoin being successful in many cases. Blood tests should be performed on a regular basis during drug treatment to watch for bone marrow suppression and liver function changes. In the atypical neuralgias and those arising after trauma or surgery, the patient may experience numbness in the area associated with the pain. This condition, described as *anesthesia dolorosa*, is severe and produces much suffering. For the atypical neuralgias, carbamazepine or phenytoin may be helpful, and baclofen and clonazepam should also be considered, sometimes in association with a tricyclic antidepressant.

II. In the primary neuralgias, if medical management is unsuccessful, then surgical treatment may be considered. Although peripheral neurectomy, cryosurgery, and peripheral phenol or alcohol blocks have been used in the past to denervate the area, in many instances, the origin of the pain is more central. The retrogasserian radiofrequency rhizotomy selectively destroys the trigeminal pain fibers specifically supplying the trigger zone without necessarily impairing sensory function. This is a relatively benign procedure and has excellent long-term results. Other neurosurgeons favor the intracranial approach to the trigeminal ganglion, in which vascular structures are stripped off the ganglion. They report good results despite the risks of a more major intervention.

Secondary neuralgias

I. Secondary neuralgias are the result of pain arising from the nerve trunks and central pathways in which abnormal central nervous system signs are present and in which the lesion is pressing on the nerve. The etiology may be extracranial (e.g., trauma, osteomyelitis, Paget's disease, or tumor) or intracranial (e.g., space-occupying lesions in the cerebellopontine angle or middle cranial fossa). Treatment is directed at the underlying cause.

Pain arising from outside the face

I. Pain perceived in the face may be secondary to lesions outside the area. Among the common ocular causes of pain are refractive errors, convergence insufficiency, extraocular muscle imbalance, trauma, arteritis, and narrow-angle glaucoma.

II. Coronary artery disease may refer pain to the left side of the neck and left mandibular area. Typically, this is brought on by physical exertion, emotional upset, or the ingestion of food, and is rapidly relieved by rest or sublingual nitroglycerin.

III. The dorsal roots of cervical nerves II and III supply an area of skin over the angle of the mandible and the posterior scalp to above the ear. Cervical sprain, degenerative arthritis, ankylosing spondylitis, or muscle spasm may irritate these nerves and cause pain, which, because of its distribution, may be confused with TMJ. Treatment is directed at the underlying cause.

Burning Mouth Syndrome (Glossodynia)

I. This is a condition largely affecting older female patients and was thought to be of hormonal or psychogenic origin. The pain is described as burning and may primarily affect the tongue or may involve the oral mucosa, lips, and oropharyngeal mucosa. The pain is aggravated by hot and spicy foods and may be ameliorated by cold liquids. Frequently the patient makes considerable changes to his or her diet to accommodate the discomfort. Most patients complain of the personal and social disability that results, and the incidence of depression in these patients is high. Characteristically the patient may be relatively pain free upon awakening, but the pain may increase as the day progresses. The etiology is unknown. Patients with clinically significant iron deficiency anemia, diabetes, or other deficiency diseases may manifest this condition, but in the majority of cases all laboratory tests, including biopsy specimens and images, are within normal limits. Recent experimental work has suggested that there may be a neurologic basis for this complaint, in that some patients have a subtle neuropathy of thermal sensitivity in the tongue.

Atypical facial pain

I. This type of pain is usually chronic in nature and is often associated with various psychiatric disorders. The nature and location of the pain may change over time and on occasion may have features consistent with myofascial, vascular, or neurogenic pain. In a review of 420 patients who were referred to a multidisciplinary facial pain group because of intractable pain of over 6 mo duration, 36% of patients had symptoms attributable to the masticatory system (TMJs and muscles of mastication), 29% had neuralgic pain of the trigeminal nerve, and 14% had facial pain of vascular origin. Fifty percent had associated psychiatric diagnoses (DSM-III-R criteria), of which depression and anxiety were most frequent. Somatoform disorder, psychosis, and pain behavior were also encountered. Because of the vague descriptions, emotional overtones, and equivocal physical finds, diagnosis and treatment are difficult.

II. These patients are offered the best treatment in a setting in which other specialists (such as psychiatrists, psychologists, physical therapists, social workers, neurologists, and neurosurgeons) can, in combination with dental specialists, address the complex issues involved. Every effort should be made to determine the organic basis of the pain while recognizing that psychiatric, neurophysiologic, and behavioral mechanisms can amplify and perpetuate the pain experience. By means of this combined approach, patients who are frustrated, angry, or despairing because of multiple failed attempts to relieve their pain can be rehabilitated. Pain programs (either inpatient or outpatient) may be helpful in redirecting the patient whose life has become centered on the pain.

Temporomandibular Disorders and Diseases

DIAGNOSIS

I. Although they are the most common cause of facial pain, temporomandibular disorders (TMDs) nevertheless require a thorough history and examination so that other potentially more serious diagnoses will not be missed. The clinical examination should include:

Palpation of the muscles of mastication (temporalis, masseter, medial pterygoid, lateral pterygoid)
Observation of mandibular motion (opening, closing, lateral excursion, protrusion)
Palpation and/or auscultation for joint noises
Examination of the dentition and occlusion

II. Masticatory system disorders have been classified in many ways. Because of the difficulty encountered in establishing a precise etiology, these disorders are often defined on the basis of symptoms and signs. The following are some broad categories:

Masticatory muscle spasm
Internal derangement
Chronic hypomobility
Trauma
Degenerative joint disease
Growth disturbances
Infections
Tumors

CLINICAL DISORDERS

I. Masticatory muscle spasm (myofascial pain dysfunction syndrome)
   A. Epidemiologic studies from many countries have clearly shown that the signs and symptoms of TMDs are widespread and that 28%–88% of people will have clinically detectable manifestations of dysfunction. Fewer individuals (12%–59%) will be aware of the symptoms, and fewer still (5%–25%) will require treatment.

1. It is generally agreed that patients with TMD will exhibit one or more of the following signs:
   a. Decreased range of mandibular motion
   b. Impaired TMJ function (e.g., deviation, sounds, sticking)
   c. Pain on palpation of the masticatory muscles or TMJs or on movement of the joint
2. They may also have one or more of the following symptoms:
   a. TMJ sounds
   b. Fatigue or stiffness of the jaws
   c. Pain in the face or jaws
   d. Pain on opening the mouth wide
   e. Locking
3. Radiographic studies of the TMJ will show no evidence of disease.
4. The etiology of this clinical complex is multifactorial—the factors most commonly cited being functional, psychological, and structural (i.e., occlusal). It is important to appreciate that, for any individual patient, one clear etiologic component is rarely apparent. More often, several possible components will be identified, including predisposing, initiating, and perpetuating factors. On the basis of this, the oral surgeon should formulate treatment goals bearing in mind the several likely etiologic factors.

B. The vast majority of patients will respond to simple, noninvasive treatment. These should include, but need not necessarily be limited to, the following:
   1. Reassurance—it is important that patients realize they are not alone with their symptoms, that they are essentially self-limiting, and that no disease exists. The role of muscle spasm and its benign nature should be carefully explained.
   2. Rest—Although it is not prudent to immobilize the mandible entirely, the patient should be instructed to have a mechanically soft diet for 2 wk and to avoid yawning and laughing with his or her mouth open. Habits such as chewing gum and biting fingernails should be strenuously resisted.
   3. Heat—the application of heat to the sides of the face by means of a heating pad, hot towel, or hot water bottle will be comforting and will relieve muscle spasm. More vigorous treatment can be achieved with ultrasound or shortwave diathermy heat treatments, which are widely available in physical therapy departments.
   4. Medications
      a. Nonsteroidal anti-inflammatory analgesics are of value in the acute stage. Ibuprofen, naproxen, and indomethacin at a low dose for 10 da are usually prescribed.
      b. Muscle relaxants are widely used but have not been proven efficacious. They are contraindicated for a chronic problem.

   c. Narcotic analgesics should be rigorously avoided.

   d. Antidepressants have a long history of effectiveness in the treatment of chronic pain, and in view of the strong association between TMD and psychological factors, their use is often justified, especially when the dysfunction is part of the complex of overall muscle pain with other signs and symptoms of depression. Tricyclic antidepressants are most widely used, and a bedtime-only schedule of 25–75 mg of norpramin or doxepin can be expected to relieve symptoms in 1–2 wk. Treatment is maintained for 2–4 mo and tapered to a low maintenance dose.

5. Occlusal therapy

   a. Appliances

      (1) A plethora of interocclusal appliances exist, and their mutiplicity suggests that the optimal design has yet to be found. The devices are usually made of processed acrylic and do the following:

         a) Improve TMJ function

         b) Improve the function of the masticatory motor system while reducing abnormal muscle function

         c) Protect the teeth from attrition and adverse occlusal loading

      (2) A full arch occlusal stabilizing appliance is the type that has proven to be most effective. Partial-coverage appliances tend to produce significant and irreversible changes in the dentition. It has been shown that an appropriate appliance can be effective in the majority of patients (70%–90%) and will both reduce masticatory muscle pain and control attrition and adverse tooth loading.

   b. Occlusal adjustments—there have been numerous claims that occlusal interferences of various types are the chief cause of masticatory muscle pain and that their elimination will result in improvement. Because masticatory dysfunction is a multifactorial problem, this is not likely to be true. The negative influence of malocclusion, loss of teeth, and occlusal interferences on masticatory function is not well supported by the evidence. However, on general principle, occlusal disharmony (including premature contacts) should be eliminated and missing teeth replaced in an effort to achieve optimal occlusion.

   c. Repositioning splints—the long-term efficacy of these appliances in the adult's nongrowing jaws has not been satisfactorily proven.

6. Behavioral modification—relaxation techniques, stress management, work pacing, imaging, biofeedback, and other

      modalities have all been shown to be advantageous. However, the most important technique undoubtedly is the therapeutic interactions of the dentist with the patient.

    7. Physical therapy is helpful when other muscle groups are involved and when conditioning and retraining of the masticatory muscles are indicated.

II. Internal derangement of theTMJ

  A. The techniques of arthrography, MRI, and diagnostic arthroscopy have demonstrated that the meniscus can be displaced or deformed and may account for the patient's symptoms of pain and limitation.

  B. The main categories of internal derangement are:

    1. Anterior displacement with reduction. This occurs when the meniscus is displaced in the closed mouth position and reduces (with a click) to the normal relationship some time during opening. In these circumstances, the patient complains of the click with a variable amount of pain. On opening, the jaw deviates toward the affected side until the click occurs and then returns to the midline. Preventing the mouth from fully closing with a splint, tongue blade, or dental mirror handle eliminates the click. The arthrogram or MRI scan will demonstrate the displaced meniscus, which reduces on opening. This situation may worsen and include intermittent locking and then finally closed lock.

    2. Anterior displacement without reduction (closed lock). If muscle spasm has been adequately relieved, pain may be minimal, but opening may be limited to 25–30 mm with restricted motion to the contralateral side. There may be a history of clicking with intermittent locking. The arthrogram or MRI scan will demonstrate a displacement without reduction (closed lock) and may also demonstrate degenerative changes. In such cases, the signs and symptoms of degenerative joint disease may also be present.

  C. Initial treatment for internal derangement consists of the same noninvasive therapies used for the myofascial pain dysfunction syndrome. In the patient who has anterior displacement with reduction (intermittent locking), these strategies are often successful. In the patient with a closed lock, especially one of long standing, these treatments may reduce muscle spasm and pain and restore some motion, but the underlying displacement may remain. When noninvasive treatment has been attempted and the patient remains restricted, interventions such as arthrocentesis or arthroscopy should be considered.

III. Chronic hypomobility (ankylosis)

  A. Anklyosis is the persistent inability to open the jaws. It may be caused by pathologic involvement of the joint structures (true ankylosis) or limitation produced by extra-articular causes (false anklyosis).

B. Infection and trauma are the primary causes of true ankylosis. The finding is severe limitation of opening, possibly with mandibular retrognathism if mandibular growth has been restricted. False ankylosis may be caused by a variety of disorders that can be categorized as:

   1. Myogenic (e.g., contracture of the masticatory muscles)

   2. Neurogenic (e.g., tetanus)

   3. Psychogenic (e.g., conversion reaction)

   4. Osteogenic (e.g., impingement of an enlarged coronoid process)

   5. Histiogenic (e.g., following TMJ surgery, temporalis muscle flaps, trauma)

   6. Neoplastic (e.g., nasopharyngeal carcinoma)

C. Radiographs show destruction of the joint surfaces, loss of joint space, and, in extreme cases, ossification across the joint.

D. The key to successful treatment is identifying the cause of hypomobility and addressing that as aggressively as possible. However, true ankylosis with fibrosis and calcification can be recalcitrant to treatment.

IV. Degenerative joint disease

A. Degenerative joint disease (osteoarthritis) of the TMJ may be the end point of several different insults to the joint structure, exceeding its capacity to remodel and repair. These insults include trauma (acute or chronic), chemical injury, infections, metabolic disturbances, and previous joint surgery.

B. The patient complains of pain on moving the jaw and of limited movement, with deviation to the affected side. There may be acute tenderness over the joint itself. Joint sounds are described as grating, grinding, or crunching, but not as clicking or popping.

C. Radiographs will demonstrate degenerative remodeling changes and loss of joint space.

D. There is a strong predilection for females. A significant number of patients are in their third or fourth decade. A few will manifest generalized osteoarthritis.

E. The natural course of the disease suggests that the pain and limitation may "burn themselves out" after several months in some individuals. The majority of patients can be kept comfortable until remission with the noninvasive techniques outlined above.

F. Some patients require injections of corticosteroids into the joint. This treatment is generally reserved for older patients and is limited to two or three injections. (The technique is similar to that for arthrography.) In persons who prove refractory to these techniques, surgery may be indicated to remove loose fragments of bone ("joint mice") and reshape the condyle. Attention should also be directed toward the meniscus, since its displacement may be a primary reason for the degenerative changes.

G. Rheumatoid arthritis can also affect the TMJ. The disease may afflict individuals of any age. In young persons, an associated micrognathia may be noted; in older persons with advanced cases, ankylosis may be the presenting complaint. Radiographic findings are of joint destruction possibly involving both the condyle and the articular eminence. Other stigmata of the disease will be evident. If medical management is ineffective, treatment of the degenerative joint disease or ankylosis, as outlined above, may be necessary.

V. Growth abnormalities

A. Studies of facial growth have demonstrated the major contribution made by the mandibular condyle to the adaptive growth of the mandible within the functional soft-tissue matrix. Several conditions can reduce this growth, including hypothyroidism, hypopituitarism, and nutritional deficiency (e.g., vitamin D deficiency). In gigantism, all the skeletal structures are enlarged, and in acromegaly, a marked prognathism is produced.

B. Several local conditions (trauma, infection, rheumatoid arthritis, radiation, scarring from burns or surgery) are causes of reduced postnatal growth.

C. In congenital abnormalities, the complex and coordinated growth of facial structures necessary for the achievement of normal form and function is altered and malformations occur. It is beyond the scope of this chapter to review all the possible anomalies that are encountered in clinical practice; suffice to say, most abnormalities of the TMJ occur in conjunction with recognized syndromes (e.g., lateral facial dysplasia, Treacher Collins syndrome). A full clinical and radiologic work-up is necessary for evaluation of the defect and to plan treatment with other specialists.

VI. Infections

A. Infection of the TMJ can be due to an open wound or to direct extension from adjacent structures (e.g., osteomyelitis of the mandible, suppurative otitis media). More rarely, it may be due to hematogenous spread from a distant site.

B. With improved medical care, better nutrition, and the introduction of antibiotics, infections of the TMJ have diminished in frequency.

C. Septic arthritis usually affects one joint, which becomes acutely painful, warm, and swollen. Characteristically, the swelling in the joint prevents the posterior teeth from meeting. Diagnostic features are the systemic indications of an infection and bacteria in the joint fluid. As sequelae of acute infection, arthritis with ankylosis and growth retardation may develop. Treatment is directed at the underlying cause.

VII. Tumors

    A. Tumors of the TMJ are rare, but clinicians need to maintain a high index of suspicion because the signs and symptoms of neoplastic disease can mimic those of other, more common TMJ disorders.

    B. Tumors may arise from the native cell population of the joint and invade the adjacent structures or they may metastasize from distant primary sites.

    C. The benign connective tissue tumors (osteoma, chondroma, osteochondroma) are most common. They present with pain or limitation of opening and an open bite on the affected side.

        1. In osteoma, a globular expansion of the condyle (as opposed to an elongation or overall enlargement seen in condylar hyperplasia) is noted on radiographs, which should be taken in both the lateral and posteroanterior planes.

        2. In synovial chondromatosis, foci of cartilage develop in the synovial membrane, and occasionally radiopaque masses are seen within the joint.

    D. Malignant tumors are rare and may be indicated by pain, swelling, and hearing loss (as the neoplasm expands into the external auditory meatus). Tumors may spread from surrounding structures or metastasize from distant sites. Radiographic changes are osteolytic or osteoblastic, depending on the tumor type.

REFERENCES

Alling CC, Mahan PE: *Facial pain*, ed 3, Philadelphia, 1991, Lea & Febiger.

Bell WE: *Orofacial pains*, ed 4, Chicago, 1989, Mosby.

Braun T: Temporomandibular joint surgery, part I. Surgical treatment of internal derangement, *Selected Readings in Oral and Maxillofacial Surgery* 1:3, 1989.

Dalessio DJ: *Wolff's headache and other head pain*, ed 5, 1987, Oxford University Press.

Hackett TP: The pain patient: evaluation and treatment. In Hackett TP, Cassem NM, eds. *Handbook of general hospital psychiatry*, St. Louis, 1978, Mosby.

Helms CA et al: *Internal derangements of the temporomandibular joint*, Radiology Research and Education Foundation, San Francisco, 1983.

Keith DA, ed: *Surgery of the temporomandibular joint*, ed 2, Cambridge, Mass, 1992, Blackwell Scientific.

Laskin DM et al, eds: The president's conference on the examination, diagnosis and management of temporomandibular disorders, *J Am Dent Assoc* 106:75, 1983.

Merrill RG, ed: *Oral and maxillofacial surgery clinics of north america*: 1. Disorders of the TMJ 1: Diagnosis and Arthroscopy, Sept 1989, 2. Disorders of the TMJ II: Arthrotomy, Dec 1989.

Okeson JP: O*rofacial pain. diagnosis: guidelines for assessment and management*, Chicago, 1996, Quintessence.

Oleson J: Classification and diagnostic criteria for headache disorders, cranial neuralgias and facial pain, *Cephalalgia* 8 (Suppl 7), 1988.

Sarnat BG, Laskin DM: *The temporomandibular joint. a biological basis for clinical practice*, ed 4, Philadelphia, 1992, WB Saunders.

Sweet WH: The treatment of trigeminal neuralgias (the douloureux), *N Engl J Med* 315(3):174–177, 1986.

Orthognathic and Reconstructive Surgery

10

DAVID H. PERROTT

Orthognathic Surgery

Preparation of a patient for elective surgical correction of a dentofacial deformity differs from that required for the evaluation and treatment of an acute problem. The patient who needs orthognathic surgery is usually many months away from the actual operation. However, to provide a successful outcome, meticulous attention must be given to developing a diagnosis and treatment plan with input from other health care providers (i.e., orthodontist, prosthodontist, periodontist, general dentist, speech pathologist). After a treatment plan has been developed, the surgeon must follow the patient's progress in preparation for the operation (see Algorithm 8).

This chapter discusses basic information on the treatment of patients with dentofacial deformities. It is recommended that one refer to the vast amount of literature on this topic for a more complete understanding of the management and treatment of these patients.

INITIAL EVALUATION

I. A thorough medical history is the essential first step. In this phase of the evaluation, it is critical to determine the following:
   A. The chief complaint, which must be recorded. The patient's major concern in seeking treatment may not coincide with the accurate diagnosis of or treatment plan for the deformity. When a discrepancy exists, one must carefully evaluate the patient's understanding and expectations of treatment.
   B. Significant etiologic factors of the deformity (e.g., acromegaly, birth injury, drug exposure, trauma, juvenile arthritis).
   C. Medical conditions that would contraindicate or require modifications to orthognathic treatment.
   D. The patient's history must include recent growth experience, past dental history, and previous orthodontics or operations.
II. Complete diagnostic records must be obtained. These consist of 1) a clinical examination, 2) facial and intraoral photographs, 3) radiographs, and 4) dental study casts, bite registration, and face bow registration for articulator mounting.

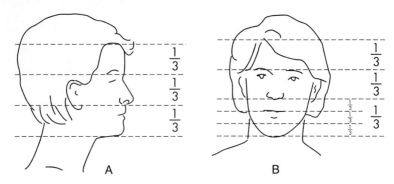

Fig. 10-1 Lateral (A) and frontal (B) proportional facial relationships.

A. The clinical examination is the most critical part of the diagnostic process. In preparation for obtaining the following information, the patient should be positioned as follows:

1. The patient should be standing with his or her head oriented so that the Frankfort horizontal is parallel to the floor.
2. The mandible should be in centric relation to the condyles properly seated in the fossae.
3. The teeth should be lightly touching.
4. The lips should be in a relaxed, nonrestrained position.

In this position, the following should be evaluated and documented:

a. Facial thirds (Fig. 10-1)
b. Frontal view
   (1) Facial form—long, short, symmetry
   (2) Eyes–intercanthal distance (28 to 44 mm), cant, and amount of visible sclera (1 to 2 mm)
   (3) Malar—flat, prominent
   (4) Nose—relationship to midsagittal plane, alar base width (should equal intercanthal distance), tip form, columella form, alae form
   (5) Upper lip length (22 ± 2 mm) and symmetry in function
   (6) Lower lip length (42 ± 2 mm) and symmetry in function
   (7) Interlabial gap when relaxed
   (8) Chin—length and symmetry
   (9) Maxillary incisor exposure at rest (2–4 mm)
   (10) Maxillary incisor gingival exposure when smiling (entire tooth and 1–3 mm of gingiva)
   (11) Maxillary occlusal plane to interpupillary plane
   (12) Maxillary and mandibular dental midline relationship to midsagittal plane
   (13) Soft- and hard-tissue midline relationship to midsagittal plane
   (14) Vermilion display

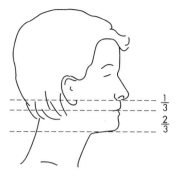

Fig. 10-2   Lower facial proportions—upper lip to lower lip = 1:2.

    c. Lateral view
        (1) Eyes—enophthalmos, exophthalmos
        (2) Malar—flat, prominent
        (3) Nose—dorsal form, tip projection, columellar length, tip to upper lip angle
        (4) Upper lip—procumbence, nasolabial angle
        (5) Lower lip—length = 2 times upper lip length (Fig. 10-2)
        (6) Chin—labiomental fold, chin-throat angle, lip competence, form, and relationship to base of nose
    d. Intraoral
        (1) Oral hygiene
        (2) Periodontal condition
        (3) Missing, decayed, crowding, tipping, rotated, or mobile teeth
        (4) Prostheses
        (5) Tongue—function and posture
        (6) Curve of Spee
        (7) Curve of Wilson—buccal tilting of posterior teeth
        (8) Occlusion (Angle's classification)
        (9) Transverse discrepancies—crossbites
      (10) Overbite, overjet, midline shifts
      (11) Freeway space
      (12) Centric relation versus centric occlusion discrepancies—if >2 mm, then photographs and radiographs must be taken in each position
      (13) Maximal incisal opening and deviation on opening
    e. Temporomandibular joint (TMJ) pain, limitation of motion, crepitus, popping, clicking, or muscle tenderness
  B. Facial and intraoral photographs. Photographs play a very important role in the treatment planning process, especially when using a computer analysis system. Therefore, the photographs must be obtained by a standardized, reproducible

method with good lighting and background illustrating the head and neck area. The following reproducible photographs are required:

1. Frontal views
   a. Lips relaxed and in centric occlusion
   b. Full smile in centric occlusion
2. Lateral view(s)
   a. Right or left with lips relaxed in centric occlusion
   b. Right and left may be necessary in severe facial asymmetries
3. Submentovertex view
4. Three-quarter profile views
   a. Right and left
5. Intraoral views
   a. Frontal in occlusion
   b. Buccal in occlusion
   c. Mirror view of maxillary arch
   d. Mirror view of mandibular arch
6. If major centric relation and centric occlusion discrepancies exist, additional lateral photographs in each position must be obtained.

C. The following radiographic studies are always required:
1. Lateral cephalogram with the teeth in centric occlusion and the lips in repose with good soft-tissue definition
2. Posteroanterior cephalogram
3. Orthopanograph of the jaws, which includes full view of the TMJs
4. A complete set of periapical and bite wing radiographs
   The following additional radiographic studies may be necessary:
1. CT scans for evaluating precise anatomic abnormalities of the midface, orbits, skull base, or condyles. TMJ tomograms may be used instead of CT scans.
2. MRI scans in the presence of TMJ disease
3. Radionuclide bone scans when the clinical history suggests the possibility of hyperplastic or neoplastic condylar growth
4. Hand-wrist film for assessment of the growth potential remaining in adolescent patients, in whom further growth may play an important role in the eventual size and position of the jaws and for whom appropriate timing of the surgery would be critical in maintaining a stable result.

D. Dental study casts, bite registration, and face-bow registration for articulator mounting. Accurate, well-trimmed dental study casts are essential to the development of a treatment plan. Duplicate casts should be poured in dental stone. They must be indelibly marked with the patient's name and the date on which they were obtained. The bases must be of sufficient size to allow monoplane trimming of the posterior cast surfaces when the casts are held in the patient's present centric occlusion. One set of casts is retained for the patient's permanent record; the other may be used for articulator mounting and any necessary model surgery.

All patients undergoing orthognathic surgery treatment planning should have a set of dental study casts mounted in centric relation using a face-bow transfer on a semiadjustable articulator. This documents for the surgeon and orthodontist the true occlusal relationships. Model surgery may be necessary to develop a treatment plan in cases of two jaw skeletal deformities or dental asymmetries.

INITIAL DIAGNOSIS

I. The problem list is developed and enumerates the various diagnoses or conditions pertinent to the patient.

A. Nonmedical problems (e.g., socioeconomic conditions, motivation for treatment) must be included if they might influence the eventual treatment or outcome.

B. Only problems that are current or that contribute to the presently contemplated treatment should be listed.

C. In the orthognathic portion of the problem list, soft tissues, teeth, and TMJs, in addition to each jaw, must be addressed and considered as a three-dimensional structure with potential problems to be found in any of the three planes.

The initial diagnostic process is now complete and all pertinent problems are listed and must be addressed in the treatment planning phase.

TREATMENT PLAN

I. Most often an orthodontist and surgeon will develop the treatment plan. However, in special situations, a prosthodontist, periodontist, speech pathologist, and others may also be required. A master problem list is developed with input from all members of the team. Each of these problems should be addressed in the treatment plan. The following is a simplified overview of the analysis leading to a treatment plan and is not meant to be comprehensive.

A. Clinical examination and photographic findings. From the clinical data obtained and documented with photographs, the treating team will have a master problem list. Not all problems listed will be addressed in the radiographic or model analysis (e.g., a deviated nose). Therefore, problems identified from the clinical examination and photographs must be addressed in the comprehensive treatment plan, which will be developed and presented to the patient.

B. Radiographic analysis. A variety of radiographic analysis techniques have been described, each having advantages and disadvantages. However, one must always remember that they are to be used as an adjunct in developing a treatment plan.

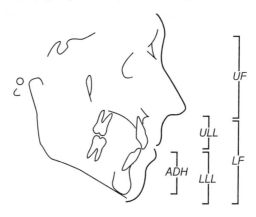

Fig. 10-3 Vertical facial dimensions. Upper face (UF) to lower face (LF) height = 5:6. Upper lip length (ULL) = 20–22 mm. Lower lip length (LLL) = 44 to 52 mm. Anterior dental height (ADH) = 40–44 mm.

The use of computers to analyze the radiographic findings and to illustrate surgical and orthodontic treatment is a major advancement. This, in conjunction with video imaging, has moved treatment planning into a new era. Figures 10.3–10.5 are common radiographic analysis landmarks used to develop a treatment plan.

The surgical treatment objective (STO) is a visual projection of the changes in skeletal, dental, and soft tissues as a result of surgical-orthodontic treatment. According to Wolford et al. (1985), the STO was designed as both a diagnostic and a treatment planning aid to 1) present a simple and accurate method of predicting results of surgical-orthodontic treatment, 2) establish the surgical movements necessary to cor-

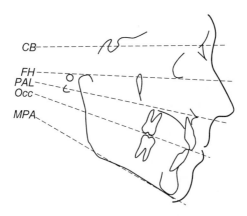

Fig. 10-4 Horizontal facial planes. CB = cranial base; FH = Frankfurt horizontal; PAL = palatal plane; Occ = occlusal plane; MPA = mandibular plane.

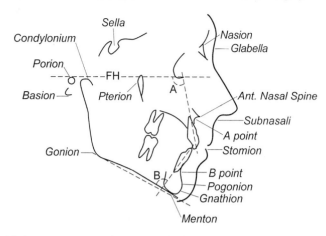

Fig. 10-5 Important cephalometric landmarks. Incisor inclination. Upper incisor angulation—angle A = 112° relative to Frankfurt horizontal. Angle B = 90° relative to mandibular plane.

rect the deformity, 3) accurately predict the resultant facial profile, and 4) provide a visual aid with a single overlay. The last two points are made much easier and more predictable with the use of computers.

Wolford recommended that the STO be divided into the initial and final. The initial STO is prepared before commencement of treatment to determine the orthodontic and surgical goals, whereas the final STO is prepared before the operation to determine the exact vertical and horizontal skeletal and soft-tissue changes to be achieved. As part of the STO, radiographic analysis is required. The following radiographic parameters should be evaluated:

1. Upper tooth to upper lip relationship—1-4 mm
2. Soft tissue thickness—upper and lower lip and chin = 1:1:1
3. Upper lip length—20-22 mm (see Fig. 10-3)
4. Overjet—0-4 mm
5. Overbite—0-4 mm
6. Vertical bony height of face—upper-lower = 5:6.
7. Lower anterior dental height—40-44 mm (see Fig. 10-3)
8. Mandibular depth—FH to NB = 88° (see Fig. 10-5)
9. Maxillary depth—FH to NA = 90° (see Fig. 10-5)
10. Upper incisor angulation to NA—22°; incisor tip—4 mm in front of NA (see Fig. 10-5)
11. Lower incisor inclination to NB = 20° (see Fig. 10-5)
12. SNA—80°-84° (see Fig. 10-5)*
13. SNB—77.50°-81.50° (see Fig. 10-5)*

---

*Steiner analysis.

14. ANB—1.50°-3.50° (see Fig. 10-5)*
15. Maxillary unit length—83.20-89.00 mm (see Fig. 10-5)†
16. Mandibular unit length—107-116 mm (see Fig. 10-5)†
17. Mandibular plane angle to FH—25° (see Fig. 10-4)
18. Occlusal plane angle—8° ± 4° (see Fig. 10-4)

   These parameters can also be analyzed using other analysis systems such as Ricketts or Bjork-Jarabak.

C. Once the clinical and radiographic data have been obtained, the surgeon can begin movement of the jaws using acetate tracing paper or a computer analysis system. The following systematic approach is recommended:

1. All dental compensations, extractions, and tooth movements must be addressed before any surgical movements can be attempted.

2. The next step of the plan begins with the incisal tip of the maxillary central incisor. The position of this tooth relative to the upper lip is the keystone of the architecture of the jaws. Therefore, one first looks to the problem list to determine whether any vertical or horizontal malposition of the maxilla exists. If so, a new position for the maxilla must be chosen.

3. Reposition the maxilla so the tip of the central incisor is positioned correctly in relation to the upper lip. This will usually place the incisal edge 2-3 mm below the drape of the upper lip at rest. This must correspond to the clinical findings. The horizontal position is chosen from the desired nasolabial angle and midfacial prominence based on clinical and radiographic analyses.

4. Using the midpoint of the mandibular condyle as the axis of rotation, rotate the mandible in a clockwise direction until the mandibular incisors are in 2-3 mm of overbite. Positive or negative overjet is temporarily ignored.

5. Without moving the tip of the maxillary central incisor, rotate the maxilla until the maxillary occlusal plane is aligned with the occlusal plane of the mandible, as established in the preceding step.

6. Determine whether the mandible requires advancement, retropositioning, or change to achieve a normal overjet.

7. The chin is evaluated and movements equating to a genioplasty osteotomy are completed to obtain optimal chin form.

8. Make a new tracing or a computer printout with the maxilla and mandible in the newly chosen positions. The two tracings can be superimposed to demonstrate clearly the amount and direction of movements that have

---

*Steiner analysis. †Harvold analysis.

been chosen. For this reason, a different color for each tracing is recommended.

9. In the presence of facial asymmetry, tracings correcting the deformity should be made from the posteroanterior cephalometric film.

10. Other areas to be addressed in developing the STO include the effects of bony and tooth movement on the soft tissues (i.e., nose, lip, neck).

D. Orthodontic analysis and treatment plan. Input from an orthodontist is critical to develop a successful treatment plan. Orthodontic treatment is designed to obtain a stable occlusion postoperatively. Issues to be addressed by the orthodontist include:

1. The presence of dental compensations

2. The significance of interarch problems (crowding, spacing, or rotation of teeth)

3. The nature of interarch incompatibilities related to transverse width discrepancies, mismatch of the maxillary and mandibular occlusal curves, or discordance in the shapes and circumferences of the two arches

To assist in formulating the treatment plan, the orthodontist and surgeon may need to perform model surgery on duplicate sets of dental casts. Several "rules" must be followed:

1. Indelible reference marks should be placed on casts before the casts are cut.

2. All cuts on casts should be realistic; root positions must be carefully estimated so the model surgery will reflect clinical reality.

3. A minimal amount of stone should be removed in areas of simulated osteotomies, thereby more accurately depicting the clinical situation at the time of surgery.

4. Fewer osteotomy sites is better. One large segment is surgically and biologically preferable to two or four smaller segments. Segmental surgery should not be thought of as a substitute for orthodontic treatment.

5. Repositioning of dentoalveolar segments should take into account the periodontal and dental stability of the new position. Large steps horizontally or vertically at the level of the crestal alveolar bone are unacceptable and would indicate the need for orthodontic rather than surgical movement of the teeth in question.

E. Presentation of treatment plan. After the development of a treatment plan, the patient should return to the surgeon and orthodontist for a presentation. This presentation should include the proposed treatment plan, alternative treatment plan(s), risks and benefits, and total time for treatment. Financial arrangements for the proposed treatment plan is addressed at this time.

Once presurgical orthodontic treatment has been started, the surgeon and orthodontist should be in regular communication. The surgeon should evaluate the patient every 3–4 mo to monitor the changes from orthodontic treatment. As part of this analysis, interim dental casts will be necessary.

After completion of the presurgical orthodontic treatment, the steps of clinical evaluation, cephalometric prediction, tracings, and model surgery are repeated. The patient is evaluated as a new candidate, since changes in position of the teeth relative to the underlying bone and to the overlying soft tissues may necessitate significant revisions in the original treatment plan. A new or revised problem list is developed, and a final surgical treatment plan is formulated.

Completion of the final surgical treatment plan requires a thorough familiarity with the various surgical procedures available, as well as their indications, contraindications, and limitations. Full details of the surgical techniques can be found in the references at the end of this chapter. The following discussion regarding treatment is based on the assumption that the reader is knowledgeable in these areas.

I. Maxillary deformities (see Algorithm 9)
   A. Vertical maxillary excess
   1. When the excess is confined to the anterior region of the maxillary arch, implying a reversed curve of Spee with an acceptable posterior occlusion, an anterior segmental osteotomy (Wassmund or Wunderer technique) or a Le Fort I osteotomy is indicated.
   2. When the excess is confined to the posterior maxilla, producing an anterior open bite with a normal relationship of the upper lip and upper central incisors, either posterior segmental osteotomies or a Le Fort I osteotomy is required. The position of the mandible produced by its autorotation following the maxillary movement may require inclusion of a mandibular osteotomy in the final surgical plan.
   3. Vertical maxillary excess involving both anterior and posterior areas, whether accompanied by an anterior open bite or not, requires a Le Fort I osteotomy. Model surgery will demonstrate the need for segmental osteotomies in conjunction with the total maxillary procedure. Also, the possibility must be considered that mandibular surgery will be necessary as a result of the maxillary change.
   B. Vertical maxillary deficiency
   1. When the deficiency is confined to the anterior maxilla (with an exaggerated curve of occlusion and acceptable posterior intercuspation), an anterior segmental osteotomy using a Le Fort I osteotomy approach is recom-

mended. Placement of a bone graft may be necessary to stabilize the movement and permit bony contact.

2. Vertical deficiency involving either the posterior or the entire maxilla may be corrected by a Le Fort I osteotomy and interpositional bone graft.

C. Horizontal (sagittal) maxillary excess

1. Premaxillary prominence with a satisfactory posterior occlusion is corrected with an anterior dentoalveolar segmental osteotomy; this procedure will usually require removal of the first premolars. The technique of Wunderer (palatal incision, labial soft-tissue pedicle) is suggested. However, this solution is usually contraindicated when the premolars have been removed previously and all spaces have been closed; extraction of additional premolars and placement of the canines adjacent to the first molars by means of this osteotomy will generally result in unacceptable periodontal and aesthetic configurations of the arch.

2. When an anterior segmental osteotomy is contraindicated or when the entire maxillary arch requires posterior movement, a Le Fort I osteotomy is chosen.

D. Horizontal (sagittal) maxillary deficiency

1. The Le Fort I osteotomy is preferred for advancement of the entire maxillary arch. Bone grafting to maintain the stability of the advancement is usually not necessary.

2. Advancement of malar areas may be accomplished simultaneously by performing horizontal osteotomies high on the lateral maxillary walls or by implanting onlay bone grafts or alloplastic materials. True advancement of the infraorbital rims will require an osteotomy of the Le Fort II type.

E. Transverse maxillary deficiency

1. The problem of a narrow maxilla will most often be addressed during the presurgical orthodontic phase of treatment. In adults, when conventional orthodontic appliance therapy for rapid palatal expansion is not successful, a minor surgical procedure may be necessary. A lateral maxillary osteotomy through the zygomatic buttress on each side will usually suffice, although separation of the midpalatal suture will be required in some patients for the palatal expansion appliance to be effective. Separation of the pterygomaxillary sutures or the interincisal bone is not necessary. This technique is known as *surgically assisted rapid palatal expansion.*

2. When expansion of all or portions of the maxilla is needed, either in the absence of orthodontic treatment or in cases of incomplete orthodontic expansion, segmental osteotomies can be planned in conjunction with a Le Fort I osteotomy. Unilateral expansion of a posterior

maxillary segment can be accomplished with a segmental osteotomy if there is no other concomitant need for a Le Fort I osteotomy.

F. Transverse maxillary excess. When the maxillary arch needs to be narrowed, a palatal ostectomy can be performed at the time of a Le Fort I osteotomy.

III. Mandibular deformities (see Algorithms 10 and 11)

A. Horizontal mandibular excess

1. If the entire mandible is prominent and the mandibular dental arch requires posterior movement, a mandibular ramus osteotomy is indicated. The vertical or oblique osteotomy, extending posterior to the inferior alveolar neurovascular bundle from the sigmoid notch to the angle of the mandible, is the procedure associated with the least morbidity. Alternative treatment methods include the sagittal ramus osteotomy or the inverted L osteotomy. Posterior body or ramus ostectomies are rarely used or indicated.

2. When the posterior occlusion is satisfactory and the prognathic relationship is confined to the anterior segment, an anterior segmental osteotomy is the treatment of choice. Extraction of two premolars is required unless a preexisting space within the dental arch can be used for retropositioning the anterior dentoalveolar segment. The position of the mental foramina must be considered in planning the procedure.

3. When the occlusion is satisfactory but the lower third of the mandible is disproportionately long, the chin requires treatment. Reduction of the lower third of the jaw can be done by contouring the bone or ostectomy of the lower border of the mandibular body.

B. Horizontal mandibular deficiency

1. If the entire mandible and lower dental arch require advancement, the sagittal ramus osteotomy is the most reliable procedure; clinical stability can be anticipated as long as there is no elongation of the height of the ramus resulting from the procedure.

2. Advancement of the mandible and closure of a small (3–4 mm) anterior open bite may be accomplished with a sagittal ramus osteotomy. However, the segments must be adequately stabilized. Alternatives to the sagittal ramus osteotomy include the inverted L and the C osteotomies. The inverted L requires a bone graft and the C osteotomy is performed from an extraoral approach, thereby making them relatively less desirable than the sagittal osteotomy.

3. When the occlusal relationship of the mandibular arch with the maxilla is acceptable, advancement of the lower third of the mandible can be achieved by means of ad-

vancement genioplasty. Implantation of bone grafts or alloplastic materials are occasionally used, but the long-term results are not as satisfactory as those obtained with the sliding genioplasty.

C. Vertical mandibular deficiency

   1. Advancement of the mandible will usually result in lengthening of the lower third of the face, the amount of vertical change being dependent on the mandibular plane and the steepness of the occlusal plane. Sometimes a posterior open bite is created to increase vertical dimension. Careful postoperative orthodontic care is required when using this approach to increase vertical dimension.

   2. Attempts to elongate the vertical dimension of the mandible by total alveolar osteotomy give unstable results, so this procedure is not recommended.

   3. Horizontal genioplasty with interpositional bone grafts for lengthening the chin may be considered for correction of vertical mandibular deficiency.

D. Vertical mandibular excess

   1. Elongation of the lower third of the face may be corrected by intrusion of the maxilla and thus requires no mandibular surgery.

   2. When no surgery is required in the maxilla or when the maxillary correction produces insufficient change in the lower third of the face, reduction genioplasty or contouring ostectomy of the lower border of the mandible may be included in the treatment plan.

E. Transverse mandibular deficiency

   1. If the mandibular dental arch is too narrow for the maxillary arch, orthodontic treatment is the primary method for increasing the circumference of the arch. If the teeth are appropriately situated over basal bone and a transverse deficiency is still present, the discrepancy will usually require maxillary surgery to narrow the upper jaw. Surgical procedures to widen the lower dental arch are unsatisfactory.

   2. If the occlusion is acceptable, transverse mandibular deficiency is generally managed by the use of onlay bone grafts or alloplastic materials to improve the contour of the jaw. This procedure is most often needed in cases of severe asymmetry.

F. Transverse mandibular excess

   1. If the occlusion is satisfactory, excessive width of the mandible is corrected by reduction contouring of the jaw.

   2. Relative excess of mandibular width may be corrected by altering the sagittal relationship of the jaws. If this relationship has been corrected and transverse discrepancy

remains, one must consider either widening the maxilla or narrowing the mandible. Ostectomy in the symphyseal area, often in conjunction with an anterior dentoalveolar segmental osteotomy or together with extraction of an anterior tooth, will enable the mandible to be narrowed. Simultaneous "relaxing" osteotomies of the ramus may be needed, particularly if the posterior portion of the dental arch must also be narrowed either unilaterally or bilaterally.

F. Stabilization techniques. Stabilization of the bony segments for the aforementioned procedures can be categorized as nonrigid or rigid. Nonrigid methods require a period of maxillomandibular fixation (MMF), whereas rigid techniques require no period of MMF. Studies indicate that rigid techniques provide improved short-term stability and improved long-term predictability, in addition to patient comfort. Guiding elastics (1 or 2 per side) are often used after rigid fixation techniques during the first 1-3 wk following the operation. However, they do not restrict jaw movement.

PREADMISSION PREPARATION

I. The medical history obtained at the time of initial evaluation must be updated at the final preadmission visit so that any changes in the patient's health status can be determined. If indicated by this history, whatever medical consultation is necessary should be arranged in anticipation of the patient's being admitted to the hospital. The physician must be apprised of the nature of the planned surgery, the anesthesia requirement, and the specific medical assistance being requested.

II. If there is the potential need for transfusion of blood products during the planned surgery, arrangements with the hospital's blood bank should be made. Whenever possible, donation of the patient's own blood for autologous transfusion should be scheduled. One unit of blood may be obtained every 7-10 da, with the last unit collected at least 2 wk before the scheduled surgery. The patient must be given a prescription for ferrous sulfate, 300 mg tid., from the time of the initial collection until admission. Two units of blood obtained in this manner will usually be adequate for use in uncomplicated orthognathic procedures.

III. A final presurgical orthodontic visit 3-4 wk before the operation is necessary to place surgical arch wires with some type of hooks to be used for intraoperative or postoperative MMF or guiding elastics.

IV. The surgeon's presurgical records, including photographs and radiographs, should be obtained within 3 wk of the operation. One week before the operation, the surgeon should obtain final dental impressions to make dental casts. If a maxillary operation or a two-jaw operation is planned, the cast must be mounted on a semiadjustable articulator. Careful model surgery for maxillary operations or two-jaw operations will provide the surgeon with preoperative data to be used during the operation. From these dental casts, the surgeon must construct the surgical acrylic splints. In two-jaw operations, an intermediate splint and final splint are required. Meticulous attention to the model surgery and splint construction is necessary to achieve a successful outcome.

INPATIENT MANAGEMENT

I. Patients are usually admitted on the day of operation. Therefore, before the operation, the following is usually completed on an outpatient basis:

A. A complete history is obtained and a physical examination is performed according to the prescribed format of the hospital or surgical center.

B. The patient's informed consent to the planned surgical procedure is obtained and documented in the record.

C. Preoperative laboratory studies, as required by the hospital or surgical center and the needs of the patient, are ordered. A complete blood count and urinalysis will usually be the minimal complement of tests. Other test and studies are conducted based on the presence of other pathologic conditions and their relevance to the operation and anesthesia.

D. The anesthesiologist will conduct a preoperative assessment of the patient. Close cooperation between the surgeon and the anesthesiologist is essential so the latter knows the nature, extent, and special needs of the planned procedure. Hypotensive anesthetic techniques are favored by some surgeons. This minimizes the amount of operative blood loss, makes the surgical field cleaner, and reduces the need for transfusion of blood products.

II. The following additional preoperative orders are recommended:

A. Antibiotics. Most surgeons prescribe prophylactic antibiotics and a short duration of postoperative antibiotics. Two million u of penicillin is given IV just before beginning the operation and is continued during the operation every 4 hr. Postoperatively, 2 million U of penicillin is given IV every 6 hr for the next 6–24 hr. For patients allergic to penicillin, cephalosporin or clindamycin may be used. If a bone graft is used (bank or autogenous), a broader coverage antibiotic, such as cephalosporin or nafcillin, is recommended. In addition, the length of postoperative antibiotic administration should be increased to 4–7 da.

B. Steroids. Corticosteroids are commonly ordered at the time of surgery in the belief that they will lessen postoperative edema and thus reduce airway embarrassment for the patient whose jaws are immobilized. A common dosage schedule is 8–12 mg of dexamethasone at the time of surgery and a tapering regimen during the next 48 hr.

IMMEDIATE POSTOPERATIVE MANAGEMENT

I. A nasogastric tube may be placed just before extubation to empty the stomach of secretions and swallowed blood. This will usually aid in reducing postoperative nausea and vomiting. The tube is removed before extubation, unless there is active bleeding.

II. Immediate postoperative orders are for analgesics, antiemetics, antipyretics, and antibiotics. For patients who have undergone maxillary surgery, nasal decongestants and antihistamines may also be prescribed to aid in clearing the nasal airway and to promote drainage of the paranasal sinuses.

III. Ice packs are used in the first 24–36 hr to help minimize postoperative edema.

IV. Airway management is of paramount importance in the perioperative period. Close monitoring is necessary both in recovery and after the patient returns to his or her room. If the operation is planned as an outpatient procedure, proper postoperative management must be explained to the patient.

If the nursing staff is unfamiliar with the needs of a patient who has had MMF, it may be necessary to place the patient in intensive care for immediate postoperative recuperation before returning the patient to the regular hospital ward. However, with improved surgical techniques, anesthesia, and the use of rigid fixation, many patients are discharged following adequate recovery or within 23 hr of the operation.

For the patient in MMF and with nasal, buccal, and labial edema, the placement of plastic syringe barrels between the cheeks and the teeth may make the patient more comfortable. Providing humidified air or oxygen through a loose or open face mask will often aid in loosening or preventing crusting of secretions in the airway.

V. In patients who have had ribs harvested for grafting, a postoperative chest radiograph should be obtained to rule out the possibility of pneumothorax.

VI. The hematocrit is usually checked in the recovery room or within 12 hr after completion of the operation. The test may be repeated as indicated if there is continued bleeding or if transfusions have been administered. Replacement of RBCs is not usually necessary if the hematocrit is greater than 30% and the patient shows no evidence of postural change in vital signs. Transfusion protocols vary between institutions.

VII. If the patient is in MMF, scissors or wire cutters must be readily available for use in an emergency. The patient's family must be both reassured with regard to and instructed in the release of MMF before the patient is discharged from the hospital.

VIII. Suction apparatus must be available at the bedside in the immediate postsurgical days, but is not generally necessary after the patient has left the hospital.

IX. To minimize edema in the immediate postoperative period, the head is elevated above the level of the heart.

X. Oral nutritional intake is encouraged as soon as possible, starting with clear liquids and progressing to a high-protein, high-calorie, fully blenderized diet. Even in the presence of rigid fixation, a soft diet is recommend for the first 3–4 wk. Consultation with the dietitian is recommended for patient and family to assist in nutritional management after discharge.

XI. Early ambulation is urged and should be started as soon as possible.

XII. Oral hygiene for the patient in MMF is achieved with the use of half-strength hydrogen peroxide rinses and the help of mechanical devices such as a Water-Pik. The latter must be used with caution in the early postoperative period, however, lest the intraoral incision lines be disrupted. The use of chlorhexidine rinses is also recommended.

XIII. Appropriate postoperative radiographs, usually consisting of a lateral and posteroanterior cephalometric film and a panoramic view, are obtained within 24–48 hr of the surgery. The mandibular condyles must be well visualized on these films, because any malpositioning would necessitate a return to the operating room at the earliest opportunity.

XIV. The patient must clearly understand the limitations on physical activity, instructions regarding nutrition and hygiene, and how to reach the surgeon in case of an emergency.

OUTPATIENT POSTOPERATIVE MANAGEMENT

I. Patients are usually seen weekly for postoperative care during the first 3–4 wk after the operation. If elastics were used for MMF, they are changed at each visit. For patients with rigid fixation, guiding elastics may also need to be changed.

II. MMF is maintained for 4–6 wk and the splint is removed at that time. For patients with rigid fixation, the splint may be removed at 2–4 wk, depending on the operation performed. After removal of the splint, the patient can begin the final phase of the orthodontic treatment.

III. The patient must be instructed in the gradual progression from a soft to a regular diet during the seventh and eighth postoperative weeks. Mouth opening exercises may be instituted during this time for any patient who demonstrates trismus.

IV. In the absence of any complications, routine follow-up visits with the patient are scheduled at 3, 6, and 12 mo after the operation. At each of these visits, the surgeon should obtain photographs and radiographs. These data should be reviewed and compared to the preoperative and immediate postoperative records to determine the achievement of treatment goals and stability of the operation.

Reconstructive Surgery (see Algorithm 12)

I. Reconstructive surgery is viewed as the restoration of form and function lost because of an acquired condition such as trauma or tumor resection. Reconstruction may involve bone or soft tissue, or both.

II. The specifics of care for the patient who requires reconstructive surgery relate to the location of the defect, the type of tissues to be reconstructed, and the donor sites to be employed. These patients have many of the same preoperative and postoperative needs as do patients undergoing major oral and maxillofacial surgery. The principles of blood and fluid management, diet regulation, respiratory care, and wound management differ only to the degree that the reconstructive procedure is more complex than other operations.

Soft-Tissue Reconstruction

I. Replacement of missing soft tissue is indicated whenever there is insufficient local tissue to achieve adequate primary closure, when primary closure of the local tissue would compromise function, and when the quality of the local soft tissue would jeopardize the success of primary closure (e.g., tissues that have previously been irradiated). An additional indication for soft-tissue reconstruction is the need to prevent or minimize wound contracture in areas that would otherwise be allowed to heal by secondary intention; such an indication is described in detail in the discussion of split-thickness skin and mucosal grafts for pre-prosthetic vestibuloplasty.

II. Choices for soft-tissue reconstruction include the following:

Split-thickness skin or mucosal grafts
Full-thickness skin or mucosal free grafts
Local composite flaps (e.g., tongue, pharyngeal, Estlander, Abbe)
Distant pedicled flaps of the axial type (e.g., deltopectoral, temporal, or trapezius)
Myocutaneous flaps (e.g., pectoralis major, sternocleidomastoid, latissimus dorsi, platysma)
Free composite flaps requiring microvascular anastomosis at the recipient site

III. The choice from among these alternatives will be made based on the indications listed. The first two types are usually employed only when the objective is to minimize scarring and wound contracture. Local composite flaps are reserved for specific anatomic locations where relatively small amounts of soft-tissue replacement are required. Both axial and myocutaneous flaps can replace large volumes of soft tissue; the latter is more often used today because of the greater certainty of its blood supply and, hence, the viability of the transferred tissue. Microvascular free grafts are employed when 1) large volumes of tissue are needed in areas where muscle-based flaps have been already used or are not anatomically accessible, and 2) large amounts of soft tissues and bone are required in previously irradiated sites.

IV. Preoperative care for the donor site is limited to thorough cleaning. To minimize bacterial colonization of the skin, shaving of hair from the donor sites is not recommended until immediately before or during the surgical procedure; microscopic shaving defects in the skin become heavily populated with bacteria if the shaving is done several hours before surgery.

V. Postoperative donor site care
   A. Care for skin graft donor sites is discussed in Chapter 6.
   B. Flaps whose viability depends on unimpeded circulation through a pedicle, whether the pedicle is composite tissue or a muscle body, must be protected from pressure. Both tension and compression are to be avoided, and the flaps should be inspected frequently in the immediate postoperative period.
   C. Some surgeons recommend the use of anticoagulants (either intravenous dextrans or low-dose heparin) to aid in the circulation in myocutaneous or microvascular free flaps.
   D. Suture lines at the recipient site should be kept meticulously clean; extraorally, they should be swabbed daily with diluted hydrogen peroxide. Intraoral recipient sites are cared for with mouth rinses of half-strength hydrogen peroxide four times daily. Activities with the potential for disrupting the flap-recipient interface (e.g., positive-pressure inhalation therapy) are contraindicated.

Osseous Reconstruction

I. Restoration of osseous continuity is almost always a procedure directed at defects of the mandible. In the maxilla the ability to restore both form and function with a prosthesis makes the need for bone grafting rare, even after extensive ablative surgery.

II. The indications for osseous reconstruction of the upper jaw are usually limited to situations in which there is nonunion or malunion following trauma, or a discontinuity defect of the alveolar process has resulted from trauma, severe atrophy, ablative surgery, or congenital deformity. Mandibular discontinuities require reconstructive surgery in almost all cases where there is a need to restore form and function and to allow construction of a functional prosthesis.

III. The principles of osseous reconstruction require that there be:
   A. Sufficient numbers of viable osteocytes or cells capable of inducing osteogenesis at the host site
   B. A form or shape to the bone graft consistent with that which is being replaced

    C. The ability of the graft to function in a manner similar to that of the missing part

    D. Stability at the graft-host interface during the period of healing

    E. Adequate blood supply from surrounding soft tissues, even if this requires the insertion of vascularized soft-tissue flaps, as described above

    F. Closure of soft tissues over the graft without tension or leakage

    G. Meticulous attention to hemostasis at the host site to minimize or eliminate the formation of hemotoma

IV. Several substitutes for bone grafts have been popular for reconstruction of jaw defects. However, it must be recognized that the use of materials such as metal, acrylic, silicone, or hydroxyapatite alone does not fulfill the principles. Similarly, cadaveric bone alone is inadequate as a bone graft material. Only autologous cancellous bone is capable of meeting the first requirement for successful bone grafting.

    A. The autologous bone must be freshly obtained at the time of the reconstructive procedure.

        1. For cancellous bone, the iliac crest is the usual donor site. The anterior ilium is most commonly used, but the posterior ilium provides more volume for reconstruction of large defects. The tibia can also be a source of large amounts of cancellous bone. Small amounts can be harvested from the mandibular symphysis, ascending ramus, and maxillary turberosity area. Some surgeons have successfully mixed cancellous bone with other materials, giving additional quantity, with the former providing the osteogenic stimulus.

           Cortical bone, which may be taken from the donor site with the cancellous into the chosen bone, serves the purpose of providing form and stability to the graft, but it is not critical to the success of the graft. Alternative means of providing shape and a solid bed for the grafted marrow include metal plates, metal or Dacron-polyurethane trays, and freeze-dried cadaver bone; in each case, fresh autologous cancellous bone is a densely packed vehicle.

        2. The usual donor sites for cortical struts of bone or for grafts of both central and cancellous material are the calvarium, the ribs, and the iliac crest. The mandibular symphysis may serve as a donor site in limited cases.

V. The requirement for stability at the graft-host interface during healing is met in ways not unlike those used for fixation of fractures.

    A. Internal fixation by means of bone plates or rigid trays that span the grafted defect and that can be solidly attached to the adjacent host bone are most frequently used and are recommended. MMF is not required when true rigid fixation is utilized.

B. MMF can be employed whenever there are adequate teeth or when intraoral prostheses can be used without the risk of pressure necrosis of the soft tissues overlying the bone graft.

The duration of MMF differs from that of fracture patients and will depend on the size of the graft, the blood supply of the recipient bed, and the method of graft fixation employed. When graft replacement of the TMJ has been done, with either a costochondral graft or an alloplastic prosthesis, early mobilization of the mandible is desired (10–14 da). In the absence of internal fixation, 6–8 wk is recommended for immobilization after grafting of a mandibular continuity defect.

C. No immobilization of the jaw is required when onlay bone grafts have been placed or when rigid internal fixation techniques are employed.

D. Extraoral biphasic pin fixation can be used as a means of providing stability, when rigid internal fixation is not possible.

VI. Meticulous hemostasis of the graft recipient site must be obtained before careful closure of the overlying tissues in anatomic layers. To minimize the potential for hematoma or serous accumulation at the graft site, a low-pressure vacuum drainage system may be used in the first 48 hr or until adequate hemostasis has occurred.

OSSEOUS DONOR SITES

I. Rib grafts

A. Any patient in whom a rib is to be harvested for a graft should have a preoperative radiographic series taken of the chest. This will allow the surgeon to assess the degree of osteoporosis that may be present, which might dictate another choice of donor site. In addition, the chest films will serve as a baseline study if respiratory problems develop postoperatively as a consequence of the rib harvesting.

B. Optimal pulmonary toilet should be attained preoperatively, and the patient should receive instruction in the routine chest physiotherapy that will be expected postoperatively.

C. The location of the incision for the harvesting of the rib graft should be chosen so as to be as cosmetic as possible. The inframammary fold provides good access for the harvesting of as many as three ribs. No more than two consecutive ribs should be harvested without leaving one rib intact before harvesting the third rib, or the chest wall mechanics may be compromised.

D. Intraoperative management of the rib donor site is the most critical factor in preventing postoperative problems.

1. Careful attention to operative technique will allow the rib to be harvested in a completely subperiosteal fashion,

thus avoiding any violation of the pleural space or disruption of the intercostal neurovascular bundle.

2. Before closure of the wound, there should be a thorough inspection for pleural leaks. If no obvious tears in the pleura are found, the wound should be flooded with normal saline and the anesthesiologist should then apply positive pressure via the endotracheal tube.

   a. If no bubbling is observed in the saline-filled wound, there can be reasonable certainty that no pneumothorax has occurred.

   b. If there are lacerations of the parietal pleura, they should be repaired with a 2-0 chromic suture on an atraumatic needle with a small-bore catheter brought out through one end of the tear. As the last suture is tied, suction is applied to the catheter and positive-pressure ventilation is given; the suture is secured as the catheter is withdrawn. The saline bubbling test is then performed again to check the adequacy of the repair.

E. Postoperatively a chest film should be obtained to reveal the possibility of undetected pneumothorax. A small one (compromising 10%–20% of lung volume) may be treated by observation. A larger pneumothorax will necessitate placement of a chest tube for evacuation of the air.

F. Pain and splinting in the area of the rib donor site may contribute to poor respiratory excursions, with increased potential for atelectasis or pneumonia. Rather than large doses of parenteral narcotics, which might decrease respiratory drive, an injection of a long-acting local anesthetic (e.g., bupivacaine) can be given to block the intercostal nerves of the affected area. This will provide excellent patient comfort and promote good respiratory toilet.

II. Iliac crest grafts

A. The iliac crest is a favored donor site for large corticocancellous grafts and pure cancellous bone, because in most patients either type of graft can be readily obtained without functional deformity.

B. Intraoperative techniques must adhere to the standard surgical principles of anatomic dissection, careful hemostasis, and protection of neighboring structures. Actual violation of the peritoneal cavity is rare, even when both inner and outer cortical tables of the ilium are taken as part of the graft, but simple mechanical irritation of the peritoneum cannot always be avoided.

C. A drain, usually of the closed-system, low-vacuum type (e.g., Hemovac), is often employed because of the tendency of the exposed cancellous portion of the ilium to bleed into the dead space of the wound after the graft has been harvested. As with all drains, this should be removed as soon as it is no longer collecting significant amounts (less than 10–20 ml in a 24-hr period).

D. Postoperatively, the patient who has had iliac crest bone harvested must be examined for adequacy of bladder and bowel function. It is not uncommon for the patient to experience bladder spasm or adynamic ileus as a result of local peritoneal irritation. Catheterization of the bladder is necessary if the bladder becomes distended and the patient is unable to void spontaneously.

E. The patient should not be given any oral food or drink until it has been determined that there is normal bowel function, as determined by the presence of normal bowel sounds and the passage of stool. If ileus is detected, nasogastric suction is instituted to aid in decompressing the adynamic bowel; the suction should be continued until bowel sounds have returned to normal. The fluid and electrolyte losses associated with the gastric suctioning must be taken into account during intravenous fluid management.

F. Physical therapy to aid in the early ambulation of the patient after harvesting of an iliac crest graft should be instituted. Use of a walker or a cane may be necessary.

III. Calvarial bone grafts

A. Use of the outer table of the calvarium has been advocated because of its proximity to the operative field, its membranous origin, its accessibility via an inconspicuous scar when done as an independent procedure or via the major operative incision when a coronal flap is used for approaching the face, and its minimal morbidity.

B. The parietal bone is the preferred donor site. The thickness of the bone is 4 to 6 mm, allowing for careful harvesting of the outer table of bone. The donor site must be located far enough lateral to avoid the superior sagittal sinus.

C. Full-thickness harvesting of the calvarium, whether deliberate or inadvertent, will require careful attention to the repair dural lacerations and will necessitate an additional donor site (usually additional outer table calvarium) for reconstruction of the skull defect.

D. When there is concern for a palpable or visible depression in the scalp resulting from the outer table harvest, reconstitution of the defect may be accomplished most simply with particulate hydroxyapatite or other alloplastic materials.

E. Postoperative morbidity is reported to be low with the use of calvarial donor sites, but the patient should be carefully evaluated for any changes in neurologic signs or symptoms.

IV. Vascularized bone grafts

A. For mandibular reconstruction, the most common donor sites for vascularized bone grafts are the tibia, ilium, and scapula. Postoperative management of the donor site is similar to that described above.

B. The success of these grafts is dependent on several factors, including limited primary ishcemia, choice and careful anastomosis of recipient vessels, limited distortion of pedicle, minimal postoperative pressure on the graft, and use of antithrombotic therapy.

C. These grafts can support the use of immediate endosseous implant placement, even in the presence of previous radiation sites.

GENERAL REFERENCES

Bell WH: *Modern practice in orthognathic and reconstructive surgery*, vols 1–3, Philadelphia, 1992, WB Saunders.

Bell WH: *Surgical correction of dentofacial deformities*, vol 3, New Concepts, Philadelphia, 1985, WB Saunders.

Bell WH: Le Fort I osteotomy for correction of maxillary deformities, *J Oral Surg* 33:412, 1975.

Bell WH, Proffit WR, White RP: *Surgical correction of dentofacial deformities*, vols 1, 2, Philadelphia, 1980, WB Saunders.

Dimitroulis G, Dolwick MF, Van Sickels JE: *Orthognathic surgery: a synopsis of basic principles and surgical techniques*, Oxford, 1994, Butterworth-Heinemann.

MacIntosh RB: Autogenous grafting in oral and maxillofacial surgery, *Oral Maxillofac Surg Clin N Am* 5:4, 1993.

Peterson LJ, Indresano AT, Marciani RD, Roser SM: *Principles of oral and maxillofacial surgery,* vols 1–3, Philadelphia, 1992, JB Lippincott.

Pogrel MA: Malignant tumors of the maxillofacial region, *Oral Maxillofac Surg Clin N Am* 5:3, 1993.

Trauner R, Obwegeser HL: The surgical correction of mandibular prognathism and retrognathia with consideration of genioplasty, *Oral Surg* 10:677, 1957.

West RA: Orthognathic surgery, *Oral Maxillofac Surg Clin N Am* 2:4, 1990.

Salivary Gland Disease

11

R. BRUCE DONOFF

GENERAL CONSIDERATIONS

I. Swelling in the submandibular or preauricular area often is a patient's presenting complaint. It may or may not be accompanied by pain. The diagnosis and treatment of such patients often include diseases of the parotid and submaxillary salivary glands (Table 11-1).
   A. The major differential diagnostic problem is separating lymph node enlargement from salivary gland enlargement.
   B. Other general diagnostic considerations include odontogenic infections in cases of submandibular swelling and bony diseases of the ramus of the mandible in cases of preauricular swelling.
II. The patient's history is most important to the differential diagnosis. An acute enlargement in the submandibular or preauricular areas, particularly when related to eating, suggests an obstruction in salivary flow; a progressive enlargement suggests a neoplastic process. Bilateral enlargement places the diagnosis in a different category of diseases, which includes Sjögren's syndrome, sarcoidosis, and other more esoteric metabolic problems.

DIAGNOSTIC PROCEDURES

I. Clinical examination is performed to determine whether any of the following pertain:

Swelling is tender
Enlargement is firm, soft, or rubbery
Seventh nerve function is intact
Salivary flow is adequate from Stensen's duct
Fluctuant material can be milked from the duct
A stone can be palpated in the duct

II. A history is taken to reveal the duration, any fluctuation in size, the presence of pain, etc.
III. Laboratory tests are performed to differentiate tumor from lymph node disease.
   A. Sialography is often helpful in demonstrating a filling defect.

Table 11-1　SALIVARY GLAND DISEASES BY MAJOR CATEGORY

Disease	Location	Comments
Submaxillary sialadenitis	Submandibular	Acute enlargement, tender, fluctuates with meals; palpable stone in floor of mouth; pus from Wharton's duct: occlusal radiograph shows stone (rarely radiolucent); usually penicillin sensitive, but pus should be cultured
Parotitis	Preauricular	Acute enlargement, less common than sialadenitis; fluctuates with meals; pus from Stensen's duct; stone palpable in cheek or seen on periapical radiograph positioned over duct; frequently due to *Staphylococcus;* may not be associated with stone, but with decreased secretion as in Sjögren's syndrome; secondary ascending infection
Parotid tumor	Preauricular	Slow growth, usually painless; unilateral, but Warthin's may be bilateral; majority are benign; pain and seventh nerve involvement suggest malignancy
Submaxillary tumor	Submandibular	Less common; slow growth
Minor gland tumor	Any area of mucosa but palate and bucal mucosa usual	Slow growth; may appear as lump or ulcer; on palate it must be differentiated from maxillary sinus tumor and from necrotizing sialometaplasia

B. Computed tomography (CT) with contrast often shows enhancement of a benign mixed tumor; it is most useful for assessing tumor involvement in both superficial and deep parotid portions.

C. However, the status of CT with sialography is controversial.

IV. Parenchymal salivary gland disease must be differentiated from lymph node disease. Major considerations include parenchymal disorders (e.g., Sjögren's syndrome, sarcoidosis) and infiltrative processes that invade the periparotid lymph nodes (e.g., tuberculosis, leukemia, lymphoma). The latter fall in the group of diseases termed Mikulicz's syndrome (Table 11-2).

MANAGEMENT PROCEDURES
Bacterial sialadenitis or parotitis

I. Whether preauricular or submandibular, bacterial sialadenitis and parotitis have a rapid onset of firm, tender swelling. A history of

Table 11-2 LYMPH NODE DISEASE MIMICKING SALIVARY GLAND DISEASE

Disease	Location	Comments
Cat scratch disease	Submandibular	Matted nodes, history of cat scratch; no evidence of pus from Wharton's duct; skin test available
Lymphoma	Submandibular or preauricular	Progressive enlargement; may be localized disease; firm, nontender; may cause secondary gland obstruction; skin test for anergy
Leukemia	Submandibular	May be localized; WBC elevated
Metastatic tumor	Either	From fossa of Rosenmöller
Infectious diseases	Submandibular	Tuberculosis, coccidioidomycosis; skin tests available

swelling with meals is often elicited. Pus can usually be expressed from either Stensen's or Wharton's duct on the involved side.
  A. Both stricture and stone may contribute to the onset and must be sought.
  B. Extensive probing of either duct and sialography especially are contraindicated in a sick patient with purulent drainage.
 II. Bacterial infections of the salivary glands usually occur in the debilitated, dehydrated, or postoperative patient. Any systemic condition like Sjögren's that leads to decreased flow of saliva also predisposes to retrograde glandular infection.
III. Before the advent of antibiotics and simple means of intravenous fluid administration, these conditions were life threatening.
IV. Before beginning treatment, the clinician must determine:
  A. The patient's status in terms of toxicity—temperature, state of hydration, malaise
  B. Whether an obstruction is present—palpation for stones in the ducts, periapical films of Stensen's duct and mandibular occlusal views to search for a stone in Wharton's duct
  C. The status of the gland secretion—purulent, inspissated (thick), or ropy saliva
 V. Appropriate culture of purulent material must be made, and laboratory tests (including WBC count) should be done.

Bacterial infections of the salivary glands
  I. If the patient with a bacterial infection is free of systemic signs or symptoms, is afebrile or has only a low-grade temperature, gives a history of recurrent swelling with meals, and now has a tender swelling, thick or purulent duct drainage, and a demonstrable stone in the duct, there are several considerations to bear in mind:
  A. Such a patient is best managed by:
    1. Culture of saliva
    2. A prescription for dicloxacillin 500 mg qid for 7 da

  3. Instructions to drink plenty of fluids

  4. Use of sour lemon candies to promote saliva flow

  5. Application of moist heat to the swelling

 B. Close follow-up is advised.

 C. Attempts to remove the stone should be instituted once antibiotic treatment is under way.

II. If the patient feels sick, has a temperature of 101° F or above, has a very tender swelling, appears dehydrated, has pus in the salivary drainage with or without a demonstrable stone, and has an elevated WBC count, the following should be done:

 A. The patient should be admitted for intravenous fluid therapy, antibiotics, and supportive care.

  1. An IV is started with D_5W at 100 ml per hr unless a cardiac or renal condition exists.

  2. Oxacillin is given in standard IV dose because *Staphylococcus* is an important pathogen in many cases.

  3. Sour lemon candies or swabs are used to promote saliva flow.

 B. The usual course will be improvement in the systemic condition, defervescence, and a drop in the WBC count within 1–2 da. Failure to show improvement within 4 da should arouse a suspicion of abscess formation. (This would be unusual.)

III. Attempts to remove a stone surgically and/or perform sialography to locate a duct stricture when no stone is demonstrable should be deferred until infection is under control and the patient's general condition warrants it. Sialography may also be indicated as part of the workup for a patient suspected of having Sjögren's syndrome, which may present as a secondary infection of the salivary gland.

Sjögren's syndrome

 I. Currently several forms of Sjögren's syndrome are recognized (Table 11-3):

  A primary form

  A secondary form associated with rheumatoid arthritis or another connective tissue disease

  A form characterized by lymphocytic aggressive behavior, which in rare cases results in lymphoma

 II. Classically, xerostomia, keratoconjunctivitis sicca, and rheumatoid arthritis form the originally described triad. Lymphocytic infiltration of salivary gland and lacrimal gland tissue characterizes the disease. Decreased salivary flow and/or tearing may be associated with enlarged parotid glands in one third of patients.

 III. Workup for a patient suspected of having Sjögren's will include the following:

  Lupus erythematoses (LE) prep

  Antinuclear antibodies

  Serum amylase

Table 11-3 PRIMARY AND SECONDARY FORMS OF SJÖGREN'S SYNDROME

Characteristics	Primary	Secondary
Rheumatoid arthritis or other connective tissue disease	No	Yes
Lymphocytic infiltration of organs	+++	+
Risk of lymphoma	++	+
Rheumatoid factor in serum	Yes	Yes
Antinuclear antibodies	Species-specific B	Rheumatoid arthritis precipitin
Histocompatibility typing	HLA-BB HLA-DR3	HLA-DR4

+ Moderately likely
++Likely
+++Very likely

Rheumatoid factor
Ophthalmologic examination for eye signs
Schirmer's test for tearing
Fluorescein
Sialography for sialectasia
Minor salivary gland biopsy (of the labial glands in the lower lip is
   most convenient)

Biopsy technique

1. In the lower lip a small anteroposterior incision is made, hemostasis being provided by the assistant (who holds both sides with a sponge).
2. Scissors are used for blunt dissection of several small glands, which are submitted to biopsy. Usually no bleeding requiring clamping is encountered. The incision must be away from any superficial vessels in the mucosal tissue.
3. The wound is closed with interrupted 3–0 catgut sutures.
4. The patient should apply pressure to the wound with a sponge for 5 min.

IV. Treatment of Sjögren's syndrome is generally supportive.
   A. Artificial saliva and tears may be helpful.
   B. teroids have a beneficial effect on salivary gland enlargement but not on xerostomia.
   C. Radiation of 400 cGy* has been implicated in the development of pseudolymphoma or true lymphoma and is contraindicated.
   D. Parotidectomy is indicated only when there is excessive enlargement of the salivary gland.

*The designation centigray (cGy) is used instead of rad.

Sarcoidosis

I. Sarcoidosis is a poorly understood disease characterized by Langhans' giant cell granulomatous inflammation. It is frequently brought to attention because of pulmonary symptoms or abnormalities in pulmonary function tests. It can be related to interstitial lung parenchymal involvement or to hilar adenopathy. Cutaneous and uveal tract manifestations are not uncommon. About 6% of patients have parotid involvement, characterized by enlargement, xerostomia, and often fever (Heerfordt's syndrome [uveoparotid fever]).

II. A specific skin test (the Kveim test) is often used. However, it provides a diagnosis only of exclusion unless a biopsy of lymph node, liver, lung, or skin shows the characteristic histopathologic features.

III. Laboratory findings of significance are hypercalcemia (often responsive to steroids), a mildly elevated alkaline phosphatase, an elevated serum gamma globulin, and possibly an elevated serum amylase. The xerostomia of sarcoidosis often responds to steroids, unlike that of Sjögren's syndrome.

IV. Open biopsy of the periparotid or parotid tissue is usually required for confirmation.

Salivary gland tumors

I. Workup of a suspected salivary gland tumor includes the following:
  A. Major gland (parotid the most common site)
    1. Clinical examination
      a. Location and consistency are important. Benign mixed tumors are usually firm but rubbery. Suspicion of fluid may suggest Warthin's tumor, which is often cystlike. Lack of fixation suggests a benign lesion.
      b. Examination for adenopathy is necessary.
      c. The most critical differential point is distinguishing between a parenchymal and a nodal problem.
    2. Laboratory examination. Blood workup is virtually noncontributory unless there is a question of infection. Tumors almost never have associated infection, unlike Sjögren's syndrome, which has involved glands. Less common submaxillary gland tumors may be confused with infected submandibular nodes or an obstructed gland.
    3. Radiologic examination
      a. Plain films are used to rule out a stone, and sialography to determine parenchymal versus nodal disease.
      b. CT may replace sialography if the question of ductal pathology is not important or if there is a question of deep lobe involvement.
    4. Special test
      a. Despite early interest and promise of the technique, radionuclide imaging is not helpful in the diagnosis of major gland tumors.

  b. Ultrasound may be useful if a vascular or cystic lesion is suspected.

B. Minor gland (palate the most common site)

  1. Clinical examination. Benign mixed tumors of the palate rarely ulcerate, although adenoid cyst and mucoepidermoid often present in such a fashion. One must ascertain whether there is nasal obstruction or whether the sinus symptoms for palatal lesions are the result of carcinoma of the maxillary sinus.

  2. Radiographic examination. Maxillary occlusal radiographs or, more commonly, tomograms of the hard palate are important in determining osseous involvement.

Table 11-4   TUMORS OF THE SALIVARY GLANDS

Type	General	Clinical
Benign tumors		
Pleomorphic adenoma (benign mixed tumor)	90% of tumors of all salivary glands	Firm but rubbery; recurrent lesions may show subcutaneous growth; no seventh nerve signs; treatment includes parotidectomy or excision
Warthin's tumor	Papillary cystadenoma lymphomatosum	May be cystic; rarely seen in minor glands; males are involved more often than females; found especially in men over 55; treatment is excision or superficial parotidectomy
Oncocytoma	Small, rare, encapsulated	Rare
Malignant tumors		
Malignant mixed tumor	Relatively rare; due to transformation of benign tumor	Very firm, often with skin fixation, seventh nerve signs; parotidectomy with neck dissection indicated if adenopathy is present; postoperative radiation is useful in selected cases

Continued

Table 11-4 TUMORS OF THE SALIVARY GLANDS—*cont'd*		
Type	General	Clinical
Malignant tumors—cont'd		
Adenocarcinoma Acinic cell	Very rare	Hard; treatment includes wide excision of tissue if in minor gland; hemimaxillectomy may
Adenoid cystic	Cylindroma; slow growing but with early neural invasion	be necessary if neural invasion is suspected; treatment is total parotidectomy, with or without nerve sacrifice, with possibility of nerve grafting; postoperative radiation has definite place in management; one must consider maxillary sinus origin in palatal lesions; use of polytomes of palate and midface or CT scans can show extent
Mucoepidermoid carcinoma	Age of patient variable; low to high grade based upon mucous cell/ epidermoid cell ratio	Treatment is based on age of patient, lesion location, histology; can infiltrate and metastasize; wide excision for mucosal lesions superficial to total parotidectomy based upon tumor extent; necrotizing sialometaplasia considered in a differential diagnosis

C. The most important part of the workup is obtaining a tissue diagnosis. A sufficient index of suspicion for parotid or submaxillary gland tumor often is an indication for surgery with biopsy at the same time. Accessibility makes possible biopsy of minor gland lesions before definitive treatment.

II. A listing of salivary gland tumors is found in Table 11-4.

III. Lesions mimicking salivary gland tumors include the following:
- A. Nasal fossa tumors. Those in the fossa of Rosenmüller may spread to the parotid lymph nodes and look like parotid tumors.
- B. Antral carcinoma. This sometimes presents as a minor salivary gland tumor of the palate. Sinus radiographs and polytomes of the palate may show osseous changes or lesions. These radiographs are also helpful in planning treatment of palatal minor gland tumors.
- C. Lymphadenopathy of the submaxillary area (Hodgkin's, leukemia).
- D. Branchial cleft cyst. These are usually posterior to the submaxillary gland and are nontender; no history of enlargement with meals is reported.
- E. Necrotizing sialometaplasia. This usually appears on the palate as an ulcerative lesion. It can be confused with a minor salivary gland tumor, especially a mucoepidermoid carcinoma, since it occurs in younger patients.
- F. Parotid enlargement with HIV infection.

GENERAL REFERENCES

Carlson ER, ed: The comprehensive management of salivary gland pathology, *Oral Maxillofac Surg Clin N Am*, August 1995.

Gorlin RJ, Goldman HM, eds: *Thoma's oral surgery*, ed 6, St Louis, 1970, Mosby.

Mason DK, Chisholm DM: *Salivary glands in health and disease*, Philadelphia, 1975, Saunders.

Moutsopoulos HM et al: Sjögren's syndrome: current issues, *Ann Intern Med* 92:212, 1980.

Facial Trauma

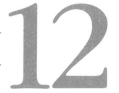

DAVID H. PERROTT

GENERAL CONSIDERATIONS

I. The patient who sustains facial trauma should be evaluated for other potential injuries, which are often much more severe and may be more life threatening. Attention to the general overall management of the trauma patient is thus the first objective of this review. Trauma management is a team effort.

II. The primary trauma survey ABCs must be followed:
   A. The airway is assessed and if found to be obstructed, a passage secured.
   B. Breathing must be adequate.
   C. The circulation must be sufficient to maintain life.

   Usually the adequacy of vital signs is ensured simultaneously with other assessments. For example, respiratory distress can be observed while the pulses are being checked, and the general condition of the patient can be noted after clothing has been removed. It is very important that there be NO movement of the neck until the status of the cervical spine has been evaluated.

PRELIMINARY ASSESSMENTS
Airway and breathing

I. One must establish the presence of respiration. If breathing is labored or stridorous, immediate intervention is required. Many of these actions are performed simultaneously.

II. The procedure for airway assessment is as follows:
   A. Inspection. Check the oral cavity for dentures, loose teeth, blood (including that from open mandibular fracture), etc.
   B. Debridement. Remove any obstructing bodies and/or suction the nasal and oral cavities.
   C. If these measures do not improve respiration, attempt a jaw thrust maneuver (keeping in mind the possibility of cervical spine injury) or placement of a soft rubber nasopharyngeal airway.
   D. During examination of the chest, check for symmetrical chest movement and the presence of bilateral breath sounds on auscultation to rule out pneumothorax. Note any paradoxical mo-

tion, since multiple rib fractures can cause flail chest, which has dire hemodynamic consequences as well as marked respiratory importance.

E. Placement of an oral airway may be helpful.

F. If the mandible has fallen posteriorly as a result of fracture, temporary stabilization with wire may bring the jaw and tongue forward, relieving obstruction.

G. If no measures improve the situation, intubation may be indicated. Oral endotracheal intubation is more rapid, but a nasal endotracheal tube may be more efficacious in the patient with facial trauma. There are few real contraindications to nasal endotracheal intubation in these patients. Nasal bone fracture and cerebrospinal fluid (CSF) rhinorrhea are often cited, but in fact they are not contraindicated if one considers that the nasal tube runs posteriorly in a horizontal direction, not in a superior direction. Fiber optic intubation is recommended if there is concern about midface fractures.

H. Tracheotomy is almost never indicated or required in an emergency room setting. Cricothyroidotomy is the preferred and indicated approach for an emergency airway.

Pneumothorax

I. An injury that permits air to enter the space between the outer covering of the lungs and the inner lining of the chest wall creates a negative pressure that collapses the lung on the ipsilateral side.

A. This typical pneumothorax results in a hyperresonant chest because the entire pleural cavity, not just the lungs, is filled with air. Breath sounds are decreased or absent depending on the extent of the collapse.

B. The chest film shows collapsed lung parenchyma and a lack of vascular markings out to the periphery of the lung field.

II. Treatment is directed at evacuating the air from the pleural space. In an emergency a needle may be placed just above the superior border of the second rib (to avoid the intercostal vessels at the inferior rib margin), midclavicular line so air can escape. If converted to a Luer-Lok at the distal end, the needle may prevent reentry of air until a regular chest tube is inserted and placed to water suction.

Flail chest

I. Fracture of several ribs or other bony chest wall components leads to paradoxical motion of the chest wall with inspiration and expiration. There are hemodynamic consequences, since paradoxical chest motion impairs venous return, which in turn reduces cardiac output. Treatment is positive-pressure respiratory support, which maintains the ribs in position.

Hemothorax

I. Hemothorax usually occurs together with collapse of lung parenchyma. Blood, along with air, is found in the pleural cavity.

II. Drainage is performed with a chest tube placed in the fifth inter-costal space, anterior to the midaxillary line. This tube lies poste-riorly and drains fluid and air when the patient is recumbent.

Cardiac tamponade

I. Blood in the pericardium prevents normal cardiac filling, making the heart an ineffective pump. The heart is enlarged, heart sounds are distant, and there is a paradoxical pulse.

II. Treatment is evacuation of fluid from the pericardial space.

Hypotension

I. The trauma patient with decreased systolic and diastolic blood pressure and thready rapid pulse presents a common diagnostic and management problem.

II. Management of the hypotensive patient is as follows:

A. Do the general appraisal and take a history if the patient is awake and alert. The patient's clothes must be removed for the examination. A family member may be the best source of information.

B. Airway patency is assured.

C. Start a secured peripheral IV with a two large-bore (16-gauge) catheters. If these lines cannot be secured, cut down at the saphenous or arm veins is recommended. Insert a Foley cathe-ter to monitor urine output. A urine sample is sent for analy-sis, particularly for occult blood or hematuria.

D. Begin lactated Ringer's solution at full rate to provide rapid volume replacement.

E. Draw blood samples for type and crossmatch, electrolytes, amylase, and CBC simultaneously with line placement.

F. After the airway is secure and fluids are started, monitor vital signs frequently and begin the general physical examination of the patient.

1. Head—lacerations, contusions, Battle's sign (ecchymotic area behind the ear); great care must be exercised during examination of the neck until cervical spine injury can be adequately assessed radiographically.

2. Chest—obvious injuries, rib fractures, and paradoxical chest motion; auscultate to assure adequacy and symmetry of breath sounds; auscultate the heart for abnormal sounds; the back should also be included in this examination.

3. Abdomen—tenderness and guarding may indicate an in-jured viscus; if high suspicion of internal abdominal injury exists, complete a paracentesis (insert an Intracath via a stab incision just below the umbilicus into the peritoneal cavity and run in 1 liter of Ringer's lactate, withdrawing the fluid through a large syringe; assess its redness visually or perform a hematocrit; if newspaper print cannot be viewed through the withdrawn fluid, significant internal bleeding is likely and the patient needs exploration) or take an abdominal CT scan.

4. Flank—tenderness may indicate renal injury or retroperi-
   toneal bleeding; examination of the urine is important in
   this assessment.
5. Extremities—lacerations, contusions, and fractures; pelvic
   and humerus injuries are often causes of major blood loss;
   make sure that all pulses are present and symmetrical.

G. When the physical examination is completed and if the patient's condition permits, a proper radiographic examination
can be performed. This will include a skull series, facial bone
series, cervical spine films, chest films, abdominal (KUB) films,
and extremity films (as needed). Often, CT scans are completed in the head and neck area to evaluate intracranial and
spinal injuries. The maxillofacial surgeon can request CT
scans of the facial area to evaluate facial injuries.

MANAGEMENT PROCEDURES
Suspected head injury

I. All of the aforementioned preliminary assessments should be
done for the patient with suspected head injury. Special attention
must be given to differentiating the effects of alcohol and other
drugs from those of serious neurologic injury.

II. The patient's level of responsiveness is assessed: Can the patient
be aroused easily, or only with painful stimuli? Can the patient an-
swer simple questions appropriately? Is the patient oriented to
time and place? The Glasgow coma scale is useful for this (see
box below).

The Glasgow Coma Scale

EYE OPENING
Spontaneous—4
To speech—3
To pain—2
None—1

BEST VERBAL RESPONSE
Oriented—5
Confused (conversation)—4
Inappropriate (words)—3
Incomprehensible (sounds)—2
None—1

BEST MOTOR RESPONSE
Obeying (follows commands)—6
Localizing—5
Normal flexion—4
Flexing (abnormal posture)—3
Extending (abnormal)—2
None (no movement)—1

A. The development of equipment for monitoring various functions in critically ill patients has not altered the need for assessing the level of consciousness.

B. The Glasgow coma scale evaluates three aspects of behavioral response: eye opening, verbal, and motor. The Glasgow coma scale: 1) provides a simple grading of arousal and functional capacity of the cerebral cortex; 2) assesses brainstem function by observation of the pupil and ocular motility; 3) is limited in localizing brain dysfunction on the basis of decorticate and decerebrate postures to the extent that posturing does not always mean brainstem damage; and 4) is not intended as a prognostic indicator; nevertheless, the level of responsiveness and the duration of a patient's remaining at a given point on the scale correlate closely with outcome.

III. A general examination is performed:

A. Pupils for reactivity and symmetry; also gross vision

B. Any lateralizing signs, weakness or asymmetry of deep tendon reflexes

C. Abnormal reflexes, e.g., Babinski

IV. Frequent monitoring of neurovital signs is important. Increasing intracranial pressure may be seen as the Cushing reflex (with increasing blood pressure, bradycardia, and bradypnea).

V. A cranial nerve examination is performed. Normal findings, or tests needed in the unconscious patient, are as follows:

Cranial Nerve	Conscious Patient	Unconscious Patient
I	Gross vision	Consensual light reflex (optic nerve intact when light into right eye causes left pupil to constrict)
II	Gross smell	Not testable
III	Pupillary constriction to light	As above for CN I
IV	Upward and outward gaze	
V	Sensation in face	Corneal reflex
VI	Lateral gaze	Centralizing of eye when head turned to either side
VII	Facial expression	Changes with painful stimulus (grimace)
VIII	Hear finger snap	Vestibular portion tested by doll's head maneuver or caloric test (cold water placed in uninjured ear causes eyes to move toward side of test)
IX	Gag reflex	Gag reflex
X		
XI	Shoulder shrug	
XII	Tongue movement	

VI. All patients with midface fractures should be evaluated for possible CSF leaks. CSF rhinorrhea or CSF leakage from the ear is not uncommon.

   A. Rhinorrhea is often found with Le Fort injuries of the maxillofacial complex. It is difficult to diagnose with certainty. Low sugar content of the CSF and the clarity of CSF on a piece of linen versus the cloudiness of mucus are often said to be helpful in the differentiation. In fact, the appearance of fluorescein dye in nasal secretions after its central injection (via lumbar puncture) is the best way of demonstrating CSF rhinorrhea. The vast majority of such injuries heal with reduction and fixation of the facial fractures. The presence of a pneumoencephalocelic aerosol on skull film or CT scan in the area above the cribriform plate suggests a large dural tear, which may require more than facial fracture fixation for treatment.

   B. CSF leakage from the ear is usually associated with temporal bone fractures, often with condylar injuries not resulting in fracture of the condyle itself. Blood from the ear may be an associated finding.

VII. Management of increased intracranial pressure includes one or more of the following:

   A. Drugs
      1. Diuretics such as osmotic mannitol or furosemide
      2. Steroids

   B. Intubation with rapid ventilation blows off carbon dioxide, which has a vasoconstricting effect on the cerebral vessels; induced respiratory alkalosis is thus helpful.

   C. Surgery—bur holes are placed to relieve tension.

   D. Monitoring
      1. Subarachnoid bolt (measurement of intracranial pressure)
      2. Subdural catheter
      3. Intraventricular catheter

Facial fractures

   I. Foreign bodies, dentures, tooth fragments, and bone fragments are removed from the oral cavity and upper airway. Any missing teeth should be accounted for by examination or radiographs, including a chest radiograph to rule out aspiration.

  II. Care is taken to guarantee an adequate airway, especially in the semiconscious or unconscious individual. This may involve the use of oropharyngeal, nasopharyngeal, or endotracheal intubation or cricothyroidotomy. Tracheotomy is done in controlled operating room settings.

 III. If there is active intraoral or extraoral bleeding, hemostasis is obtained by pressure. Ligation should be done judiciously to avoid nerve injury.

  IV. Temporary stabilization of fractures with wires, particularly in the mandible, is helpful in reducing bleeding and providing comfort.

V. Severe nasal bleeding may be controlled by packing with petrolatum gauze. Uncommonly, anterior nasal packing may require additional posterior nasal packing. This is conveniently placed by means of gastric catheters threaded through the nose to the pharynx and led out through the mouth; gauze packs are attached by sutures through the perforations at the catheter tips; when the catheters are withdrawn through the nose, the packs are brought securely to the posterior nasopharynx; the sutures are tied externally at the nose so the packs will not be aspirated. An alternative means of controlling bleeding is the use of Foley catheters placed into the nasopharynx area, inflated and advanced to occlude the posterior nasal cavity.

A. CSF rhinorrhea is not a contraindication to anterior nasal packing, since the cribriform plate is superior to the pressure packs.

B. Similarly, nasal endotracheal intubation is not contraindicated, since the nasal tube traverses the lower portion of the nasal cavity and will not block the leak. Obviously each case must be appropriately managed on an individual basis. Fiberoptic intubation is recommended to assist in proper tube placement.

VI. A thorough eye examination must be done in all patients, particularly in those with suspected zygomatic and maxillary injuries.

VII. Teeth in the line of a fracture must be checked. Any that are mobile or show evidence of root fracture or severe crown injury should not be maintained. If erupted, third molars in the area of angle fractures should be considered for removal, since this will permit satisfactory intraoral open reduction to be performed. Third molar removal remains controversial and the choice of treatment should be on an individual case selection.

Mandibular fractures

I. Radiographic assessment of mandibular fractures includes:

A. Lateral oblique and posteroanterior (PA) views of the mandible (good for general appraisal)

B. Reverse Towne's view (particularly good for condylar fractures)

C. Panoramic radiograph (better than oblique and PA views for overall diagnosis)

D. Base view or occlusal view (for judging the symphyseal region)

II. Treatment alternatives for mandibular fractures are:

A. Closed reduction

1. In the dentulous patient, alignment of teeth in proper occlusion and application of maxillomandibular fixation (MMF). Erich arch bars can be used to achieve MMF. If gaps in the dentition exist, firmer Winter arch bar material is helpful for construction of a splint.

2. In the edentulous patient, use of dentures or splints placed via circummandibular wires is appropriate. In certain eden-

tulous mandibles, an external fixator (i.e., Joe Hall Morris) permits stabilization of the fracture without disruption of the tissue in the area of the injury.

B. Open reduction and internal fixation
  1. Intraoral. Most mandibular fractures can be stabilized through an intraoral approach. Nonrigid fixation using wire osteosynthesis and MMF is one technique. Rigid internal fixation (RIF) techniques use plates and/or screws and usually do not require MMF.
  2. Extraoral. This is the most versatile approach to mandibular fractures. However, the presence of a scar and potential nerve injury are major disadvantages. It provides the opportunity to use wire osteosynthesis or RIF techniques.
  3. External fixators. Use of an external fixator (i.e., Joe Hall Morris) can be used for severely comminuted fractures or when an external or intraoral approach is not possible.

III. Considerations in the choice of method include:
  A. Site of the fracture and its position relative to the teeth
    1. A fracture through a dentulous area, especially if it is not displaced, may be treated by closed reduction with arch bars and MMF or with a splint and no MMF. If the fracture is displaced, the treatment of choice may be intraoral or extraoral open reduction with arch bars and MMF, with a splint and no MMF, or with RIF and no MMF. Splints may be necessary to establish proper occlusion in patients with severe fractures and in patients with limited or poor dentition.
    2. If the fracture is distal to the last tooth and undisplaced, MMF with arch bars may suffice. Because there are no teeth distal to the fracture, a dental splint is useless. If the fracture is displaced, MMF may be combined with either intraoral or extraoral open reduction; rigid fixation may eliminate the need for MMF.
  B. Degree of displacement and mobility. In general, the greater the displacement and/or mobility of the fracture segments, the greater is the indication for an open as opposed to a closed technique of reduction.
  C. Adequacy of the dentition and occlusion. Closed reduction requires adequate dentition and occlusion. In condylar fractures associated with inadequate posterior occlusion, it may be necessary to use a splint to prevent collapse of the posterior facial vertical dimension, which may lead to anterior open bite if both condyles are fractured.
  D. Type and duration of anesthesia required of a given procedure and the age, condition, and suitability of the patient for a general anesthetic
  E. Requirements imposed by concurrent acute problems, other injuries, or preexisting medical conditions

1. If a mandibular fracture accompanies extensive midface injuries, open reduction of the fracture may be indicated to establish and maintain the facial vertical dimension in treatment of the maxillary injuries.

2. Similarly, in a head-injured patient, treatment may be geared toward more rigid fixation because of the lack of cooperation, abnormal movements, and intensive care and nutritional requirements. Frequent delay in the onset of treatment in this group of patients can lead to a higher complication rate.

F. Patient compliance. Noncompliant patients who may not tolerate a period of MMF are best treated with RIF and no postoperative MMF.

IV. Considerations in formulating a treatment plan include:

A. Condylar fractures (see Algorithm 6)

1. Most condylar fractures are best treated by a conservative approach, closed reduction, and immobilization with MMF, especially if there is malocclusion or pain at the time of the initial examination. If the patient is comfortable and can occlude satisfactorily, a liquid to soft diet may be all the treatment that is needed.

2. If MMF is used, it is maintained for 10–14 da. Then, if the patient is comfortable and able to occlude, physiotherapy is instituted to rehabilitate joint function. A soft diet, analgesics, and local heat are prescribed. If the patient is unable to occlude, continuing MMF for 4–6 wk is not contraindicated. However, this is usually not needed and only adds the problem of limited jaw motion to management.

3. In children, a high condylar fracture can lead to excessive hematoma formation and ankylosis. Therefore, prolonged MMF is contraindicated. Ankylosis can result from involuntary splinting without MMF, and thus physiotherapy must be encouraged.

4. Specific indications for open reduction of a condylar fracture are:

a. Limited jaw motion following MMF that appears to be due to obstruction by a displaced condylar fragment.

b. Anterior and laterally displaced fractured condyles that are outside the fossae.

c. Bilateral fracture with severe midface injuries and loss of vertical dimension. Open reduction is done to reestablish facial vertical dimension.

d. Bilateral fracture in the presence of cervical spine injury requiring brace treatment. The brace may force the mandible posteriorly, and thus open reduction can maintain the jaw position.

e. Failed therapy (i.e., open bite) following closed reduction.

      f. Access to the condyle can be through a preauricular incision or a parotid tumor type incision.

  B. Multiple fractures

    1. Body plus condyle. Because early mobilization is desirable for the condyle, the body fracture should be repaired with a fixation method that does not depend entirely on MMF. Thus, condylar fracture may be an indication for open reduction of a body fracture that, alone, would have been treated by closed reduction and longer MMF.

    2. Bilateral body and body plus angle. In such multiple fractures there can be a tendency toward a "bucket-handle" deformity, because the anterior fracture segment is distracted downward by the infrahyoid muscles. In horizontally unfavorable parasymphyseal fractures there can be inward collapse of the anterior segment with loss of anterior anchorage of the tongue, leading to airway obstruction. In these instances, open reduction with RIF is indicated to resist muscle pull.

  C. Comminuted fractures. Open reduction may involve the risk of detaching fragments of bone from the blood supply. However, if this is done in the presence of RIF, this is not a major concern. Therefore, these fractures can be treated with closed reduction, external fixators, or open reduction with RIF.

V. Postoperative orders for the patient with mandibular fracture(s) include:

  A. Drugs

    1. Pain medications (e.g., meperidine) and antiemetic medications (e.g., prochlorperazine maleate [Compazine]) are used during the immediate postoperative period.

    2. IV fluids and rate based on patient requirement.

    3. Antibiotics are usually used preoperatively and for a short period following stabilization. Penicillin or clindamycin for penicillin-allergic patients is recommended.

  B. Nursing orders for the patient after open reduction of a fractured mandible (condition satisfactory, no allergies) include the following:

    1. Head of bed elevated 30°

    2. Petrolatum to lips

    3. Scissors or wire cutter taped to the bedside when MMF is used

    4. Bed rest with bathroom privileges; ambulation is begun the morning after surgery

    5. High-protein, high-calorie liquid diet; dietary consultation

    6. Deep breathing and coughing exercises

    7. Water-Pik for oral cleansing if MMF is used

    8. Chlorhexidene rinses

    9. Suction setup at bedside

C. Postoperative radiographs should be obtained before discharge.

D. The patient is discharged when his or her condition is stable, afebrile, and taking adequate fluid and nourishment by mouth, and it is determined that a home environment is adequate for care.

E. Fear of vomiting is unwarranted after the initial postoperative period, but the patient should be instructed in how to cut and release MMF. A wire cutter should be at the bedside and with the patient if wire ligatures were needed for MMF.

F. Follow-up should be within 1 wk. Occlusion should be checked, sutures removed, medications reviewed, and the patient reinstructed in hygiene and nutrition.

G. In general, most mandibular fractures show clinical union at 3 wk and should be tested clinically. If the fracture area is firm, a soft diet should be continued through 6 wk with maintenance of arch bars across fracture sites for at least 1 wk after MMF is removed.

Zygomaticomaxillary fractures (see Algorithm 5)

I. General considerations include all those listed earlier.
  A. In addition, a thorough eye examination is a necessity and an ophthalmologic consult is recommended. The examination should include the following:
    1. Pupils should be examined for:
      a. Traumatic mydriasis or pupillary dilation (common findings)
      b. Diplopia, especially in upward gaze, is usually caused by edema or muscle entrapment.
    2. Fundus to rule out hemorrhage and papilledema; the latter is not an acute finding of increased intracranial pressure
    3. Full extraocular motions
    4. Presence of subconjunctival hemorrhage
    5. Lacrimal drainage system for signs of epiphora
    6. Presence of enophthalmos or exophthalmos
    7. Gross vision
  B. Palpation for bony injuries—intraoral and extraoral, including infraorbital, frontozygomatic, buttress, and nasal fractures—is performed.
  C. The presence of infraorbital paresthesia is documented and recorded.
II. Radiographic assessment includes:
  A. Skull films (PA and lateral) for general appraisal
  B. Waters' views to check the antrum and zygomas
  C. "Jug-handle" (submentovertex) views for the zygomatic arches
  D. Tomograms or CT scans, particularly for blowout orbital fractures

E. CT will be used in preference to tomography and plain radiographs in many institutions

III. Treatment is, realistically, a clinical judgment based on experience and the problem at hand.

A. Most fractures of the middle third of the facial skeleton can be managed by internal fixation.

B. Treatment alternatives for zygomatic fractures include the following:

1. Gillies approach—based on the anatomic location of the temporalis fascia; this is an excellent technique for reduction of a fractured zygomatic arch and also for reducing a stable fracture of the body of the zygoma. In the latter instance, an additional incision is required to stabilize the zygoma. Although the radiographic appearance of rotation or displacement on a Waters' view may be of value in determining stability preoperatively, this is not always possible.

2. Eyebrow approach—this technique permits access to the medial aspect of the zygoma, with excellent leverage for reduction. A Rowe elevator or urethral sound is placed medial to the zygomatic arch. This approach also permits wiring or placement of a bone plate at the frontozygomatic suture for stability.

3. Supratarsal fold—this approach provides access to the frontozygomatic suture with a cosmetic result.

4. Infraorbital approach—this provides direct access for transosseous wiring of the fractured infraorbital rim. It has largely been displaced by the infraciliary approach, which is more cosmetic. The infraorbital approach is used when a laceration already exists in the skin beneath the eye.

5. Infraciliary approach—this provides excellent access to the infraorbital rim and the orbital floor. However, ectropion can be a serious complication.

6. Conjuctival approach—this provides a very cosmetic result, but it has limited access. If combined with a lateral canthal extension (canthotomy), the infraorbital rim, floor, and frontozygomatic suture can be visualized and treated.

7. Intraoral approach—this is placed in the buccal sulcus and the instrument remains beneath the zygoma and/or arch; it must not enter the sinus. This approach is used for RIF of the buttress area.

8. Transantral approach—elevation of the zygoma is accomplished through the antrum. This approach also can be used for assessment of the orbit. Antral packing may support the reduced zygoma, or an inflated Foley catheter balloon can be used. Again, there is limited access for direct wiring of an unstable fracture. Care must be taken to avoid displacement of bony floor fragments into the globe.

9. Hemicoronal incision—in severely displaced ZMC fractures with comminuted arch fractures, this approach provides excellent visualization for excellent reduction and RIF.

C. Unstable fractures of the zygoma are treated by the following:

1. Tranosseous wiring or miniplate fixation. Stabilization can be done at the buttress, infraorbital rim and/or frontozygomatic suture. RIF is generally utilized. The number of points fixated is dependent on fracture displacement and stability. This can be achieved by the eyebrow or infraciliary approach.

2. Kirschner rod—this has limited usefulness, since other, more precise methods are available, but it may have a place in certain instances. The rod is inserted from the contralateral antrum into the medial cortical bone of the fractured zygoma. The bone must be held in proper position so as not to cause overreduction.

3. Packing support—rarely will a reduced fractured zygomatic arch be unstable. In that instance, a stab incision over the arch permits placement of rubber or gauze packing for lateral stabilization.

D. Blowout fractures of the orbital floor, which commonly occur with fractures of the middle third of the facial skeleton, are controversial in terms of the need for and timing of repair.

1. A pure blowout fracture of the orbit is an isolated injury. Although the majority of orbital floor injuries occurring in conjunction with other fractures heal very well when treated as part of the other injuries, a pure blowout injury deserves special attention.

2. Relative indications for exploration of the blowout injury are as follows:

   a. It is not an emergency, unless there is retrobulbar hemorrhage or emerging proptosis and pain.

   b. Clinical examination shows limitation of upward gaze and a positive forced duction test.

   c. Observation alone may show resolution of the diplopia.

   d. Entrapment of the globe can be demonstrated at forced duction testing after local anesthesia of the globe. The tendon of the inferior rectus is grasped with forceps, and attempts to rotate the globe superiorly encounter resistance in a positive test.

   e. There is radiographic evidence of herniation of the orbital contents, using CT scanning or tomography.

   f. Enophthalmos >2 mm is often directly observable and not amenable to reconstruction later.

3. Studies show that such signs and symptoms of blowout fracture may result from edema and not from true entrapment of the inferior rectus muscle. Usually such edema re-

solves within 5–7 da, and the patient should be reevaluated at that time.

   a. If indications for exploration still exist, an infraciliary approach permits adequate exposure and insertion of a bone graft (autogenous or bank bone) or alloplastic materials.

   b. Intraoperative steroids are recommended, and care should be taken not to place too much pressure on the globe during the procedure.

  E. Treatment alternatives in maxillary fractures may include no fixation, which is usually done only for minimal injuries or in elderly patients without gross bony displacements, who are considered to be poor risks.

IV. Postoperative care of the patient is as follows:

  A. When there are no other injuries, the same orders as for mandibular fractures apply to zygomaticomaxillary injuries. In addition, the use of oxymetazoline (Afrin) nasal spray, pseudoephedrine (Sudafed) tablets, and sinus precautions will reduce sinus symptoms. Sinus precautions consist of no nose blowing, no use of straws, and no smoking, all of which can place a negative pressure on the maxillary sinus.

  B. The use of iced saline sponges is most effective in limiting periorbital edema and ecchymosis.

  C. A tongue blade or a bent finger splint taped over the injured side is most effective in reminding the patient and the nursing staff that the patient should not lie on the side of the treated fracture.

Nasal Fractures

  I. A thorough history is obtained

 II. The clinical examination must include:

  A. Skin for lacerations, intercanthal distance

  B. External bone and cartilage for asymmetry, crepitus, swelling, tenderness

  C. Intranasal-mucosal tears, CSF leaks, septal hematoma, septal deviation

  D. Associated injuries

III. Radiographs. Most nasal fractures are difficult to confirm by radiographs. A lateral nasal radiograph may be helpful.

IV. Treatment

  A. Unilateral and bilateral fractures can be treated in the emergency room.

  B. Lacerations should be closed.

  C. Unilateral fractures treated with septal and external local anesthetics. The fracture is reduced and the nose is packed. An external splint (i.e., Aquaplast) is placed. Packing is removed in 3–5 da. The splint is removed in 5–7 da.

  D. Bilateral fractures with or without telescoping segments may require general anesthetic or sedation in conjunction with local anesthetics. The bony segments and the septum are reduced and intranasal and extranasal splints are placed.

E. Serious comminuted nasal fractures may require bone grafts with open reduction.

Le Fort I, II, and III and nasoethmoidal fractures
(see Algorithm 7)

I. Clinical examination
   A. The entire midface is examined for signs of swelling, bony mobility, asymmetry, malocclusion, infraorbital paresthesia, flattened bridge of the nose, subconjunctival hemorrhage, CSF leak, and widened intercanthal measurement.
   B. The patient should be carefully evaluated for associated injuries (e.g., neurologic or ophthalmologic).

II. Radiographs
   A. Plain radiographs include lateral and PA skull, submental vertex view, Waters' view, and panoramic radiograph.
   B. CT scans are very useful in identifying the injuries and assist in treatment planning.

III. Treatment
   A. Le Fort I fractures are with MMF to reestablish occlusion and stabilization of the fracture with wire osteosynthesis and MMF or RIF and no postoperative MMF.
   B. Le Fort II and III fractures are treated with MMF to reestablish occlusion and wire suspension with MMF or open reduction with wire osteosynthesis/wire suspension and MMF or open reduction with RIF and no MMF
   C. Severe Le Fort II and III fractures often require broad exposure to reestablish facial dimensions. This is best approached through a coronal flap incision.
   D. Nasoethmoidal fractures are most often treated with open reduction.
      1. Approaches can be through an open sky incision or a coronal flap.
      2. Repositioning of the medial canthal ligament is critical. This can be done with wire, bone plates and screws, or external nasal splinting. In general, the best results are obtained with open reduction and stabilization with wires and/or RIF.
      3. In severe comminution, primary bone grafts may be required.

GENERAL REFERENCES

American College of Surgeons: *Advanced trauma life support*, Chicago, 1993, American College of Surgeons.

Andreasen JO: *Traumatic injuries of the teeth*, Copenhagen, 1972, Munksgaard.

Assael LA ed: Trauma, *Oral Maxillofac Surg Clin N Am* 2:1, 1990.

Bell WH ed: *Modern practice in orthognathic and reconstructive surgery,* vols 1-3, Philadelphia, 1992, WB Saunders.

Ellis E, Zide MF: *Surgical approaches to the facial skeleton,* Baltimore, 1995, Williams & Wilkins.

Haug RH ed: Midface Trauma I. In. *Atlas of oral and maxillofacial surgery,* 1993, Philadelphia, WB Saunders.

Haug RH ed: Midface Trauma II. In. *Atlas of oral and maxillofacial surgery,* Philadelphia, 1994, WB Saunders.

Kaban LB: *Pediatric oral and maxillofacial surgery,* Philadelphia, 1990, WB Saunders.

Peterson LJ, Indresano AT, Marciani RD, Roser SM eds: *Principles of oral and maxillofacial surgery,* vols 1, 2, Philadelphia, 1992, JB Lippincott.

Rowe NL, Williams JL: *Maxillofacial injuries,* Edinburgh, 1994, Churchill Livingstone.

Worthington P, Evans JR, eds: *Controversies in oral and maxillofacial surgery,* Philadelphia, 1994, WB Saunders.

Odontogenic Infection

13

R. BRUCE DONOFF

GENERAL CONSIDERATIONS

I. The extension of dental decay to the pulp chamber of a tooth or the presence of periodontal disease may give rise to signs and symptoms of infection. Most commonly, toothache, pain on mastication, or sensitivity to hot and cold are the presenting complaints and are usually treatable in an outpatient setting.

II. Another common odontogenic infection is pericoronitis, a purulent inflammation associated with a partially impacted wisdom tooth.

III. Management of these problems becomes complicated when the signs of generalized infection occur. This chapter discusses the management of localized dental infection, emphasizing the care of the patient who has a more serious odontogenic infection occurring with generalized symptoms. The bacteriology, use of antibiotics, and management of patients with specialized infections are also discussed.

INFECTIOUS PROCESSES
Localized abscess

I. Pain associated with a decayed tooth or a tooth that has periodontal disease may be associated with swelling. Radiographs usually demonstrate either a periapical lucency or a deep pocket. The tooth may or may not be mobile but will be sensitive to percussion in an apical direction.

II. The basic principles of management include obtaining drainage and controlling the bacterial infection with antibiotics. A most important clinical determination is the presence of fluctuant swelling.

A. In the absence of fluctuant swelling, local measures (e.g., pulpectomy or curettage of a pocket) usually provide adequate drainage. Removal of the offending tooth may be indicated, based on clinical or radiographic data, because of the inability to rebuild the tooth or the degree of bony destruction. Judicious use of the proper antibiotic is required to prevent sequelae due to the presence of infection.

B. If a fluctuant swelling is present, all of the above options exist, plus the possible need to perform an incision and drain the swelling. Abscesses presenting as intraoral swellings usually are found on the buccal aspect of the offending tooth. Incision and drainage with a blade and insertion of a ¼-in gauze drain are simple procedures. However, patient comfort may be improved by the use of nitrous oxide or diazepam (Valium) for sedation, along with the local anesthetic agent. Such adjuncts are recommended because the sole use of a local anesthetic in any surgical procedure in the presence of infection often will be inadequate.

C. The antibiotic of choice in the nonallergic patient is penicillin. Penicillin V is suggested because its use is less affected by the need for patient compliance, in terms of schedule related to meals. Erythromycin, coated to reduce gastrointestinal upset, is used in the allergic patient. Doses required for adequate coverage of localized infections, as described, are 250 mg qid, and treatment for 1 wk is suggested.

D. Controlling a localized infection with antibiotics alone is inadequate and fails to follow the basic tenets of treatment detailed in A and B above (i.e., the establishment of drainage).

III. Any infection that results in swelling beyond simple buccal or mucosal enlargement or swelling that affects the soft palate, floor of the mouth, or tongue may be serious. Constitutional symptoms of fever, malaise, or chills must also arouse clinical suspicion of a more serious problem.

A. The most important clinical decision to be made is whether the patient's swelling represents an abscess or cellulitis. An abscess demands surgical intervention, whereas cellulitis is best managed medically, at least until signs of abscess formation occur.

B. A conservative approach to the management of the sick patient with an odontogenic infection is most rewarding. Infections are not less serious because they arise from the teeth and supporting structures.

C. Radiographs to diagnose the problem may disclose osteomyelitis. In cases of clinically significant swelling, a CT scan may be informative, suggesting fascial space involvement and directing surgical drainage.

D. The decision to admit such a patient to the hospital must be based on an assessment of systemic toxicity and the adequacy of hydration. Although a temperature of 100° F is not worrisome, a fever up to 102° F and higher may be observed and warrants direct attention.

E. Indications for hospitalization include:
  1. Signs of severity
    a. Fever
    b. Dehydration
    c. Rapid progression of swelling
    d. Trismus

      e. Marked pain

      f. Quality or location of swelling

      g. Elevation of tongue

      h. Swelling of soft palate

      i. Bilateral submandibular swelling—possibility of Ludwig's angina

  2. Symptoms of severity

      a. Marked pain

      b. Malaise

      c. Chills

      d. Difficulty swallowing

      e. Difficulty breathing

  3. Laboratory tests

      a. Elevated temperature ($>101°$ F)

      b. Elevated WBC count ($>10,000$)

      c. A shift to the left on differential count (increase in immature leukocytes)

  4. Associated problems

      a. Diabetes mellitus

      b. Patient taking steroids or other immunosuppressive drugs

      c. Prosthetic valve or other prosthesis

E. Reasons for hospitalization are to provide:

  1. An antibiotic dosage that cannot be achieved orally with patient comfort

  2. Adequate hydration

  3. Relief of pain

  4. Extraoral surgical drainage if indicated

  5. Appropriate monitoring of life-threatening symptoms

F. Admitting orders for the patient include the following:

  1. Medications

      a. D_5W, 1000 ml at 100 ml/hr

      b. Piggyback 6 million U of aqueous penicillin in 500 ml D_5W; give 83 ml q6h

      c. Meperidine (Demerol) 50 mg PO or IM q4h prn.

  2. Procedures

      a. Routine vital signs

      b. Head of bed elevated $30°$

      c. Nothing by mouth

      d. Moist heat to facial swelling

Actinomycosis

I. Infection by *Actinomyces israelii* occurs in the head and neck region. The clinician must always be alert to the finding of "sulfur granules" on incision and drainage. Appropriate cultures must be ordered. The organisms are extremely fastidious, and growth usually takes 4 wk. Clinical suspicion is thus very important. Penicillin is required in a dose of 20 million U/day for an extended time (4–6 mo).

II. Clinically the term "lumpy jaw" is used for this condition. The patient usually has a tender facial swelling that is difficult to distinguish from the swelling of any other odontogenic infection. Chronicity by history will guide the astute clinician to search for the organisms on culture.

Osteomyelitis

I. Infection of bone secondary to odontogenic infection is, fortunately, uncommon. In children the cause is often difficult to determine. Osteomyelitis is a chronic infection, and therefore patients usually do not have acute pain or swelling but rather have insidious discomfort.

II. The diagnosis is made by finding osteolytic areas of sequestrum formation. In the jaws the use of tomography is very helpful in defining the full extent of disease; bone scanning may be helpful in the edentuous patient, but often periodontal disease limits its applicability. This is particularly important in planning the area of surgical debridement.

III. Decortication of the mandible is the treatment of choice. The maxilla is rarely involved. The proper use of antibiotics requires a determination of bactericidal levels based on culture and sensitivity testing. Although high-dose intravenous treatment for 1 mo is suggested, testing often permits such levels to be maintained by combinations of IM and PO penicillin and probenecid (Benemid) to limit renal excretion. The use of external irrigation with antibiotics has neither scientific nor clinical merit.

IV. Work-up of suspected osteomyelitis includes the following:
   A. Clinical examination for exposed bone, the causal tooth, or other disease
   B. Radiographic examination, including tomography, to define the extent of disease properly
   C. Appropriate culture of purulent material and bone from debridement; previous antibiotic treatment may affect results

ODONTOGENIC INFECTION IN THE COMPROMISED HOST

I. Although the vast majority of patients with odontogenic infection usually have mixed infections sensitive to penicillin, odontogenic infections in the patient compromised by chemotherapy often present unusual bacterial and fungal indications.

II. A number of studies of patients receiving chemotherapy for leukemia have shown that gram-negative infections occur in this group. Such patients are usually immunosuppressed by steroids or other antimetabolites, and under these circumstances *Pseudomonas* and *Proteus* infections occur. A higher than usual rate of *Candida* infections also occurs in these patients.

III. The clinician must be astute in recognizing an infection that is completely altered in its presentation because of leukopenia. In a patient whose WBC count is 1000, pericoronitis may appear without opercular swelling or purulence. Careful attention to the re-

Table 13-1 ODONTOGENIC INFECTIONS		
Examination	Normal	Compromised host
Bacteriological	Mixed infection, rarely gram-negative	Increased presence of gram-negative organisms
Clinical	Swelling, pain, pus, fever	Innocuous findings, no pus, often little swelling; may have dark papules of gingiva in *Proteus* infections
Laboratory	Elevated WBC count, fever	Depressed WBC count, often no fever

sponse of the patient to any prescribed antimicrobial is a must. (See Chapter 4.)

IV. A comparison of odontogenic infections in the normal and the compromised host is given in Table 13-1.

TREATMENT PROCEDURES
Antibiotics (Table 13-2)

I. General considerations

  A. Selection of an antibiotic is based on the following considerations:

    1. Antibiotics treat infections, not fever.

    2. One must identify the nature of the infection.

      a. What organ system—history, physical examination, laboratory findings

      b. What organism—Gram stain, culture

    3. The choice of antibiotic depends on

      a. Need to treat specifically (i.e., antibiotic sensitivity testing)

      b. Host factors

        (1) Hypersensitivity

        (2) Organ dysfunction—renal, hepatic

        (3) Immunosuppression

      c. Drug pharmacology

        (1) Route and dose

        (2) Tissue distribution

        (3) Toxicity

        (4) Cost

    4. Reevaluation is needed to look for alteration of flora and superinfection

  B. Disadvantages of antibiotics include the following:

    1. Antibiotics do not prevent infection.

    2. There is inherent drug toxicity.

    3. Patient sensitization may occur.

Text continued on p. 314

Table 13-2 ANTIBIOTICS USEFUL IN TREATING ODONTOGENIC INFECTIONS

	Dose	Clinical considerations and toxicity
Penicillins		
Penicillin	250 mg PO q6h for 7 da	Adequate for most infections
	500 mg PO q6h for 7 da	For more severe infections and infections in patients without toxemia, with diabetes, etc.
	500,000 U IM aqueous, 600,000 U IM procaine, 6–10 million U IV aqueous	For immediate coverage if needed, followed by oral dose schedule; used for severe infections in hospitalized patients; side effects include GI upset with oral treatment; possibility of allergic reaction, urticaria being most common; aqueous penicillin contains 1.7 mEq of potassium per million units; in cardiac patients volume and dose may be important
Methicillin	1 g IM (1 g diluted in 50 ml of sterile saline injected over 15 min q4h)	Penicillinase resistant; used only against penicillinase-producing staphylococci; better agents are available
Oxacillin	0.5–2.0 g q4–6h IV, 0.5–2.0 g q6h IM, 0.25–1.0 g q4–6h PO	Oral absorption unpredictable; oxacillin, dicloxacillin, and nafcillin all more effective than methicillin against nonstaphylococcal gram-positive organisms
Dicloxacillin	0.125–1.0 g q4–6h PO	Oral drug of choice because of its good absorption; good also for sialadenitis of suspected staphylococcal origin

Extended spectrum penicillins

Amoxicillin	0.25–1.0 g q8h PO	Amoxicillin is similar to ampicillin but has superior GI tract absorption; potential advantages are in situations requiring high peak levels or when tid schedule is preferred; amoxicillin equal to ampicillin for pneumococci, streptococci, staphylococci (nonpenicillinase producers), *Neisseria, Hemophilus influenzae, Escherichia coli, Proteus mirabilis*; slightly more effective than ampicillin against enterococci and *Salmonella*
Ampicillin	0.5–2 g q4–6h IV, 0.5–2.0 g q6h IM, 0.25–1.0 g q6h PO	
Amoxicillin clavulanate	0.25–0.5 g q8h PO	May reduce effectiveness of oral contraceptives
Metronidazole	250–500 mg PO qid, 500 mg IV q6h	Presumably an anaerobic-specific antimicrobial

Penicillin alternatives

Erythromycin	250 mg PO q6h, 500 mg PO q6h for 7 da	Adequate for most infections; larger dose for more severe infections or sick patients; not recommended for IM or IV use because of local tissue irritation
Clindamycin	0.6–2.7 g/da IV in 2–4 doses, 300 mg q6–8h IM, 150–300 mg q6h PO	Spectrum similar to that of lincomycin and erythromycin; useful against nonenterococcal gram-positive organisms and most anaerobes (including *Bacteroides fragilis*, which is often resistant to penicillin); diarrhea may occur in 1%–10% of patients and may progress to pseudomembranous colitis due to toxic product of *Clostridium difficile.*

Continued

Table 13-2 ANTIBIOTICS USEFUL IN TREATING ODONTOGENIC INFECTIONS—cont'd

	Dose	Clinical considerations and toxicity
Cephalosporins and cephamycins		
Cephalothin	4–12 g/da IM or IV	Main advantage is its activity against gram-positive cocci, including penicillinase-producing staphylococci, about 95% of *E. coli*, most *Salmonella* and *Shigella*, and many *Proteus mirabilis* and *Klebsiella pneumoniae*; *Enterobacter* and indole-positive *Proteus* species are not sensitive to first-generation cephalosporins but are sensitive to cefamandole and cefoxitin; cephapirin and cephacetrile are similar new drugs
Cefazolin	1–4 g/da IM or IV	More effective against *E. coli*, less effective against staphylococci; main advantages are its higher blood levels, longer halflife, and relative lack of pain with IM use
Cephalexin	0.25–1.0 g q6h PO	Oral drug of choice; cephradine and cefadroxil are similar but more expensive
Second generation		
Cefamandole	1–3 g q4–6h IV, 0.5–1.0 g q4–6h IM	Newer drug with enhanced spectrum against gram-negative organisms, primarily *H. influenzae, Enterobacter,* and indole-positive *Proteus;* less effective against staphylococci and streptococci; unlikely drug for usual odontogenic infections
Cefoxitin	1–2 g q4–8 h IV, 1 g q6h IM	New semisynthetic cephamycin; more resistant to beta-lactamases of gram-negative organisms; not more effective against *Pseudomonas* or most *Enterobacter;* also active in vitro against most anaerobes, including *B. fragilis;* because of its higher cost, its recent use as prophylactic drug in major head and neck surgery does not appear justified

Tetracyclines

Tetracycline	250–500 mg q6h PO	GI toxicity, contraindicated in pregnancy
Oxytetracycline	250–500 mg q6h PO	GI toxicity
Doxycycline	100 mg q12h PO	Excellent absorption; does not accumulate in serum of patients with renal failure
Minocycline	200 mg initially, 100 mg q12h PO	Long acting, but little use in odontogenic infections; main use is in *Nocardia* infections
Chloramphenicol	0.5–1.0 g q6h IV, 0.25–1.0 g q6h PO	Bacteriostatic, effective against wide variety of gram-positive and gram-negative bacteria; drug of choice for *Salmonella* and ampicillin-resistant *H. influenzae*; no use in odontogenic infection but often useful combined with penicillin for prophylactic coverage in facial trauma patient; used intravenously; main toxic effect, aplastic anemia

Aminoglycosides

Streptomycin	0.5–1.0 g q12h IM	Rarely used alone because of rapid development of resistance; based on its synergistic effect, it was earlier used with penicillin against staphylococci
Kanamycin		Because of its ototoxicity and nephrotoxicity, this agent has been largely supplanted by gentamicin
Gentamicin	1–2 mg/kg q8h IV, IM	Effective for *Proteus* and *Pseudomonas* infections resistant to other drugs; reduced dose necessary with impaired renal function
Tobramycin	1–2 mg/kg q8h IV, IM	Less expensive; *Pseudomonas* more sensitive to it; thus should be reserved for serious infections with *Pseudomonas* or gentamicin-resistant organisms

4. Selection may result in resistant organisms, causing:
   a. Superinfection
   b. Alteration of microbial world

II. Penicillins
   A. Numerous studies of the bacteriology of odontogenic infection suggest that better than 95% of the offending organisms are appropriately treated with penicillin. Routine culture and sensitivity are not recommended unless there is clinical suspicion of an unusual causal bacterium. Such situations exist for all extraoral incision and drainage procedures, any compromised host, and any clinically resistant infection.
   B. In general, penicillin, erythromycin, cephalosporin, and clindamycin are most useful. The specific application of each is based on the clinical setting, need for an intravenous or intramuscular route of administration, and potential toxicity.

III. Cephalosporins and cephamycins
   A. Cephalosporins and cephamycins are comparable to the extended-spectrum penicillins. Their advantage lies in their resistance to inactivation by the beta-lactamases produced by staphylococci and many enteric bacteria. There is some cross-reaction (10%–20%) in penicillin-allergic patients. There is no advantage in using a third or fourth generation drug in the treatment of odontogenic infection.
   B. The major use of cephalosporins and cephamycins in odontogenic infection is when it is suspected that an infection, particularly of the salivary glands, is staphylococcal and cloxicillin cannot be used.

IV. Tetracyclines
   A. The tetracyclines were the first true broad-spectrum antibiotic. They are bacteriostatic and active against a wide range of gram-positive and gram-negative organisms, being most valuable in treating mixed infections.
   B. Tetracyclines are the most widely prescribed drug for odontogenic infections and are as good a choice as penicillin.

V. Aminoglycosides
   A. Streptomycin, kanamycin, gentamicin, and tobramycin are discussed only briefly because of their limited need in the treatment of odontogenic infection and other infectious diseases treated by the oral and maxillofacial surgeon. Some knowledge of these drugs are useful.
   B. These drugs share several pharmacologic and therapeutic properties:
      1. They are bactericidal.
      2. They have wide-spectrum activity.
      3. Development of bacterial resistance to them is slow, except for streptomycin.
      4. They have poor GI absorption.
      5. They are nephrotoxic.
      6. They are ototoxic.

Table 13-3   ANTIBIOTIC SENSITIVITY TESTING

Cocci	Rods
Gram positive	
Streptococcus—penicillin	*Actinomyces*—penicillin
Staphylococcus (penicillinase resistant)—penicillins	*Clostridium* (anaerobic)—penicillin
Peptostreptococcus (anaerobic)— penicillin	
Gram negative	
Neisseria—penicillin	*Pseudomonas*—gentamicin, carbenicillin
Veillonella (anaerobic)—penicillin	*Hemophilus*—ampicillin
	Enterobacteriaeceae—aminoglycosides or ampicillin
	Bacteroides (anaerobic)—clindamycin, penicillin

VI. Antibiotic sensitivity testing. Table 13-3 presents the usual organisms of odontogenic infection grouped according to their appearance by Gram stain.

   A. Anaerobic culture method. Special tubes are available and are far better than culturing plates in an atmosphere free of oxygen. Two tubes are used; thus the first swab is placed in a second special tube containing materials, ensuring anaerobic conditions.

   B. The method of Gram staining material is as follows:

     1. Smear the material as a thin transparent film on a clean slide.

     2. Gently heat the slide in a flame to fix.

     3. Flood the slide with an alcoholic solution of crystal violet for 5–10 sec; pour off.

     4. Flood the slide with Lugol's iodine solution for 5–10 sec.

     5. Wash with acetone or acetone-alcohol solution rapidly until the color comes off.

     6. Pass briefly (2–3 sec) under water to wash.

     7. Counterstain with safranin for 5–10 sec and rinse with water.

     8. Dry.

VII. Summary of antibiotics

   A. Standard (narrow-spectrum) antibiotics for penicillin-susceptible organisms:

     1. Penicillin G

     2. Penicillin V

   B. Standard (narrow-spectrum) antibiotics for penicillin-resistant organisms:

1. Methicillin
2. Oxacillin
3. Cloxacillin
4. Dicloxacillin
5. Nafcillin

C. Extended-spectrum antibiotics for penicillin-susceptible organisms:
   1. Amoxicillin
   2. Ampicillin

D. Extended-spectrum antibiotics for penicillin-resistant organisms:
   1. Cephalosporins
   2. Cephamycins

Incision and drainage

I. The important clinical decisions to be made revolve around when to drain and what to drain. Because an abscess represents dead white blood cells, antibiotics do not penetrate this hypoxic area, and surgical drainage is a must.

II. Fluctuance of a swelling (a soft spot within the swelling) is the most reliable physical sign.

III. Appropriate aerobic and anaerobic cultures should be obtained. Culture and sensitivity are requested, as should be cultures for fungi and tuberculous organisms.

Follow-up studies

I. In a retrospective review of 175 admissions for facial infection (158 patients), clinical signs, daily temperature course and WBC count, and all culture data were compiled and analyzed by computer. Follow-up of more than 1 wk was obtained in 103 patients; in most of the remaining patients the dental infection resolved completely and there was no need for follow-up appointments.

A. The average age of the patients was 36.9 ± 17.1 (SD) yr (range 7–95), and the male to female ratio was 1.3 : 1.

B. The average hospital stay was 9.7 ± 9.0 (SD) da (range 1–46).

C. The majority of infections (60%) were odontogenic. Others were related to soft tissues (including salivary glands) (17%), trauma (10%), and irradiation for tumor (8%). Only three followed major elective surgery.

II. Of the 302 cultures taken, 101 were reported as mixed flora, and there were 398 bacterial strains identified.

A. Sensitivity testing was performed in 64 cases. Most infections were composed of mixed aerobic and anaerobic flora.

B. Penicillin (or clindamycin) was the antibiotic of choice in most cases, except for those confined exclusively to the soft tissues, where coverage against *Staphylococcus aureus* was necessary. This was true even when sensitivity testing in vitro showed penicillin resistance.

C. Aerobic gram-negative organisms were uncommon in dental infections (2 of 90 patients) and were best correlated with a long hospital stay (average 21 da). No cases of *Bacteroides fragilis* were identified.

III. The presence of fever (>99.5°F), when combined with clinical suspicion, was the most accurate predictor of both the need for incision and drainage and the success of antibiotic treatment. In clinically similar groups, febrile patients had an 88% chance (71 of 81 patients) of having undergone a productive incision and drainage, whereas afebrile patients had only a 30% chance (7 of 23).

A. After successful incision and drainage, most patients (41 of 45) defervesced within 36 hr and remained afebrile until discharge. There was no difference in short-term follow-up between patients discharged between 12 and 36 hr and those discharged more than 2 da after becoming afebrile. Nine of eleven patients who required readmission had osteomyelitis. There was no difference in the clinical course during follow-up of 40 patients switched to oral antibiotics on the day before discharge, as compared with other patients in the study.

B. The policy is thus reinforced: early admission, incision and drainage for febrile patients with significant clinical signs, discharge of patients after an afebrile period of 24–48 hr.

IV. Although some reports of *Bacteroides melaninogenicus* resistant to penicillin have appeared, this has not been found in our institution. Furthermore, the possible occurrence of *B. fragilis* has not been a problem.

REFERENCES

Chow AW et al: Orofacial odontogenic infections, *Ann Intern Med* 88:392, 1978.

Sabiston CB et al: Bacterial study of pyogenic infections of dental origin, *Oral Surg* 41:430, 1976.

Sanford JP, Gilbert DN, Sande MA. *Sanford guide to antimicrobial therapy.* 1995, Smith-Kline Beecham.

Socransky SS, Gibbons RJ: Required role of *Bacteroides melaninogenicus* in mixed anaerobic infections, *J Infect Dis* 115:247, 1965.

Dental Considerations in Cancer of the Oral Cavity and Oropharynx

14

R. BRUCE DONOFF

GENERAL CONSIDERATIONS

I. The oral cavity consists of the lips, floor of the mouth, oral portion of the tongue, buccal mucosa, upper and lower gingivae, hard palate, and retromolar trigone. The oropharynx includes four areas: the base of the tongue, the tonsillar region, the soft palate, and that portion of the pharyngeal wall between the epiglottic fold and the nasopharynx. Cancer can affect any of these areas.

II. Epidemiology

    A. Incidence

        1. Statistics for the United States in 1981 shows 815,000 new cancer cases; 27,710 (3.4%) of these were oral cancers.

        2. Estimates for 1996 were that 1,359,159 new cancer cases would be diagnosed, of which 29,490 would be oral cancer: 3190 of the lip, 5900 of the tongue, 9100 of the pharynx, and the remainder of the buccal mucosa, salivary glands, etc. Approximately 4% of cases would occur in men, and 2% in women.

        3. Squamous cell carcinoma of the oral cavity was diagnosed in 31,000 Americans in 1992.

        4. About half of the patients afflicted die within 5 years of diagnosis. During the period 1986–91, 36% present as localized, 43% with regional spread, and 9% with distant involvement.

    B. Histologic types

        1. Squamous cell carcinomas represent 91% of all oral cancers. In general, the less-differentiated tumors have a higher incidence of positive lymph nodes and a higher risk of distant metastasis than do low-grade lesions of comparable size and from similar anatomic sites.

            a. The local and regional control of squamous cell carcinoma by radiation therapy is not affected much by grade, but the survival rate is lower for a high-grade tumor because of the increased rate of distant metastasis. Although during a course of radiation therapy the response rate or disappearance rate of high-grade lesions is usually more rapid than that of low-grade tumors, the rate of disappearance does not correlate with radiocurability.

b. Tumors that grow in an exophytic pattern usually have a lower rate of lymph node metastasis and are more readily treated by an operation or by interstitial irradiation because their borders are well defined and the chance of missing the margins is lower. These lesions respond better to all treatments.

c. Some carcinomas, generally poorly differentiated, tend to be infiltrative, with fingers of tumor cells beyond the visible or palpable lesion. This pattern is associated with a higher rate of regional lymph node metastasis and is often more difficult to eradicate surgically. Because irradiation portals usually have a generous margin around the obvious lesion, it is less likely that the margins will be missed with radiation therapy; however, control by radiation therapy alone is also less likely to be achieved for this growth pattern than for the more discrete lesions.

d. Another point of importance is differentiating radiation necrosis from recurrent tumor histologically and identifying necrotizing sialometaplasia of the minor salivary glands in irradiated tissue. The opinion of an expert pathologist is a must.

2. Lymphoepithelioma is a carcinoma with a lymphoid stroma. It occurs at an anatomic site that has lymphoid aggregates in the submucosa (e.g., nasopharynx, tonsil, or base of the tongue). It also has a higher rate of cure by radiation therapy than does squamous cell carcinoma.

3. Verrucous carcinoma is often a confusing histologic diagnosis, being described as hyperkeratosis or pseudoepitheliomatous hyperplasia. Because it is an exophytic lesion with an indolent growth pattern, it resembles a wart. Despite reports in the literature of its poor response to radiation therapy, our experience with this modality has been good over long periods of follow-up. If the morbidity of surgery is minimal, surgery remains a first choice of treatment, but radiation is a satisfactory alternative.

4. Spindle cell carcinoma, a squamous cell lesion with intermixed spindle cells resembling sarcoma, occurs in an estimated 2%–5% of malignant specimens taken from the upper digestive tract. The degree of spindle cell component varies. Most important, there are no data to suggest that this histologic type is important in treatment decisions.

5. Leukemias and lymphomas:
   a. Leukemias
   b. Hodgkin's disease
   c. Non-Hodgkin's lymphoma
   d. Multiple myeloma

      e. Burkitt's lymphoma

      f. Midline granuloma

  6. Other cancers of the head and neck:

      a. Malignant salivary gland tumors

      b. Major glands

      c. Minor glands

      d. Malignancies involving the jaw bones

      e. Carcinoma

      f. Metastases

      g. Sarcoma

      h. Ameloblastoma

      i. Maxillary sinus cancer

      j. Giant cell tumors

      k. Laryngeal carcinoma

      l. Nasopharyngeal carcinoma

      m. Malignant melanoma

      n. Skin and lip cancers

C. Age and gender (Tables 14-1 and 14-2)

D. Sites of distribution (percentage by location) of oral cancer include the following*:

Lip, 44.9%
Oral tongue, 16.5%
Floor of mouth, 12.1%
Mandibular gingiva, 12.1%
Palate and maxillary gingiva, 4.7%
Buccal mucosa, 9.7%

E. Mortality. Cancer is the second major cause of death, after heart disease, nationwide. The age-adjusted mortality rate per 100,000 population in 1978–79 from all cancers was 216.9 for men and 132.7 for women, and from oral cancers alone it was 5.8 for men and 1.9 for women.

III. Etiology and predisposing factors

  A. Tobacco

  B. Alcohol and cirrhosis

  C. Leukoplakia. Although hyperkeratotic lesions have traditionally been thought of as clinically suspicious, recent reviews (Tables 14-3 to 14-6) suggest some association with carcinoma, but not an overwhelming one. Based on these data, white lesions should be managed by observation and periodic biopsy, not by aggressive surgery.

  D. Erythroplasia (erythroplakia)

    1. The red, or red and white, oral mucosal lesion is far more likely than the solely white lesion to manifest a dysplastic or malignant change or to transform itself into one of these pathologic states.

---

*Data from MD Anderson Hospital.

Table 14-1   AGE AND SEX DISTRIBUTION OF ORAL CANCER*

Age (yr)	Male	Female
<19	1	1
20–39	3	5
40–49	12	14
50–59	29	27
60–69	30	24
>70	25	29

*Based on cancers diagnosed and/or treated during the period 1969–71 in seven metropolitan areas and two states.

Table 14-2   AGE AND SEX INCIDENCE OF ORAL CANCER PER 100,000 POPULATION

Age (yr)	Male	Female
40–49	11	4
50–59	29	9
60–69	43	11
70–79	49	12
>80	59	20

Same basis as in Table 14-1.

Table 14-3   LEUKOPLAKIA ASSOCIATED WITH CARCINOMA

Site of carcinoma	No. of patients	No. with leukoplakia (%)
Buccal mucosa	35	8 (23)
Gingival (alveolar) mucosa	43	9 (21)
Lip	249	38 (15)
Tongue	261	37 (14)
Floor of mouth	126	17 (13)
Oropharynx	160	18 (11)
Total	874	127 (15)

From Chierici G, et al. *J Oral Med* 23:91, 1968.

Table 14-4   MALIGNANCIES AND PREMALIGNANT CHANGES IN BIOPSY SPECIMENS CLINICALLY DIAGNOSED AS LEUKOPLAKIA

Source (country), year	No. of patients	Findings (%)
Renstrup (Denmark), 1963	185	Carcinoma (3)
		Dysplasia (12)
Waldron (U.S.), 1975	3256	Carcinoma (3)
		Dysplasia (17)
Banoczy (Hungary), 1976	500	Carcinoma (10)
		Dysplasia (24)
Hahn (Germany), 1961	152	Carcinoma (10)
Silverman (U.S.), 1968	117	Carcinoma (10)

Table 14-5   MALIGNANT TRANSFORMATION IN ORAL LEUKOPLAKIAS OBSERVED OVER TIME

Source (country), year	No. of patients	Incidence (%)	Observation period (yr)
Einhorn (Sweden), 1967	782	4.0	1–44
Pindborg (Denmark), 1968	248	4.4	1–9
Kramer (England), 1969	187	4.8	—
Banoczy (Hungary), 1977	670	5.9	1–30
Silverman (U.S.), 1968	117	6.0	1–11

Table 14-6   PROGRESSION IN CLINICAL LEUKOPLAKIA FROM DYSPLASIA TO CARCINOMA

Source (country), year	No. of patients	Cancers (%)	Time (yr)
Mincer (U.S.), 1972	45*	5 (11)	1–8
Banoczy (Hungary), 1976	69†	9 (13)	1–20
Pindborg (Denmark), 1977	21‡	3 (14)	7

*Of these lesions, 38% persisted, 7% disappeared spontaneously, and 44% were excised (about half recurring).

†Of these, 45% were excised (8 of the 9 malignant changes were in the 23 lesions not subjected to surgery).

‡In a control group of 40 dysplasias not associated with leukoplakia, only one became malignant.

    2. Additionally, the differential diagnosis broadens to include candidal and other infections, traumatic ulcerations, and inflammatory disease.

  E. Oral lichen planus. Erosive chronic lichen planus has been associated with carcinoma.

  F. Syphilis

  G. Herpes simplex virus

  H. Dentures. Denture irritation can, at most, be only a carcinogenic cofactor in specifically predisposed individuals. This supposition is based on the fact that more than 35 million Americans over 30 yr of age wear one or two complete dentures, and yet carcinoma of the palate and alveolar mucosa accounts for less than 11% of all oral cancers. Still, the frequently observed denture sore spot must be observed carefully and all attempts must be made to minimize denture irritation.

  I. Dental radiation

  J. Fluoridated water

IV. Diagnosis

  A. Delay in diagnosis

  B. Signs and symptoms:

    1. Ulceration or erosion

    2. Chronicity

    3. Erythema

    4. Lymphadenopathy

    5. Induration

    6. Leukoplakia

    7. Fixation

  C. Biopsy

  D. Exfoliative cytology

  E. Fine needle biopsy

  F. Toluidine blue

V. Spread of tumor (Tables 14-7 and 14-8)

  A. Local extension

  B. Lymphatic spread

  C. Hematogenous spread

  D. Metastases to the mouth

VI. Prognosis

  A. Staging and reporting of end results. The TNM classification system is used as the basis for staging (see the box on page 329):

    1. Stage IT1, N0, M0

    2. Stage IIT2, N0, M0

    3. Stage IIIT3, N0, M0; T1 or T2 or T3, N1, M0

    4. Stage IVT4, N0 or N1, M0; any T, N2 or N3, M0; any T, any N, M1

  B. Cause of death

    1. In a study of 94 deaths at M.D. Anderson Hospital from head and neck cancer, 43 (46%) were due to infection and 12 (12%) to hemorrhage.

Table 14-7   LYMPH NODE PALPATION GUIDELINES

Cause	Texture	Sensitivity	Mobility
Acute infection or inflammation	Soft	Tender	Movable
Malignancy	Firm	Nontender	Movable or fixed

Table 14-8   DISTRIBUTION OF CERVICAL LYMPH NODE METASTASES IN 1155 PATIENTS WITH OROPHARYNGEAL SQUAMOUS CARCINOMA

Site of primary tumor	Percentage of regional lymph nodes involved	Nodal regions most commonly involved	
		First	Second
Nasopharynx	87	Subdigastric	Postcervical
Base of tongue	78	Subdigastric	Midjugular
Tonsillar fossa	76	Subdigastric	Midjugular
Oropharynx	59	Subdigastric	Midjugular
Retromolar pillar	45	Subdigastric	Submaxillary
Soft palate	44	Subdigastric	Midjugular
Oral tongue	35	Subdigastric	Submaxillary
Floor of mouth	31	Submaxillary	Subdigastric

TNM system of classification and staging

T	=	Primary tumor
N	=	Lymph node involvement
M	=	Distant metastasis
TIS	=	Carcinoma in situ
T1	=	Greatest diameter <2 cm
T2	=	Greatest diameter 2–4 cm
T3	=	Greatest diameter >4 cm
T4	=	Massive tumor >4 cm with deep invasion
N0	=	No clinically massive nodes
N1	=	Single clinically positive homolateral node <3 cm
N2	=	Single clinically positive homolateral node 3–6 cm (N2a) or multiple clinically positive homolateral nodes <6 cm (N2b)
N3	=	Massive homolateral node(s), bilateral nodes, or contralateral node(s)
M0	=	No evident metastasis
M1	=	Distant metastasis present

Table 14-9   ORAL CANCER END RESULTS IN 1570 CASES (% OF 5-YR SURVIVAL RATES)

Tumor site	Cancer stages			
	I	II	III	IV
Hard palate	93	40	16	8
Oral tongue	90	64	34	6
Soft palate	73	48	32	5
Buccal mucosa	72	61	42	0
Floor of mouth	68	70	50	9
Mandibular gingiva	64	49	37	10
Maxillary gingiva	62	64	36	29
Posterior tongue	50	44	26	1

2. Hypercalcemia may occur in advanced head and neck cancers and complicates management by causing gastrointestinal complaints, confusion, and dehydration.
3. Carcinomatosis is an infrequent cause of death.
4. Distant spread occurs in over 10% of patients.

C. Table 14-9 demonstrates the importance of detection at an early stage in reducing mortality. These data further document an improved survival rate for localized as compared with advanced metastatic disease. Increased survival was noted when the figures for 1969-73 were compared to those for 1942-66, reflecting advances in treatment techniques rather than increases in detection at an early stage.

MANAGEMENT PROCEDURES

I. Surgery and radiation are the only curative treatment for carcinoma arising in the head and neck. Chemotherapy used alone is not curative, and its role as an adjunct to surgery or radiation, or both, is under investigation. The decision as to which modality to use depends on such factors as the functional and cosmetic results, the general stage of the patient's health, and the preference of the patient and his or her family.

II. Primary lesion
   A. Surgery. Given comparable cure rates, the following represent advantages of surgical intervention:
      1. A limited amount of tissue is exposed to treatment.
      2. Treatment time is shorter.
      3. The risk of immediate and late radiation complications is avoided.
      4. Irradiation can be reserved for a subsequent head and neck primary tumor that may not be treatable by surgery. (The need for irradiation in this situation is quite low.)

5. Pathologic examination may show more extensive involvement, which may then be treated by immediate irradiation.
B. Radiation. The following are the advantages of radiation treatment (assuming comparable cure rates):
1. The threat of a major operation can be avoided. Even though operative mortality is only 1%–2%, this may appear high because there is no immediate threat from radiation therapy.
2. No tissues are removed.
3. Elective irradiation of the lymph nodes can be included with little added morbidity, whereas if surgery is the primary modality one must either monitor the neck for disease or perform an elective neck dissection.
4. The salvage of failed irradiation by surgery is more likely to succeed than the salvage of a surgical failure by reoperation or irradiation, or both.
5. Multiple primary lesions can be treated simultaneously.
III. Cervical lymph nodes
A. The incidence of subclinical disease in the regional lymphatics when the neck is clinically negative ranges from 16%–54%, and the risk of subclinical disease for any single primary lesion may be estimated by the size (or T stage) and the differentiation of the lesion. Nasopharyngeal and supraglottic lesions are exceptions to this rule.
B. To avoid unnecessary intervention, a policy of "wait and see" may be followed for the N0 neck, and treatment may be started later (often successfully) if clinically positive nodes appear. However, even though such a policy may prove successful, these patients are at an increased risk of distant metastasis and have a poorer prognosis. Elective neck treatment is therefore indicated when the associated morbidity is low; also, it has the added advantage, because of its high success rate, of eradicating the lesion initially and thereby simplifying follow-up examinations.
C. Management of the clinically negative neck is as follows:
1. Radiation treatment
a. There is a large volume of data supporting the success of radiation therapy in eradicating subclinical diseases of the regional lymphatics. Given the presumed 25% overall risk of subclinical disease in the regional lymph nodes, the efficacy of neck irradiation is 90%.
b. If the primary lesion is to be treated by irradiation, then elective neck irradiation incurs little or no added cost and little added morbidity. Elective neck irradiation is usually not recommended, however, for small superficial T1 lesions, in which the risk of subclinical disease in the lymph nodes is small, because the portals required for this include a large amount of normal mucosa and the majority of both parotid glands.

2. Elective neck dissection
   a. It is a difficult decision to recommend full radical neck dissection, with the resulting cosmetic and functional losses, unless the potential benefit is considerable. Recent operative modifications reduce this morbidity.
   b. The Bocca operation (or functional neck dissection) preserves the spinal accessory nerve, jugular vein, and sternocleidomastoid muscle and works as well as radical neck dissection for subclinical (N0) disease.
   c. The supraomohyoid neck dissection differs from the Bocca procedure in that the lower internal jugular nodes below the omohyoid muscle are not removed, because of the insignificant risk of metastasis to them in certain oral cavity lesions.
   d. An elective supraomohyoid neck dissection on one or both sides may be better thought of practically as a staging procedure. If the nodes are negative, no further treatment is given. If the nodes are positive, the neck dissection is completed or postoperative radiation therapy is used.
   e. Functional supraomohyoid neck dissection is not sufficient treatment for lesions of the oropharynx because it will miss tumor in the lower neck. It is a more difficult and longer procedure than the standard radical neck dissection.
D. Management of the clinically positive neck is as follows:
   1. Radical neck dissection is satisfactory treatment for the ipsilateral nodes in a patient with N1 or N2a disease.
   2. Radiation therapy is added for other N stages and/or for control of contralateral subclinical disease. Radiation therapy alone is sufficient for lower limit N1 disease but should usually be combined with a neck dissection for upper limit N1, N2a, or N3 disease. In practice, it is always safer to add a neck dissection immediately after radiation therapy, because the detection of neck node recurrence after high-dose irradiation is difficult because of fibrosis. Salvage is generally unsatisfactory.
IV. Combined surgical and radiation treatment
   A. The cure rates for early carcinomas of the oral cavity and oropharynx (T1 and T2) are good. The rates for advanced tumors (T3 and T4) are less satisfactory whether treatment is by surgery alone or by radiation therapy alone. At our institution twice-a-day radiation therapy is used. Early results suggest improvement in T3 tumors. In these more extensive lesions, failures of surgical treatment are usually due to marginal recurrences, whereas failures of radiation therapy are primarily the result of the inability to control either the radioresistant nidus at the primary site or the nodal disease. Therefore, a combined program of surgery and radiation therapy is frequently em-

ployed. This permits surgical resection of gross disease, even when the resection margins are inadequate, followed by irradiation for subclinical or occult disease. Such an approach also allows effective palliation and even occasional cure of many patients who are not otherwise salvageable or who are faced with functionally and cosmetically crippling alternatives.

B. Preoperative radiation therapy
1. The aims of preoperative radiotherapy are to:
   a. Prevent marginal recurrences
   b. Control subclinical disease in the primary site or in the nodes
   c. Convert technically inoperable tumors into operable ones
2. Preoperative irradiation has the theoretical advantage of treating cancer cells in their maximal state of oxygenation.
3. The disadvantages of preoperative radiation therapy are that:
   a. The extent of tumor is obscured at the time of surgery.
   b. There is a delay in the surgery.
   c. There is an increased risk of postoperative complications.
4. Conventional protocol. The dosage used is subcancericidal, consisting of 4500 cGy in 1 mo. Radical surgery follows 1 mo later and is performed as if radiation therapy had not been given. Such an approach is applicable to medium-sized or advanced tumors, which have poor radiotherapeutic or surgical cure rates and are not associated with significant postoperative function and cosmetic morbidity.
5. Postoperative or sequential postradiation resection. Dosage is cancericidal, 6000 to 6500 cGy in 6–7 wk delivered to the primary site as well as to the first-echelon lymph nodes. In contradistinction to the conventional protocol, radiation therapy is followed by limited surgical resection with only the residual nidus of the primary lesion in the muscles and bone excised. This method assumes that the peripheral superficial disease has been controlled by high-dose irradiation.

C. Postoperative radiation therapy
1. The advantages of postoperative radiation therapy are that a higher dosage of radiation can be delivered and the clinician has a better understanding of the known sites of residual disease, as well as the extent of pathologic involvement. The aim of such treatment is to eradicate residual cancer at the resection margin and any subclinical disease implanted in the wound or in the neck nodes.
2. Postoperative radiation therapy is usually performed approximately 3–4 wk after surgery, when the wound has healed. A dose of 5500 cGy at 6 wk is used if the surgery was radical. If the surgery was primarily a debulking proce-

dure, high-dose radiotherapy for gross residual disease must be given.

D. Radiation effects:
  1. Mucocutaneous changes
  2. Loss of taste
  3. Loss of salivary function
  4. Nutritional deficiencies
  5. Dental caries
  6. Candidiasis
  7. Osteoradionecrosis (Table 14-10)
     a. The incidence of osteoradionecrosis varies depending on the reporting institution, aggressiveness of radiotherapy, and follow-up time.
     b. The risk of spontaneous osteoradionecrosis is somewhat unpredictable but is related to the dose of radiation delivered. The risk is increased even more in dentulous patients if teeth within the treatment field are removed after therapy.
     c. Careful attention to the teeth in the line of proposed therapy is most important, but extractions are not the only method of preventing sequelae. (See "Dental management of the oral cancer patient," p. 339.)
  8. Soft-tissue necrosis

V. Chemotherapy
  A. Carcinoma of the oral cavity and oropharynx represents a continuing challenge to and frustration for the medical oncologist. At present, the role of chemotherapy remains to be defined; its impact on long-term survival is negligible. There is a need to find ways of improving local and regional control, avoiding deforming surgical procedures, reducing the incidence of distant metastases, treating recurrences when surgery and radiation therapy are no longer an option, and reducing the dose of radiation and risk of complications. The medical oncologist is referred patients who have advanced cancer on initial presentation or who have received surgery or radiation therapy, or both. They are elderly, cachectic, depressed, and desperate. Accordingly, data on the use of single agents and combination treatments are difficult to interpret.
  B. Drugs. Some studies of single agents suggest a modicum of success. There is no evidence that long-term survival is affected. Drugs most often used are:
     1. Methotrexate
     2. Bleomycin
     3. Cisplatin
  C. Combination chemotherapy. The response rates to combination regimens are better than those to single-agent regimens, especially in previously untreated patients. It is unclear, however, what impact these improved response rates will have on survival.

Table 14-10 REPORTED INCIDENCES OF OSTEONECROSIS IN PATIENTS IRRADIATED FOR HEAD AND NECK CANCER

Hospital	No. of patients	Years	Dose (cGy)	Cases (%)
M.D. Anderson	381	1966–71	6000–7500	54 (14)
Geisenberger	108	1948–60	5000–9500	10 (9)
Swedish	104	1939–51	4000–8500	6 (6)
Westfield	491	1940–57	4000–18,000	26 (5)
University of California	278	1961–69	5000–7000	10 (4)
Roswell Park	47	1968–72	3600–12,900	2 (4)

D. Combined modality treatment. Theoretically, the use of chemotherapy as a first treatment might control the primary site and
downgrade the primary lesion, sensitize the tumor to radiation
effects, create a situation in which a less extensive operation
was required, and reduce the risk of distant metastases. Studies
to date have failed to substantiate any of these in humans. Currently, better designed trials using more potent agents (e.g., cis-
platin) are under way.

VI. Specific considerations

A. Lip

1. Because radiation therapy and surgery yield equally high
cure rates for small limited cancers, the selection of treatment depends on the cosmetic result following the procedure. Surgery is also preferred for extensive cancer associated with bone involvement and for significant soft-tissue
involvement requiring major reconstructive surgery.

2. Radiation therapy is best for:

a. Superficial lip cancer involving more than one third of
the entire lip

b. Cancer involving the commissure and upper and lower
lips

c. Recurrent tumor

d. The patient who refuses surgery

3. Radical neck dissection with adjuvant radiation therapy is
needed for metastatic nodes, but prophylactic or elective
neck dissection or irradiation for the N0 neck is not indicated. Low-grade lip cancers rarely metastasize, and subsequent nodal metastases are also rare. Therapeutic neck dissection results are comparable to prophylactic dissection
results for occult nodes. Thus, the small group of patients in
whom metastases develop can still be cured and the majority spared of an operation.

B. Oral tongue

1. Management of carcinoma of the oral tongue is controversial and depends on the size, location, and growth pattern,
as well as the nodal status.

2. For T1 and T2 lesions, both surgery and radiotherapy are effective.

a. Small lesions can be satisfactorily treated by transoral resection, without resulting functional morbidity. This is
particularly true in older patients, who tolerate prolonged curative radiation therapy less well. Radiation
therapy is preferred for small, posteriorly situated, poorly
defined lesions, which are more difficult to approach for
surgical excision.

b. Large, superficial, exophytic T1 and T2 lesions without
much muscle involvement can be treated by radiation therapy, with high control rates and excellent cosmetic results.

c. Medium-sized tumors with involvement of the adjacent
floor of the mouth are well treated by comprehensive ra-

diation therapy to the primary site and neck nodes, with surgery reserved for salvage of residual or recurrent disease. Primary surgical treatment in these cases would have to include partial glossectomy, partial mandibulectomy, and radical neck dissection.

3. For T3 and T4 lesions with deep muscular invasion and often associated nodal metastases, a combination of radiation therapy and surgery is best.

C. Floor of the mouth

1. Obstruction of Wharton's duct may cause enlargement of the submaxillary gland, which can mimic nodal involvement. In T1 lesions nodal metastases are low, but T3 and T4 lesions are associated with a high incidence of node involvement, which may be bilateral. Evaluation of the extent must include inspection for involvement of the undersurface of the tongue and adjacent gingiva. Normal mucosa over the mandible without fixation almost always precludes mandibular involvement. Dental radiographs are best for showing bone involvement.

2. Small tumors limited to the mucosa are highly curable by radiation therapy alone. T2 and early exophytic T3 lesions may receive a trial course of radiation. If a good response is obtained, treatment should be completed and salvage surgery may be considered for residual disease at the primary site and neck nodes.

3. When the adjacent mandible is thought to be involved, surgical excision with a rim of normal inner border of the mandible is indicated, followed by postoperative radiation therapy. Large T3 and T4 lesions with marked involvement of adjacent tissue require combined radiation therapy and surgery as a composite resection. The irradiation may be preoperative or postoperative.

D. Retromolar trigone and anterior pillar can be treated by either radical surgery or radiation therapy.

1. Superficial T1 and T2 lesions are treated by radiation therapy, with surgery reserved for salvage.

2. Large infiltrating lesions (T3 and T4) with or without metastatic nodes are treated by combined high-dose, limited-field irradiation and composite resection.

E. Buccal mucosa

1. Small T1 lesions with well-defined margins can be treated by surgical removal. The lesion as well as adjacent suspicious tissue will be eradicated.

2. T2 lesions are well treated by radiotherapy, with good functional and cosmetic results.

3. T3 and T4 lesions with deep muscular invasion are poorly treated by radiation therapy. En bloc excision of the primary and regional lymph nodes is the treatment of choice.

4. Verrucous carcinoma has been discussed previously.

F. Gingivae. Treatment depends on the extent of the lesion, the status of the lymph nodes, and the presence or absence of bone involvement. Panorex or polytomes of the mandible are a minimal workup for bone involvement.

1. Small T1 exophytic lesions without bone involvement can be treated by radiotherapy alone.

2. Large lesions (T2 and T3) require high-dose radiation, and local control of disease is poor. The risk of osteoradionecrosis is high. Therefore, advanced lesions associated with destruction of the mandible with or without metastases should be treated by radical surgery. Good survival rates are obtained with partial mandibulectomy and radical neck dissection.

G. Soft palate

1. Surgical resection of the carcinoma of the soft palate is unsatisfactory and often results in marginal recurrences. Even when surgery is successful, the effects on swallowing and speech are unacceptable.

2. T1 and T2 exophytic mucosal tumors should be treated by radiation therapy.

3. Advanced T2 and T3 lesions are often associated with nodal involvement, and radiation therapy is given first for cure, with residual disease treated by local resection. Surgical resection for nodal involvement, even if bilateral, is indicated if control of the primary tumor can be achieved by irradiation. Chemotherapy with or without radiation therapy may offer some degree of palliation.

H. Hard palate

1. The hard palate is the most common site of occurrence of minor salivary gland tumors. Squamous cell carcinoma is rare and generally ulcerative with invasion of bone. There is a low incidence of nodal involvement.

2. Early lesions without bony involvement can be treated by radiation therapy, with surgery reserved for salvage.

3. Advanced, deeply ulcerated, infiltrative lesions with bone destruction are best treated by combined radiation therapy and surgery, with prosthetic rehabilitation of the defect.

I. Tonsil

1. Radiotherapy gives excellent results for T1 and T2 lesions, with far less functional and cosmetic morbidity than results from surgery.

2. Advanced tumors of the tonsil (T3 and T4) with invasion of the base of the tongue are rarely curable by either radiation therapy or surgery alone and should be managed by combined methods.

J. Base of the tongue

1. A high percentage of patients with this type of tumor have nodal involvement. Aggressive primary surgery is extremely mutilating and often followed by marginal recurrence and nodal disease.

2. T1 and T2 lesions are radiosensitive and curable by radiation therapy alone, with results comparable to those achieved by surgery.
3. Large infiltrative (T3 and T4) lesions are rarely curable by single-modality treatment. Combined high-dose radiation therapy and limited surgery offer the best treatment.
4. For totally inoperable lesions, palliative irradiation or chemotherapy is all that can be offered.

K. Pharyngeal wall
1. Early lesions are extremely rare and can be controlled by either surgery or radiation therapy.
2. Advanced tumors with nodal disease require combined therapies. Surgical procedures usually require laryngopharyngectomy with or without esophagectomy and radical neck dissection. Despite aggressive approaches, the ultimate prognosis is poor.

Dental management of the oral cancer patient

I. Problems arising in the dental management of the oral cancer patient are most often related to needed treatment procedures rather than to the malignancy itself.
II. Radiotherapy and chemotherapy are the modalities most often associated with dental and oral complications, which can include:

Mucositis
Kerostomia
Radiation caries
Osteoradionecrosis

Management of the Irradiated Patient

I. Radiation-induced oral complications can occur in:
A. Mucosa. A transient mucositis results from the direct effect of radiation on the mucosa; however, xerostomia resulting from radiation-damaged salivary glands and direct injury of bone tend to be more permanent complications.
B. Enamel. Radiation caries is thought to be not so much a direct effect of radiation on enamel as the result of a lack of natural cleaning activity associated with a dry mouth.
C. Bone. Because of its high mineral content, bone absorbs more energy than do soft tissues. This phenomenon may account for the osseous damage that occurs when soft-tissue malignancies are irradiated and also is responsible for the most severe dental complication arising from radiotherapy—osteonecrosis.
II. Osteoradionecrosis is an infection of irradiated bone that leads to pain, bone loss, functional disability, and cosmetic disfigurement.
A. The chief features are exposed bone and pain arising from either the bone itself or adjacent soft tissues that have been irritated by contact with devitalized bone. Radiation parameters that influence the occurrence of osteoradionecrosis are:

1. Quality and quantity of radiation. Before the 1960s, ortho-voltages were generally used in the treatment of oral malignancy. Such radiation was associated with a 17%–37% incidence of osteoradionecrosis. With the advent of megavoltage units, the incidence of osteoradionecrosis declined, from 2% to 5%. As a result, megavoltages have come to be perceived as "bone sparing." Doses in excess of 5000 cGy are not uncommon, yet at this level of exposure, death of bone cells and a progressive obliterative arteritis (endarteritis, periarteritis, hyalinization, fibrosis, and thrombosis of vessels) result. The consequences of cellular death are an aseptic necrosis of the portion of bone directly in the beam of radiation, with compromised vascularity in the adjacent bone. Although the irradiated bone may function normally, when microorganisms gain entry via mucosal ulcerations, the result is lacerations, scaling of teeth, compound fractures, periodontal disease, and infection necessitating endodontics or exodontics.

2. Size of portals. Portal size, dose fractionation, meticulous collimation, and shielding of normal tissues are now recognized as variables that are important in defining the risk of radiation-related oral complications. The use of intraoral cone delivery of radiation minimizes exposure of normal tissues and permits greater conservation of teeth.

3. Location and extent of lesion. The mandible is associated with a higher incidence of osteoradionecrosis than is any other bone. This is probably explained by the fact that most oral tumors are perimandibular and susceptibility is increased by the dense mandibular cortical plates, with less extensive vascular network than exists in the maxilla.

4. Condition of the teeth and periodontium. Establishing and maintaining the health of the dentition dramatically diminish the likelihood of radiation-induced complications. Guidelines for establishing and maintaining dental health are discussed later.

B. Methods for managing the patient with osteoradionecrosis are beyond the scope of this presentation; instead, we will limit ourselves to methods of preirradiation and postirradiation dental care that minimize the possibility of developing osteoradionecrosis. The following guidelines have been promulgated on the basis of collected clinical documentation and clinical and basic research; however, it should be recognized that the subject remains controversial.

  1. Guidelines for preirradiation dental care are as follows:

    a. All nonrestorable teeth and teeth with significant periodontal disease in the direct beam of radiation should be extracted before radiation therapy begins.

    b. In patients with poor oral health and poor motivation to maintain oral hygiene, complete extractions are recommended.

    c. Extensive alveoloplasty should be performed to permit a primary mucoperiosteal closure. All sharp bony margins should be smoothed (because irradiated bone will not remodel spontaneously).

    d. To allow initial healing and required restorative treatment, radiation should be delayed 10–14 da.

    e. All remaining teeth should be restored and periodontal treatment completed within this 2-wk interval. Instructions and an opportunity to practice oral hygiene should be provided.

    f. A custom tray is used for application of 0.4% stannous fluoride gel, 1% sodium fluoride gel, or 1% acidulated fluorophosphate gel. After flossing, fluoride treatment should be performed for 15 min twice a day.

2. Guidelines for postirradiation care are:

    a. Dentures should not be used for 1 yr after treatment.

    b. The need for the patient to continue oral hygiene and fluoride therapy should be emphasized.

    c. Saliva substitute can be provided (VA Oralube or Orex) if xerostomia-induced soft-tissue disorders arise. Such saliva substitutes contain minerals and fluoride and may help to reharden tooth surfaces.

    d. If postirradiation pulpitis develops and the tooth is restorable, endodontics with antibiotic prophylaxis should be instituted.

    e. Necessary extractions should be limited to one or two per sitting. Removal should be as atraumatic as possible with trimming only of sharp bone margins and without raising extensive flaps or attempting to obtain a linear closure. Antibiotic prophylaxis is important. Specific antibiotic recommendations are as follows:

        (1) Aqueous penicillin, 1 million U, given intravenously 15 min before surgery, and then oral doses of penicillin V, 500 mg qid for 10 da. The initial oral dose should be given 1 hr after the parenteral dose.

        (2) Alternatively, 1 g penicillin V given orally 1 hr before the procedure and then the same postsurgical regimen as above.

        (3) In patients allergic to penicillin, 1 g erythromycin 1 hr before surgery and then 500 mg qid for 10 da.

Management of patients receiving chemotherapy

  I. In recent years, the use of chemotherapy in managing malignant oral disease has expanded dramatically. Unfortunately, complications arising from such treatment have also increased. Oral morbidity resulting from malignant disease and its chemotherapeutic treatment is a significant and challenging problem, without completely satisfactory solutions.

  II. Pretreatment evaluation

A. Ideally, patients planned for chemotherapy should be completely evaluated by a general dentist. After chemotherapy has begun, it may not be possible to obtain radiographs or to perform other diagnostic procedures, so this initial evaluation provides an important baseline.

B. The circumstances under which chemotherapy patients are evaluated may not be optimal, because such persons may be debilitated even before the initiation of chemotherapy. Typically, the patient may have severe oral pain, limited opening, and accumulated debris or other obstructions. The use of topical anesthetic agents may be helpful in examination.

   1. Baseline and subsequent visits should include both intraoral and extraoral examinations, radiographs, if possible, and selected laboratory studies.

   2. The most important laboratory values are total WBC count, differential analysis (i.e., polymorphonuclear leukocytes [PMNs], lymphocytes, and immature forms), platelet count, bleeding time, PT, and PTT. These and other clotting parameters may be required if contemplated dental treatment will elicit bleeding.

C. After collection of an adequate database, difficult decisions need to be made regarding the type, timing, and aggressiveness of the proposed treatment. An important factor in such planning appears to be the patient's bone marrow status and predicted effects on peripheral blood counts over the next 7–10 da.

D. The need to extract all teeth in patients undergoing chemotherapy is no longer accepted; however, hopelessly nonrestorable teeth should be removed, the remaining teeth cleaned of both supragingival and subgingival deposits, and periodontal therapy instituted for peridontal pockets that the patient will not be able to keep plaque free. Additional dental treatment can then be completed to help ensure an aesthetic, functional, comfortable, and disease-free mouth.

III. Preventive therapy

A. The basic concepts involved in preventing oral complications arising from chemotherapy (i.e., bleeding, infection, pain) are similar to those outlined for the irradiated patient.

   1. Patient education is the first step in any preventive regimen. Meticulous oral hygiene resulting from both the patient's and the dentist's (or hygienist's) efforts greatly minimizes the likelihood of complications.

   2. The patient's blood count will begin to fall after chemotherapy, and professional hygiene measures must be adjusted accordingly. In general, moderately aggressive hygiene measures are appropriate if the patient is not severely myelosuppressed (WBC $>2000/mm^3$, with $>20\%$ PMNs and platelets $>20,000/mm^3$).

   3. Brushing (using a soft brush), flossing, and thorough scaling are desirable. Frequent rinsing also helps to remove debris

and bacteria. The patient's dental appliances can be worn as usual if they fit well and if he or she is closely observed for ulcer formation.

B. Active myelosuppression complicates the situation. Based on clinical impression, it seems that when the patient's total WBC count drops below 1500–2000/mm^3 with <10% PMNs, brushing and flossing should be stopped. This is a subject of controversy, however, because there are no absolute guidelines for assessing safe peripheral blood count levels.

  1. The risk of bacteremia resulting from attempts at hygiene must be evaluated in the context of bacteremias resulting from florid oral disease. In such patients, mouth rinsing and tooth cleansing using a 2 × 2-in sponge can usually be continued.

  2. Because of their ability to provoke bacteremias in an immunosuppressed patient, oral irrigation devices are not advised.

C. Oral bleeding is commonly associated with immunosuppression. Management of the underlying causes for such bleeding is the province of the hematologist; however, the dentist may be consulted on local measures to control bleeding and adjust existing appliances to minimize oral trauma. The incidence of oral bleeding increases exponentially with platelet counts <20,000/mm^3.

D. As observed for irradiated patients, fluoride is of significant benefit in preventing caries. Excellent oral hygiene, low sugar intake, and fluoride rinses can do much to minimize caries.

Management of patients receiving both radiation and chemotherapy

I. It is not uncommon to encounter a patient receiving both of these treatment modalities. Increasingly, patients who have been treated with surgery as well as with radiation and chemotherapy are seen. The basic concepts in management are essentially the same as outlined previously.

II. Some treatment regimens that have proved to be successful are as follows:

A. Individualized fluoride treatment programs can include either of the following:

  1. Brushing at bedtime with a stabilized 0.4% stannous fluoride gel

  2. Nightly rinsing with freshly prepared 0.1% aqueous stannous fluoride

B. Control of intraoral soft-tissue problems

  1. Pain: Dyclonine with diphenhydramine rinses or 2% viscous lidocaine solution

  2. Decreased salivary flow. A specific preparation (e.g., VA Oralube)

GENERAL REFERENCES

MD Anderson Hospital and Tumor Institute: *Neoplasia of the head and neck*, Chicago: 1974, Mosby.

Million RR, Cassisi NJ: *Management of head and neck cancer, a multidisciplinary approach*, Philadelphia, 1984, JB Lippincott.

Randolph VL et al: Combination therapy of advanced head and neck cancer, *Cancer* 41:460, 1978.

Shillitoe EJ et al: Immunoglobulin class of antibody to herpes simplex virus in patients with oral cancer, *Cancer* 51:67, 1983.

Silverman S, ed: *Oral cancer*, New York, 1981, American Cancer Society.

Wang CC: *Radiation therapy for head and neck neoplasms*, Hertfordshire, England, 1983, John Wright & Sons.

Cancer statistics, 1996, *Calif Cancer Clin* 46:3, 1996.

Cysts and Tumors

15

ROBERT CHUONG

GENERAL CONSIDERATIONS

I. Cysts and neoplasms of the maxilla and mandible include a variety of odontogenic and nonodontogenic, epithelial, and mesenchymal lesions. These lesions will be discussed according to their tissues of origin and will be separated into odontogenic and nonodontogenic categories.

II. Clinical features that may be of assistance in the differential diagnosis of jaw lesions include:

   A. History—signs and symptoms, mode of onset, rate of progression, age, other systemic factors

   B. Radiographic features—relative lucency or opacity, definition of borders, unilocular or multilocular outline

   C. Relationship to teeth—contiguity, tooth vitality, tooth displacement, root erosion

   D. Relationship to bony cortex—central or peripheral, or both, cortical expansion or perforation

   E. Location within the jaw—maxilla or mandible, or both, anterior or posterior jaw, inferior or superior to the inferior alveolar canal

   F. Coexistence with other diseases—e.g., giant cell lesions of the jaws with hyperparathyroidism; giant cell lesions with Noonan's syndrome, keratocysts with basal cell nevus syndrome

III. Odontogenic cysts, fissural cysts, odontogenic tumors, and nonodontogenic tumors will be discussed. Emphasis will be on differential diagnosis and treatment planning based on biologic behavior.

JAW CYSTS

I. Odontogenic cysts

   A. Apical and residual cysts

      1. These cysts derive from epithelial rests within the periodontal ligament, which may be stimulated to proliferate by chronic inflammation initiated by pulpal necrosis.

2. The apical cyst is the most common odontogenic cyst. It is attached to the apex of a pulpally compromised tooth and is also known as a radicular cyst.

3. The residual cyst is essentially the same process that is discovered after a tooth has been removed. Distinction between a residual cyst and a primordial cyst of a supernumerary tooth may be impossible.

4. Radiographic appearance of these lesions is typically a well-defined unilocular radiolucency within the alveolar bone.

5. Treatment is enucleation. Endodontic therapy alone may allow involution of a small apical cyst. Recurrence is rare.

B. Dentigerous (follicular) cyst

1. This is an odontogenic cyst that:

   a. Derives from cells of the reduced enamel epithelium after the crown of the tooth has been completely formed.

   b. Is always associated with an unerupted tooth.

   c. Is generally unilocular radiographically; when multiple cysts are encountered, the basal cell nevus syndrome should be considered.

   d. May cause cortical expansion although not perforation.

   e. Is usually associated with impacted mandibular third molars or maxillary canines, since these are the most commonly impacted teeth.

   f. Is a potential site for development of an ameloblastoma; multiple cases of ameloblastoma have been reported arising in the wall of dentigerous cysts. Fewer cases of mural squamous cell carcinoma have been reported. All dentigerous cysts should be carefully examined microscopically for associated neoplastic processes.

2. Treatment includes enucleation and removal of the associated tooth. One must rule out keratocyst. Marsupialization is rarely indicated. Recurrence rates vary with the size and location of the cyst but are usually <5% in most series.

C. Primordial cyst and odontogenic keratocyst

1. The primordial cyst derives from undifferentiated dental lamina and therefore is not associated with a tooth crown. It has a keratinizing squamous lining. All such cysts are keratocysts, but not all keratocysts are primordial.

2. The odontogenic keratocyst

   a. Derives from dental lamina.

   b. Occurs predominantly in the posterior (molar, ramus) areas of the jaws.

   c. Is often multilocular, often grows rapidly, and can induce paresthesia and cortical perforation.

   d. Recurs at a high rate; reported recurrence rates vary (range 10%–65%) depending on size and location of the cyst, treatment, and duration of follow-up. Recurrences may be discovered 10 or more yr after treatment. A high recurrence rate may be related to satellite cysts or to the higher mitotic index seen among the lining cells. Recurrences have been reported in bone grafts.

e. Contains fluid with lower protein content than serum; aspiration may therefore be helpful in preoperative assessment of suspected jaw cysts.

3. The basal cell nevus syndrome should be considered when multiple keratocysts of the jaws are detected. This is an autosomal dominant disease characterized by:

   a. Jaw cysts
   b. Multiple early-onset basal cell carcinomas
   c. Palmar and plantar pitting
   d. Skeletal abnormalities (bifid ribs, vertebral anomalies, pectus excavatum, hypertelorism)

4. Treatment is enucleation. Large or recurrent lesions may require en bloc resection with immediate bone graft reconstruction. Lesions that display aggressive clinical behavior may be best approached as a neoplasm rather than as a typical odontogenic cyst. Use of cauterizing solutions (Carnoy's solution) or excision of the overlying mucosa to minimize the possibility of recurrence has been suggested. Marsupialization is rarely indicated. Close long-term follow-up is essential because recurrences may arise 10 or more yr after initial treatment.

D. Calcifying odontogenic cyst (Gorlin's cyst)

1. This lesion is similar to the calcifying epithelioma of Malherbe and is thought to be of epithelial origin. It has characteristics of both a cyst and a solid tumor.

2. The lesion most commonly affects the mandible (70% of cases). It grows slowly and may involve soft tissue. The large majority (75%) have been central, with the remainder either entirely peripheral or accompanied by superficial bone erosion.

3. It appears typically as a radiolucency containing radiopaque foci.

4. Treatment is enucleation. Recurrence may be due to soft-tissue spread.

II. Nonodontogenic cysts (fissural)

A. General features

1. Fissural cysts form at the junction between developing structures of the face as a result of incomplete involution of epithelial cells. This aberration can result in so-called fissural cysts, which may be either laterally or medially situated. Such lesions occur within bone or soft tissue, or both.

2. Any fissural cyst in the maxilla may contain oral and/or nasal respiratory epithelium.

3. Adjacent teeth are vital and often displaced.

4. Treatment in all cases is enucleation. Recurrence is virtually unknown.

B. Lateral fissural cysts of the maxilla

Osseous Lesions and Related Clinical Findings

	Pain	Paresthesias	Growth rate	Mucosa	Palpation	Radiograph	Special tests and features
Cysts	– (unless infected)	–	Slow		Firm to springy	Circumscribed	Tooth vitality, impacted teeth, multiple Gorlin's
Odontogenic tumors	–	–	Slow	–	Firm to springy	Circumscribed	Ameloblastoma, root resorption, unilocular vs. multilocular
Benign non-odontogenic tumors	–	–	Slow (GCRG is exception)	–	Firm to springy	Circumscribed	Central giant cell reparative granuloma, AV malformation (bruit-thrill), systemic intravascular coagulopathy, myxoma

Malignant tumors	+	+ (especially lymphoma)	Rapid	– (but can be fixed or ulcerated)	Firm, spongy, crepitant	Diffuse (cortical perforation)	CT scan (to show extent of bone perforation), root resorption
Inflammatory bone disease	+	–	Days, weeks	±	Firm to spongy	Diffuse	WBC count, skin tests, tomograms (to show extent of osteomyelitis), bone scan, ESR
Primary bone diseases	–	–	Slow	–	Firm	Generalized	Paget's (alkaline phosphatase) hyperparathyroidism (serum calcium and phosphate)

Code: + Present or involved
      – Not involved

AV = atrioventricular; CT = computed tomographic; ESR = erythrocyte sedimentation rate; GCRG = giant cell reparative granuloma; WBC = white blood cell.

1. These cysts develop at the point of fusion of the globular portion of the median nasal process and the maxillary process.
2. They occur at the junction of the primary palate (lip and premaxilla) with the secondary palate (posterior to the lateral incisor).
   a. When within bone, they are called globulomaxillary cysts.
   b. When in the lip or lateral nose, they are nasolabial cysts.
   c. When eroding through labial cortex, they are nasoalveolar cysts.
3. They usually present as a swelling of the upper lip or nasal base, including the nasal floor. The differential diagnosis of swelling within the nasal floor (most commonly in blacks and females) should include the lateral fissural cyst.

C. Median fissural cysts of the maxilla
1. Nasopalatine cysts develop from paired nasopalatine ducts, which enter the mouth just posterior to the incisive papilla. They are the most common fissural cyst. Within this group are the incisive canal cyst and the cyst of the papilla incisiva. These designations are determined by location, the latter being entirely within soft tissue.
2. Median palatine cysts derive from epithelial remnants at the median palatine fissure (as a midline palatal swelling).

D. Fissural cyst of the mandible
1. This extremely rare cyst is located in the symphysis. Fewer than 10 cases have been reported.
2. The surrounding teeth are vital and may be displaced, an important feature in distinguishing this lesion from apical cysts.

III. Diagnosis and treatment of jaw cysts
A. Several clinical and radiographic features of a radiolucent lesion of the jaw that may be of assistance in diagnosis and treatment planning include:
1. Association with teeth. Are the teeth vital? If so, the apical cyst can be ruled out.
2. Composition of the cyst. Is the lesion unilocular or multilocular? The latter may suggest a keratocyst or noncystic neoplasm (e.g., myxoma).
3. Cyst fluid aspirate. Keratocysts have a relatively low protein concentration compared with serum. Blood that can be aspirated easily is consistent with a central vascular malformation or an aneurysmal bone cyst.
4. Location. Noting whether a lesion is medially or laterally situated and determining its proximity to the teeth can aid in distinguishing fissural cysts from odontogenic cysts. Lesions that appear in non-tooth-bearing areas of the jaws (e.g., the proximal ramus or inferior to the mandibular canal) are probably nonodontogenic.

B. Two general modes of treatment are employed for the various cysts of the jaws:
   1. Enucleation of the cyst in its entirety, at times with excision of overlying soft tissue at sites of perforation (see **I.C.2.,** Odontogenic keratocyst p. 346)
   2. Marsupialization, a process of exteriorizing the cyst, thus decompressing it, by making its lining continuous with the lining of the oral cavity

C. In general, enucleation is preferred because the cyst is completely removed and entirely available for histologic study. In practice, marsupialization is rarely necessary but may be indicated when a cyst is extremely large and enucleation might be incomplete or when injury to contiguous neurovascular, dental, and sinus structures is likely. Advocates of marsupialization claim that this technique is less likely to devitalize teeth and induce oroantral fistulas. With this method, consideration should be given to eventual enucleation once the cyst has contracted over time.

D. The decision to carry out primary closure of a bony cavity after removal of a cyst is a matter of clinical judgment. The incision must be planned to allow the suture line to be supported as much as possible by bone. Consideration should also be given to creating an osteoperiosteal flap (i.e., reflection of the bony cortex overlying the cyst while it remains attached to the mucoperiosteal flap). In general, the size and location of the cyst determine whether to place a dressing and thus commit the wound to healing by secondary intention.

E. Cysts up to 20 mm in size will usually heal primarily, particularly in the maxilla, where dependent drainage is advantageous. In the mandible the tendency toward blood clot liquefaction and delayed healing is exaggerated by the unfavorable influence of gravity. Trimming the bone margins of the residual defect (saucerization) will help limit dead space by allowing the reapproximated flap to partially collapse into the cavity.

F. Relative indications for placement of a dressing are:
   1. A large bony defect with unfavorable drainage
   2. A previously infected cyst
   3. When significant bleeding has been encountered

G. It is arguable that even when a large bony defect is encountered primary closure is indicated; if the original lesion is uninfected, there is a good chance of successful healing. Should the wound break down because of premature blood clot liquefaction and dehiscence of the incision, the argument continues, one can then place a dressing and proceed in a fashion similar to the planned method of healing by secondary intention.

H. If a dressing is indicated, we usually employ ½- to 1-in gauze impregnated with balsam of Peru. The pack is withdrawn either partially or totally, usually on the fifth or seventh day, and is changed regularly until the residual defect has contracted enough so that the wound can be readily managed by irrigations.

1. Autogenous bone may be placed in large cavities to promote healing by stabilizing clot and promoting osteogenesis. However, this is rarely indicated with jaw cysts.
2. Demineralized bone has been advocated for speeding osteoinduction. Its obvious advantage lies in the avoidance of potential donor site morbidity.

JAW TUMORS

I. Odontogenic tumors
   A. General features
      1. Odontogenic tumors result from the misdirection of cellular activity involved in odontogenesis.
      2. They are classified according to the embryologic process of induction (i.e., the process of change brought about by the action of one tissue type on another, specifically epithelium and mesenchyme).
      3. In the United States they comprise approximately 9% of all tumors of the oral cavity.
   B. Epithelial tumors with minimal induction
      1. Ameloblastoma
         a. This tumor derives from cell rests of the enamel organ (dental lamina) or from the epithelium of odontogenic cysts, primarily dentigerous cysts. Ameloblastoma accounts for 1% of all jaw cysts and tumors.
         b. Eighty percent occur in the mandible, 75% of these in the molar-ramus area. Most patients are in their third to fifth decade of life.
         c. The ameloblastoma grows by slow and persistent expansion. It rarely causes nerve compromise or pain. Its behavior in the maxilla may differ from that in the mandible because of the greater cortical density of the latter, which tends to confine the tumor.
         d. Radiographically the lesion is classically multilocular (multicystic [MC]), although unilocular (unicystic [UC]) lesions are encountered.
         e. A peripheral ameloblastoma has been described and has a more innocuous biologic pattern than the UC or MC forms. Most reported cases have involved the gingiva.
         f. Treatment is controversial, although there is general agreement that the peripheral form can be excised with a small margin of normal tissue without removing contiguous bone, and the UC form can be enucleated. The MC form should be excised with a margin of uninvolved bone. Immediate bone graft reconstruction is appropriate. Treatment must be tailored to tumor location and, to

some degree, to social factors. The reliable patient who will return for follow-up who has a large lesion of the mid-body of the mandible might be treated by so-called *peripheral ostectomy* rather than resection. This is a method of aggressively burring the periphery of the lesion, typically to the cortical bone. Its advantage is that it may allow preservation of mandibular continuity and has been shown to be effective in some instances of large mandibular lesions that would have been traditionally resected. Lesions of the posterior maxilla must be resected because there are no natural barriers to the spread of the ameloblastoma. Cortical bone, in general, is not invaded by ameloblastoma.

g. Radiation therapy may play a role in the treatment of some cases, although surgery is the predominant method of treatment. Radiation therapy is useful in instances in which tumor has extended into the soft tissue. It is not effective as primary treatment of intraosseous ameloblastoma. It is most likely useful in the posterior maxilla.

h. Recurrence rates have been reported to be 30%, probably reflecting the tumor's ability to penetrate bone. A small number of instances of distant metastases have been reported. A malignant form of ameloblastoma, including malignant transformation of a peripheral ameloblastoma, has been reported.

2. Adenomatoid odontogenic tumor (adenoameloblastoma)
   a. This lesion is not related to ameloblastoma.
   b. Its pathogenesis is uncertain, but it may arise from cell rests of the enamel organ, from odontogenic cysts, or from disturbances of the developing enamel organ.
   c. It usually presents as a painless swelling of the jaw.
   d. It is often associated with an impacted tooth, particularly a mandibular canine.
   e. It may contain areas of calcified material of the dystrophic type.
   f. The majority of patients are in their 20s; 65% have been female.
   g. Treatment is conservative excision. Recurrences have not been reported, even after incomplete removal.

3. Calcifying odontogenic tumor (Pindborg tumor)
   a. This is a benign neoplasm that arises from reduced enamel epithelium. It has been found to:
      (1) Occur frequently in middle age, similar to the ameloblastoma
      (2) Affect the mandible most commonly (3:1 relative to the maxilla), usually in the premolar-molar area
      (3) Often present as a painless swelling
      (4) Be associated with an unerupted tooth (in perhaps 50% of cases)

(5) Invade locally, behaving similarly to an ameloblastoma

(6) Appear as a radiolucency with radiopaque foci of either unilocular or multilocular configuration; its early radiographic appearance may be indistinguishable from that of a dentigerous cyst

b. Treatment should be similar to that for the ameloblastoma (i.e., conservative surgical excision with a margin of uninvolved bone).

C. Epithelial tumors with induction. Clinically, benign behavior is expected with induction. All tumors in this category behave accordingly, and conservative excision is the appropriate management.

1. Ameloblastic fibroma
   a. This odontogenic tumor is characterized by slow progression with possible cortical expansion but not invasion.
   b. Patients are generally in the 5–20 yr age group.
   c. Painless swelling, usually in the premolar-molar area, is the most common presentation. The mandible is affected more often than the maxilla.
   d. Histologically there is encapsulation around cords and islands of epithelial cells in a connective tissue stroma. Thus it is a true mixed tumor. The stroma, which strongly resembles the embryonal connective tissue of the primitive dental pulp, allows distinction from ameloblastoma.
   e. It presents usually as a well-defined unilocular radiolucency not associated with an impacted tooth. Occasionally it is multilocular.
   f. Treatment is enucleation. Recurrence is rare.

2. Squamous odontogenic tumor. This recently described lesion may be characterized as follows:
   a. Benign mixed tumor consisting of squamous odontogenic epithelial islands in a mature fibrous connective tissue stroma
   b. Probably arises from rests of Malassez in the periodontal ligament or from gingival mucosa.
   c. Appears as a painless swelling or loosening of teeth
   d. Occurs most commonly in the second and third decades of life, with no gender predilection
   e. Usually discovered in the anterior maxilla and posterior mandible
   f. In the maxilla, displays a more aggressive behavior than in the mandible; this is presumably related to the lesser density of bone in the maxilla
   g. A discrete radiolucency adjacent to one or more teeth
   h. Treated generally by enucleation or curettage; more aggressive maxillary lesions may best be managed by en bloc excision; recurrences have not been reported

D. Mesenchymal odontogenic tumors
   1. Myxoma
      a. This benign swelling is not clearly odontogenic but is found virtually exclusively in the jaws.
      b. It is a slow-growing and persistent tumor that is locally invasive with periods of rapid expansion. It does not metastasize. Variations in rates of expansion are often not readily explained by histology.
      c. Peak incidence is in the second and third decades of life. Both jaws are affected.
      d. Histologically the tumor is characterized by stellate cells with long anastomosing cytoplasmic processes in a mucinous matrix. It is important to distinguish this pattern from the myxoid features of other tumors.
      e. Typically a multilocular radiolucency is seen. Distinction from ameloblastoma or central giant cell lesions may be impossible radiographically.
      f. Treatment is controversial, but generally en bloc excision is recommended because local invasiveness is a feature of this lesion. Small lesions may be aggressively curetted. Large ones displaying aggressive behavior (cortical perforation, rapid expansion) should be resected. Reported recurrence rates average 25%.
   2. Odontoma
      a. The odontomas constitute a group of solid odontogenic tumors containing both enamel and dentin. Mature ones contain cementum as well.
      b. Odontomas may be classified as compound, complex, and ameloblastic.
         (1) Compound odontomas are the most highly differentiated variety. Essentially, when a calcified lesion of the jaws manifests morphologic similarity to a tooth, this designation is appropriate. Such tumors display a predilection for the incisor-canine region, and if they interfere with eruption of contiguous teeth, their removal may be indicated. Simple excision is the proper treatment.
         (2) Complex odontomas are a type of hamartoma that is intermediate in prevalence between the compound and the ameloblastic types. Their morphology is less similar to that of a tooth, and they often are associated with an unerupted tooth. They demonstrate slow growth, affecting females more often than males (2:1), and approximately 70% occur in the second and third molar areas. Conservative excision is appropriate.
         (3) Ameloblastic forms include the ameloblastic odontoma and the ameloblastic fibroodontoma, which are tumors consisting essentially of a compound or com-

plex odontoma with an associated soft-tissue component of ameloblastic tissue or ameloblastic epithelial
islands scattered in a fibromyxoid stroma. Correspondingly, they may show a cystlike radiolucency
around the calcified component. Sarcomatous transformation of ameloblastic fibroodontoma has been
reported. Nevertheless, conservative treatment (curettage) is appropriate with close, long-term follow-
up.

3. Cementoma
   a. The term *cementoma* is applied by clinicians to the le-
      sion perhaps more appropriately called *periapical ce-
      mental dysplasia* (PCD).
   b. It describes a group of lesions that contain cementum,
      including PCD, cementifying fibroma, and cementoblas-
      toma.
      (1) PCD is the most common lesion in the cementoma
          group, appearing mainly in blacks and females, rarely
          among patients younger than 25 yr of age. It is usu-
          ally discovered at routine examination as a periapical
          radiolucency continuous with the periodontal liga-
          ment (in its early stages) or as a mixed radiolucent-
          radiopaque irregular lesion (in later stages). In its ma-
          ture stage, fully calcified osteocementum is found.
          Surgery is not indicated except in the rare instances
          of chronic gingival ulceration and secondary infec-
          tion. Conservative excision is then appropriate.
      (2) Cementifying fibroma is difficult to separate from os-
          sifying fibroma and will be discussed in the next sec-
          tion (nonodontogenic tumors).
      (3) Cementoblastoma is a benign tumor that is self-limit-
          ing, attached to the root of a tooth (most commonly
          a mandibular premolar or molar), and composed of
          globules of cementum. It does not recur after simple
          enucleation.

II. Nonodontogenic tumors
   A. General features
      1. Benign nonodontogenic mesenchymal tumors make up the
         majority of jaw tumors in children.
      2. Odontogenic epithelial tumors are relatively more common
         in adults—e.g., ameloblastoma occurs overwhelmingly in
         middle-aged persons.
      3. Nonodontogenic tumors may be classified according to
         their presumed tissue of origin.
         a. Benign mesenchymal
         b. Malignant mesenchymal
         c. Vascular
         d. Hematopoietic-reticuloendothelial
         e. Neurogenic
         f. Malignant epithelial

4. Some lesions are difficult to classify in this fashion and thus are placed in conceptually convenient groups. For example, the aneurysmal bone cyst is included in the vascular group. The present discussion will consider only the *benign* categories. Malignant jaw tumors are discussed elsewhere in this text.

B. Benign mesenchymal tumors
   1. Giant cell lesions. These tumors fall into three groups—giant cell reparative granuloma (GCRG), brown tumor of hyperparathyroidism, and giant cell tumor (GCT). Distinction among them by histologic criteria may be impossible. Therefore, clinical features must be employed to categorize the lesions and determine treatment. Clinically, aggressive tumors (rapid expansion, perforation of the bony cortex, tooth erosion) are considered GCTs. There remains significant controversy, however, over whether a true giant cell tumor of the jaws can even be said to exist because such lesions of the jaws do not undergo malignant conversion, as is relatively common with GCTs of the long bones.
      a. Giant cell reparative granuloma
         (1) This tumor is clinically quiescent, affecting the mandible more often than the maxilla and females more often than males (2:1). It occurs usually in children and young adults.
         (2) It is generally located in the premolar area, rarely if ever posterior to the 6-yr molar. It is the most common central jaw tumor to cross the midline.
         (3) The patient usually has no symptoms. The lesion often is discovered as an incidental radiographic abnormality. It may be of either unilocular or multilocular configuration, sometimes with faint central trabeculations. Cortical expansion, occasionally with perforation, is common. Teeth are typically displaced rather than eroded.
         (4) Differential diagnosis of these radiographic changes should include GCRG, myxoma, central vascular malformation, central mucoepidermoid carcinoma, odontogenic keratocyst, and ameloblastoma. When the GCRG presents because of swelling or pain, the symptoms are usually slight.
         (5) Curettage or conservative excision is appropriate. Recurrences are uncommon, but when they arise and/or if the aggressive clinical features described accompany reappearance of the lesion, consideration should be given to revision of the GCT diagnosis and more aggressive resection may be indicated.
      b. Brown tumor of hyperparathyroidism
         (1) This tumor is characterized by histologic, clinical, and radiographic features indistinguishable from those of GCRG.

    (2) There are central jaw changes occurring with both primary (parathyroid adenoma or hyperplasia) and secondary (chronic renal failure) hyperparathyroidism.

    (3) Diagnosis is made from biopsy findings consistent with those in GCRG and elevated serum parathyroid hormone (PTH). Radiographs demonstrate resorption lacunae in the phalanges and loss of the lamina dura. Histologic findings interpreted as consistent with GCRG should always lead to consideration of hyperparathyroidism.

    (4) Treatment principally concerns the primary disease. Primary hyperparathyroidism requires excision of the autonomous focus of PTH production. The secondary form requires management of the renal disease, including calcium and vitamin D supplements.

    (5) Brown tumors may require resection if they are large and/or if the associated cortical expansion causes functional problems. Small lesions may involute once the primary disease has been controlled.

  c. Giant cell tumor

    (1) True GCT of the jaws is rare. We employ clinical criteria to make the designation when biopsy shows histology consistent with GCRG. Rapid expansion inducing significant pain, root resorption, rapid cortical perforation, and multiple recurrences of early onset indicate an aggressive although benign lesion that should be designated GCT.

    (2) There has been only one well-documented case of malignant GCT of the jaw. Distinction from osteosarcoma, which may contain many giant cells, is essential.

    (3) GCT of the jaws seems to be intermediate in aggressiveness between the innocuous GCRG of the jaws and the aggressive, sometimes malignant GCT of the long bones.

    (4) Treatment is controversial. En bloc resection with immediate reconstruction is appropriate for very aggressive tumors and for those that have recurred several times after curettage or simple excision.

2. Myxoma. This benign tumor was discussed in the odontogenic category, although some experts place it in the nonodontogenic group because many occur in non-tooth-bearing parts of the jaws.

3. Fibrous dysplasia

  a. This lesion of the jaws is usually monostotic, although it may be part of a generalized disease with or without endocrine abnormalities. It frequently presents as a painless, slowly progressive swelling in the first and second decades of life. Periods of rapid expansion may be seen—

e.g., during the pubertal growth spurt or during pregnancy. The lesion rarely changes significantly after 25 yr of age. When expansion of the bones of the craniofacial skeleton is significant, functional deficits may occur, particularly interference with vision and mandibular hypomobility.

b. Other important features of fibrous dysplasia include:

    (1) The maxilla is involved more commonly than the mandible, and, by extension into the orbit, the process may cause proptosis or obstruct vision.

    (2) Radiographic changes vary according to the age of the patient and the activity of the disease. In very young patients with rapidly expanding fibrous dysplasia, radiographs demonstrate a multilocular or unilocular radiolucent lesion with cortical thinning. In older patients with clinically quiescent lesions, radiographs demonstrate a mixed radiolucent-radiopaque or a simply radiopaque mass.

    (3) Serum calcium, phosphorus, and alkaline phosphatase are normal (Appendix II, p. 384).

    (4) Histology is characterized by a mixture of fibrous tissue, bone, giant cells, blood vessels, and mast cells. There appears to be a direct correlation between clinical disease activity and cellularity of the connective tissue, as well as with the numbers of mast cells.

    (5) Treatment is indicated when there is interference with vision, nasal breathing, and jaw function, as well as to improve appearance, because fibrous dysplasia may markedly distort facial skeletal form and symmetry. Surgical recontouring by excision and burring is the usual treatment and is most predictable once the patient has reached skeletal maturity. Long-term follow-up is important because rare instances of spontaneous sarcomatous change have been reported, although most of these occurred subsequent to radiation therapy, which (it is now clear) plays no role in the management of this disease.

4. Ossifying fibroma

a. This tumor is considered a variant of fibrous dysplasia and is included in the general category of fibroosseous lesions. It is characterized by:

    (1) Slow expansion, rarely causing pain or paresthesia

    (2) Occurrence more commonly in the mandible than in the maxilla, in contrast to fibrous dysplasia

    (3) Peak incidence in the third and fourth decades of life

b. A well-defined radiolucency is seen in the early stages. The lesion progressively calcifies, and, as it does so, its borders become less distinct.

    c. The ossifying fibroma may not be separable clinically, radiographically, or histologically from a cementifying fibroma.

    d. Treatment consists of local excision or enucleation. The tumor separates readily from surrounding bone. Rarely, without histologic change, an ossifying fibroma behaves aggressively. Such lesions warrant more extensive excision.

5. Cherubism

    a. This tumor has histologic features that make it inseparable from the GCRG. However, its historical and clinical features allow easy diagnosis. These include:

      (1) Autosomal dominant inheritance with 50%–70% penetrance in females and 100% penetrance in males. Expressivity is variable but usually bilateral and symmetrical; sporadic spontaneous mutations may occur.

      (2) Evident usually by 3–4 yr of age, presenting as a slowly progressive painless swelling. The mandible is affected more often and to a greater extent than the maxilla. Disease progression slows by about 10 yr of age and the lesions may regress at puberty.

      (3) Association with firm, nontender cervical lymphadenopathy is common; increased skin pigmentation is less common.

      (4) Deciduous teeth that exfoliate prematurely; multiple missing and impacted secondary teeth ("floating teeth") may be found.

    b. Radiographically, a multilocular, usually bilaterally symmetric, expansion of the jaws is seen. The cortex is thinned. The posterior mandible is most commonly involved, although the condyles are always spared. Teeth seem to be floating within the tumor and may be malformed.

    c. Treatment must be individualized. Surgical contouring is appropriate when expansion is severe, leading to functional jaw or airway disturbances, or when the disease causes social problems in the older child. If possible, intervention is delayed until growth has ceased.

6. Osteoblastoma and osteoid osteoma. These lesions are histologically indistinguishable. Both display trabeculae of woven bone and osteoid in a vascular fibrous stroma. Separation is based on growth potential.

    a. The osteoblastoma may be significantly larger than 1 cm in diameter, whereas the osteoid osteoma is rarely larger. In addition, the latter classically causes severe pain that is most intense at night.

    b. The osteoblastoma is a solitary radiolucency. The osteoid osteoma has a distinct sclerotic border around an otherwise similar lesion.

    c. Treatment of both lesions is en bloc excision. Recurrence after curettage is common. Because the calvarium is the usual site of osteoblastoma in the craniofacial skeleton and may cause trismus if the temporal bone is involved, a combined maxillofacial and neurosurgical approach may be required for excising this tumor.

C. **Vascular lesions.** Central vascular lesions of the jaws are uncommon. Distinction between hemangioma and vascular malformation is important in the understanding of these lesions. The aneurysmal bone cyst will also be discussed.

    1. The **hemangioma** is a true tumor of endothelium and is the most common benign tumor of childhood. It is usually not present at birth, exhibits a period of rapid postnatal growth, and typically involutes slowly until age 5–7 yr. Central hemangioma of the facial bones is rare (less than 100 cases). Most have occurred in the mandible. Less than 1% of hemangiomas of the maxillofacial region in one large series were of the central type.

    2. **Vascular malformations** are morphogenetic abnormalities of vascular channels that are present at birth and grow proportionately with the host. Expansion may occur secondary to trauma, infection, and bleeding. Isolated central vascular malformations of the jaws are rare; over one third of lesions affecting the maxillofacial region directly involve the underlying bone as well.

        a. Central vascular lesions may display a multilocular appearance radiographically. Hypertrophy and distortion of bone occur with lymphatic malformations. Destructive changes of bone are common with arterial malformations.

        b. Treatment must be individualized. Central jaw hemangiomas rarely bleed spontaneously and usually do not require treatment. If bleeding is a problem, selective embolization and en bloc resection may be required. Evaluation for potential chronic coagulopathies is essential in the management of vascular malformations (chronic consumption coagulopathy). Total resection of vascular malformations is often not possible. Partial resection with the assistance of selective embolization may allow control of hemorrhage.

    3. **Aneurysmal bone cyst** consists of blood-filled spaces lined by spindle cells. Multiple giant cells are also seen. Some areas may be histologically indistinguishable from giant cell reparative granuloma. There is no true epithelial lining. This is a slow-growing tumor, usually of the mandible, affecting females most commonly. Painless swelling is the general presentation, which appears as a multilocular radiolucency on further examination. Treatment is curettage, and recurrence is rare.

D. Hematopoietic-reticuloendothelial tumors. Histiocytosis X is a spectrum of diseases of unknown etiology characterized by the accumulation of cholesterol-laden histiocytes in hard and/ or soft tissues. The histiocytosis group includes eosinophilic granuloma, Hand-Schüller-Christian disease, and Letterer-Siwe disease. (Burkitt's lymphoma is discussed with this group, although it is not a true histiocytosis X.)

1. Eosinophilic granuloma is the localized form of histiocytosis, usually affecting the craniofacial skeleton (particularly the jaws). The posterior body and angle regions of the mandible are most often involved. Dental symptoms may lead to discovery of the lesions and can include loose teeth, delayed healing of extraction sites, and chronic gingival ulcers.

   a. Radiographically the teeth appear to be floating, simulating severe periodontal disease. The cortex is usually thinned and expanded. The lesion is typically well demarcated, although usually with an irregular outline.

   b. Treatment is enucleation and curettage and/or low-dose radiation (600–1000 cGy).

2. Hand-Schüller-Christian disease is the disseminated chronic form of histiocytosis, affecting multiple organ systems. Diabetes insipidus, proptosis, and dental malocclusion may be caused by tumor infiltration of the pituitary gland, orbit, and jaws. Hepatosplenomegaly, eczematoid skin changes, and deafness may be associated findings.

   a. Radiographically the individual lesions are similar to those found in eosinophilic granuloma. Jaw lesions tend to be more diffuse. Teeth are displaced as the alveolar bone is destroyed.

   b. Treatment is variable. Individual lesions may be improved by curettage or radiation, or both. Various chemotherapeutic regimens have been tried, with variable success. The disease is slowly progressive.

3. Letterer-Siwe disease is the acute, often fulminating form of histiocytosis. It usually affects children 2 yr of age or younger. The disease is relentless, as massive invasion of liver, spleen, and marrow occurs. Generalized lymphadenopathy, constitutional disturbance, pulmonary and gastrointestinal involvement, and skin changes are inevitable. Bone lesions are less prominent in this form, although central jaw involvement may lead to changes simulating severe periodontal disease. Treatment is by various chemotherapy protocols. Further discussion is beyond the scope of this chapter.

4. Burkitts's lymphoma is a disease of unclear etiology, predominantly affecting males, that may involve many organ systems, including the facial and long bones, nervous system, salivary glands, pelvic and abdominal viscera, and retroperitoneum.

    a. Jaw involvement is most common in the African form of this disease. The maxilla is affected more commonly than the mandible (2:1), and bimaxillary disease is not infrequent. Jaw presentations include premature loss of teeth and swelling.

    b. In the early stages this disease may present radiographically as a loss of lamina dura around adjacent teeth.

    c. Treatment consists of surgical debulking and high-dose administration of alkylating agents. Remission occurs in over 90% of cases.

E. Neurogenic tumors. Benign neurogenic tumors involving the jaws include the traumatic neuroma, neurofibroma, neurilemoma, and melanotic neuroectodermal tumor of infancy. We will not discuss the traumatic neuroma because it is not a true neoplasm.

  1. Neurofibroma is a tumor derived from Schwann cells. Approximately one third of persons afflicted with neurofibromatosis have abnormalities of the underlying bone, such as cystic change with cortical expansion, subperiosteal erosion, or bony hypoplasia. The last may occur without apparent central involvement. Central lesions are usually solitary rather than one of many in a person with neurofibromatosis.

    a. Central neurofibromas usually cause dull discomfort and paresthesia. Most are found in the mandible.

    b. Radiographic findings may include a fusiform expansion of the inferior alveolar canal or multilocular radiolucent changes in areas contiguous to overlying soft-tissue lesions.

    c. In contrast to the neurilemoma, neurofibromas are not encapsulated. In addition, they are known to undergo sarcomatous change in a significant number of cases, although there has been little experience with central jaw lesions. Long-term follow-up must be stressed.

    d. Treatment is local excision. Because the involved bone is very vascular, resection may result in significant blood loss. The mandibular nerve is sacrificed if involved. Immediate bone and/or nerve grafting should be considered.

  2. Neurilemoma (schwannoma) also derives from Schwann cells. The affected person usually experiences pain, swelling, and often paresthesia. The mandible is most commonly involved.

    a. This tumor is encapsulated and, consistent with this feature, appears radiographically as a unilocular or multilocular lucency with well-defined borders.

    b. Treatment is enucleation. Recurrence is rare.

  3. Melanotic neuroectodermal tumor of infancy

    a. This tumor, of neural crest origin, presents in children during the first year. Although reported in extragnathic sites, the canine area of the anterior maxilla is most commonly involved. Characteristic findings are swelling of the upper lip, usually without pain, and displacement of adjacent tooth buds.

b. The tumor has infiltrating projections within a vascular fibrous stroma. Granules of melanin are seen.

c. Treatment is conservative local excision. Recurrence rates of approximately 15% have been reported. There appears to be no malignant potential.

III. Diagnosis and treatment of jaw tumors

A. Diagnosis is based largely on history, physical examination, radiographic and laboratory investigations, and biopsy. The mature surgeon will be aware that histologic designations are sometimes ambiguous and must be carefully correlated with the clinical features that essentially summarize the biologic behavior of the tumor. The central giant cell lesions and the various forms of ameloblastoma highlight the importance of such correlations.

B. Aggressive but histologically benign lesions (characterized by rapid expansion, root resorption, paresthesias, cortical perforation, and invasion of soft tissue, as well as recurrences of early onset) may require deviation from "standard" treatment protocols. Wider resection may be appropriate. Treatment must be determined by histology and the biologic behavior of the tumor.

C. Radiolucent jaw lesions warrant routine assessment of serum calcium, phosphorus, and alkaline phosphatase.

D. Any central jaw tumor characterized by the pathologist as GCRG warrants consideration of hyperparathyroidism, because the brown tumor is histologically indistinguishable from the reparative granuloma. Appropriate laboratory studies include those just listed, as well as serum parathyroid hormone levels (perhaps serum BUN and creatinine) and screening radiographs of the jaws and hand.

E. Tumors discussed in this chapter do not metastasize, although local recurrences may arise. When discontinuity defects result from resection, immediate bone graft reconstruction is indicated. When the sensory branches of the trigeminal nerve are sacrificed, immediate interpositional nerve grafting using the sural or greater auricular nerve is indicated.

F. When children are affected by these tumors, treatment must not be compromised because of fears of interfering with subsequent facial growth. Although essential to consider, growth disturbances can be minimized by early functional rehabilitation, which can be achieved by early jaw reconstruction and, in selected instances, the aid of dental prostheses.

GENERAL REFERENCES

Batsakis JG: *Tumors of the head and neck*, ed 2, Baltimore, 1979, Williams & Wilkins.

Chuong R et al: Central giant cell lesions of the jaws. A clinico-pathology study, *J Oral Maxillofac Surg* 44:708, 1986.

Chuong R et al: The odontogenic keratocyst—an update, *J Oral Maxillofac Surg* 40:797, 1982.

Chuong R, Kaban LB: Diagnosis and management of jaw tumors in children: a ten year experience, *J Oral Maxillofac Surg* 43:323, 1985.

Katz JO, Underhill TE: Multiocular radiolucencies, *Dent Clin North Am* 38:63, 1994.

Meiselman F: Surgical management of the odontogenic keratocyst: conservative approach, *J Oral Maxillofac Surg* 52:960, 1994.

Shear M: Developmental odontogenic cysts, an update, *J Oral Pathol Med* 23:1, 1994.

Waldron CA: Fibroosseous lesions of the jaws, *J Oral Maxillofac Surg* 51:828, 1993.

Williams TP: Management of ameloblastoma: a changing perspective, *J Oral Maxillofac Surg* 51:1064, 1993.

Williams TP, Connor FA: Surgical management of the odontogenic keratocyst: aggressive approach, *J Oral Maxillofac Surg* 52:964, 1994.

Trigeminal Nerve Injuries

16

R. BRUCE DONOFF

The clinician confronted with a patient suffering from abnormal sensation needs some guidance in answering questions related to the most effective management. Diagnosis is the first priority, and this chapter provides basic information on the differential diagnosis, management, and treatment of trigeminal nerve injuries and answers some very basic questions for the clinician:

1. How significant a clinical problem is nerve injury in the orofacial regions?
2. How do trigeminal nerve injuries differ from nerve injuries elsewhere?
3. What is the relationship of trigeminal nerve damage to the genesis of chronic orofacial pain?
4. Which clinical parameters affect the prognosis following trigeminal nerve injuries?
5. How are trigeminal nerve injuries best assessed?
6. What are the indications for intervention when trigeminal nerve damage is diagnosed?
7. What techniques are most effective for repair of injured trigeminal nerves?

ETIOLOGY AND EPIDEMIOLOGY

I. Secondary to oral and maxillofacial surgical procedures
   A. Third molar surgery. Retrospective and prospective studies to date show a range of incidences for both inferior alveolar nerve (IAN) and lingual nerve injuries following odontectomy. For the lingual nerve this range is 0.06%–11%, and for the IAN it is 0.4%–5.5%. These data reflect the detection of abnormal sensation following surgery without classifying the neurosensory disturbances related to anesthesia or those of paresthesia or dysesthesia. Prognosis depends on the extent of the injury, which will be discussed later, but in general for the lingual nerve recovery occurs in 86% of patients, whereas for the IAN recovery is 97%. The better prognosis for IAN injuries is believed to be due to the fact that the injured nerve is contained

within the mandibular canal, which may act as a guide for its regeneration.

B. Orthognathic surgery. Results vary depending on the type of surgery. Sagittal osteotomies have the highest incidence of nerve dysfunction postoperatively. The simultaneous performance of a genioplasty must also be considered because the mental nerves are at risk.

C. Preprosthetic surgery. This is usually done secondary to mental nerve damage with vestibuloplasty.

D. Implant placement. This represents a special case, as the clinician is faced with the dilemma of whether to remove or back off the implant in cases resulting in sensory aberration. Clinical experience suggests about a 3% incidence of nerve dysfunction for implants placed in the posterior mandibular areas.

E. Other surgical procedures

F. Endodontic procedures. As the number of endodontic procedures increase, injuries due to extravasation of materials used during procedures have led to increased complications. In this clinician's experience, these injuries are best treated very early because chemical rather than traumatic anatomic aberrations are at the crux of this problem.

II. Needle injury. This is a controversial topic. The incidence is guessed to be about one in 400,000 inferior alveolar nerve blocks. There are certainly more patients reporting a "shock" in the tongue or lip with a block than those reporting postprocedural problems. Presumed etiologies include direct trauma to the nerve from a needle, intraneural hematoma formation, and local anesthetic toxicity due to either the agent itself or its vehicle. It is of interest that usually the lingual nerve is affected. The prognosis is guarded with return of normal sensation usually less than that for the IAN.

III. Secondary to an intracranial lesion. In any patient presenting with a neurosensory deficit, especially if it is unilateral, a unilateral peripheral tumor or intracranial lesion must be considered. A high suspicion is most important without antecedent surgical trauma, but might occur in conjunction with a surgical history and confound the picture. Proper workup with radiographs of the facial bones and even CT scans of the face and head may be indicated.

IV. Part of a posttraumatic injury syndrome (see Chapter 9)

DIAGNOSIS

I. Clinical assessment. Careful examination and reporting of the extent of a neurosensory deficit are very important. The magnitude of response and mapping of the area involved are critical in assessing recovery over time. Our experience suggests that it is most important to describe the problem in terms of anesthesia, complete loss of sensation, paresthesia, partial loss of sensation, dysesthesia, and partial loss of sensation with a painful component. In general, using these criteria, even without a detailed examination, endodontic injuries are usually dysesthetic, whereas lingual nerve injuries are rarely dysesthetic.

The basic examination schema includes the following:

A. Touch
   1. von Frey's filaments
   2. Dull and sharp touch
B. Sense of direction
C. Thermal sensitivity
D. Two-point discrimination
E. Pattern recognition
F. Tinel's-like signs
   1. Lingual nerve. Palpation over the lingual alveolus may elicit a shooting sensation along the lateral border of the tongue in cases of profound sensory loss. This is usually indicative of neuroma formation.
   2. Inferior alveolar nerve. This is seen less frequently, but pressure with a cotton swab over the healing or healed third molar socket may elicit a shooting sensation to the lip. This is due to the superior displacement of the nerve or neuromatous tissue into the mandibular socket.

II. Summary of clinical assessment. To date, the best clinical reports suggest that anesthesia of the lingual nerve (which does not change with time), especially in conjunction with a Tinel's-like sign, of the affected nerve has a poor prognosis for recovery without treatment. The suggested observation period for such problems is 2 to 3 mo.

Paresthetic conditions present more difficulty because such a high percentage of these, especially of the IAN, recover naturally. It is important to realize that all studies to date suggest that the gold standard time of 6 mo is arbitrary. Most IAN injuries recover before then, thus the clinician finds him- or herself in a most difficult situation. Communication with the patient, based on outcome data (discussed later), is recommended.

III. Laboratory testing. The goal of both examination and laboratory testing is to determine which injured nerves have a very good to excellent prognosis for natural recovery versus those that do not.

A. Electrophysiology
   1. Somatosensory evoked potentials (SEP). To date, SEP measurement has been plagued by considerable variability due to artifact. The most important issue is that evoked potentials demonstrate peripheral findings and not central findings. Thus far, the long latencies observed in human measurements suggest that peripheral abnormalities are not being recorded.
   2. Magnetic source imaging (MSI). This involves the use of a magnetic sensor and stimulation with a nonelectrical stimulus in order to monitor the magnetic activity in the appropriate cortical regions. Unlike electrical activity, magnetic

activity is not affected by passage through cranial bone. The magnetic activity is superimposed on a previously obtained MRI scan of the cortical area. Although this method is experimental and costly, it offers promise.

B. Diagnostic nerve blocks for painful conditions. In cases of dysesthesia, it is critical to ascertain that peripheral neurectomy will be successful. Thus, an IAN block that is effective in relieving pain suggests strongly that more central tracts of the trigeminal system have not been affected by the peripheral lesion—so-called deafferentation pain.

III. Radiologic and other imaging methods

A. Tomogram of the mandible. Look for disruption of the canal or root tip.

B. Magnetic resonance imaging. This may be useful in demonstrating lingual neuroma (experimental).

IV. Diagnosis

A. Correlation of clinical signs and symptoms with types of nerve injuries (types I, II, and III). Seddon (1993) described three types of nerve injury—neuropraxia, axonotmesis, and neurotmesis—based on the severity of tissue injury, prognosis for recovery, and time for recovery. Neuropraxis is a conduction block resulting from a mild insult to the nerve trunk. There is no axonal degeneration, and sensory recovery is complete and occurs in a matter of hours to several days. The sensory deficit is usually mild and characterized by paresthesia, with some stimulus detection but poor discrimination and disturbed stimulus interpretation. Axonotmesis is a more severe injury. Afferent fibers undergo degeneration, but the nerve trunk is grossly intact with a variable degree of tissue injury. Sensory recovery is good but incomplete. The time course for sensory recovery depends on the rate of axonal regeneration and usually takes several months. The sensory deficit is characterized by severe paresthesia. Neurotmesis is a complete disruption of the nerve; sensory recovery is not expected, except when the nerve courses through a canal, such as the mandibular canal. This sensory deficit is characterized by anesthesia.

B. History. It is important to ascertain the method of anesthesia used during surgery. Local anesthesia may cause injury, and the patient should be asked if a shock was experienced during anesthetic administration. With combined local and general anesthesia or sedation this information often cannot be obtained reliably from the patient.

On occasion the surgeon may see the IAN during removal of the wisdom tooth; this has little significance. The occurrence of bleeding following wisdom tooth removal may signify disruption of the canal contents. Judicious control of such bleeding without tight packing of the wound is recommended. Also, the use of antibiotic-containing dressings, especially tetracycline, should be avoided, for it has been shown to cause neuritis experimentally.

It is very rare to see the lingual nerve during third molar surgery. The anatomic variations which may predispose to injury have been described. The very low incidence of injury supports the anatomic variability theory of injury predisposition.

    C. Index of suspicion. Follow-up of nerve injuries is dependent on the surgeon's index of suspicion of an injury. Certainly it is not difficult to recognize an IAN that courses through the roots of a third molar. It is the subtle signs of concern, like bleeding, which should be noted.

  V. Outcome analysis. Results correlating clinical findings to resolution of neurosensory disturbance are important to our understanding of the Seddon classification. Neuropraxia results in complete recovery, whereas in axonotmesis there is incomplete recovery. Both retrospective and prospective studies have been reported, all strongly suggesting that recovery of IAN injuries is better than that of lingual nerve injuries, probably owing to the guidance provided by the mandibular canal. The results suggest that a certain number of IAN and lingual nerve injuries do not resolve by themselves. The task, then, is to discover which early lesions these nerve injuries represent.

Axonal recovery, cellular recovery, and even receptor recovery appear to be time dependent. Clinical results support this contention, but a lack of stratification of patients as to age, gender, race, and mechanism or type of injury confuses the picture. The best predictive outcome is for patients who have received anesthesia. Thus, clinical findings of anesthesia and Seddon's neurotmesis, particularly when combined with a Tinel's-like sign on palpation of the lingual area for lingual nerve deficits, permit surgical treatment to be carried out with confidence. It is unlikely that this type of injury falls into any of the categories of nerve damage which may show spontaneous resolution of the sensory deficit.

 VI. Management and treatment

    A. Inferior alveolar nerve. Based on the previous outline of diagnosis, prognosis, and recovery, the following recommendations are made: careful follow-up and a description of the neurosensory deficit. Anesthetic findings should be followed by an operation in 3 mo if there is no improvement.

Endodontic injuries, if painful, should be reviewed with the patient, and early decision should be made, particularly if there is evidence of material in the canal.

Paresthetic injuries should be monitored with the patient's understanding that improvement warrants further follow-up through 6 mo, but that the opportunity for intervention is lost.

Root tips that are displaced to compress the canal are a special case. Experience shows that unexpected favorable results in terms of numbness may occur even when the foreign body is removed well after 6 mo.

Dental implant injuries represent a special case. The best treatment is prevention, and careful preoperative evaluation as to proper implant placement and length is recommended. If a sensory deficit is noted after local anesthesia wears off, a decision must be made quickly. Factors that should be considered are that 1) removal may cause further damage, and 2) a successful implant, even with paresthesia, may be acceptable to the patient. There is no real information on outcomes following even early removal of implants.

The issue of nerve repositioning is somewhat easier to discuss. A comparison of nerve abnormalities following nerve repositioning and implant placement without nerve repositioning suggests that in the former group at 18 mo, 94% had normal sensation, 4% had paresthesia, and 1% were anesthetic. In comparison, in cases without nerve repositioning at a similar follow-up period, 3% had paresthesia.

B. Lingual nerve. The main indication for surgery is unchanging anesthesia of the lingual nerve with the presence of a Tinel's-like sign. This sign may not appear until a month after the procedure.

VII. Summary. There are no large-scale reports of success rates for microneurosurgery of the peripheral trigeminal nerve. The high likelihood of spontaneous recovery in the paresthetic IAN-injured patient deserves major consideration when decisions regarding treatment are made. Currently there are potential methods being developed that may help in clarifying this area of patient management that is so often complicated by litigation.

Returning to the introductory questions, some imperfect answers exist for the clinician faced with these problems.

1. How significant a clinical problem is nerve injury in the orofacial regions? Anyone who has ever had a local anesthetic block knows the feeling of numbness. It is not pleasant, and certainly if methods exist to eradicate it or improve the condition, patients should be apprised of this. In terms of its epidemiology it remains a relatively rare condition.

2. How do trigeminal nerve injuries differ from nerve injuries elsewhere? Most knowledge of nerve injury comes from study of motor nerves. Sensory nerves, particularly the trigeminal system, are part of a very complicated neuropathway. Thus, peripheral injuries in the IAN, for example, can result in changes proximal to the injury.

3. What is the relationship of trigeminal nerve damage to the genesis of chronic orofacial pain? Clinical experience strongly suggests that pain is more related to injuries of the IAN than to those of the lingual nerve. In addition, endodontic injuries appear to have a special predilection for the development of painful conditions.

4. Which clinical parameters affect the prognosis following trigeminal nerve injuries? The nerve involved is important. The IAN, for reasons discussed, has a better prognosis in general. The level of neurosensory loss is also important. Thus, anesthesia, paresthesia, and dysesthesia should be determined.

5. How are trigeminal nerve injuries best assessed? Clinical parameters remain the most important guide, with periodic examination and observation of any changes being critical.

6. What are the indications for intervention when trigeminal nerve damage is diagnosed? These are outlined in this chapter and in the algorithms.

7. What techniques are most effective for repair of injured trigeminal nerves? Epineural repair using standard microsurgical techniques are required.

GENERAL REFERENCES

Donoff RB: Nerve regeneration: basic and applied aspects, *J Crit Rev Oral Biol Med* 6:18-24, 1995.

Pogrel MA, Bryan BS, Regezi J: Nerve damage associated with inferior alveolar nerve blocks, *J Am Dent Assoc* 126:1150-1155, 1995.

Seddon HJ: Three types of nerve injury, *Brain* 112:1, 1943.

APPENDIX I
Oral Manifestations of Systemic Disease

CHRONIC INFECTIOUS DISEASES

	Clinical features	Diagnosis	Oral manifestations	Treatment
Leprosy (*Mycobacterium leprae*)	Slightly contagious granulomatous disease Skin most commonly involved	Histological exam acid-fast bacilli	Nodular lesions on mucous membranes Facial paralysis bilaterally if CN VII involved	
Fungus Actinomycosis (*Actinomyces israelii*)	Chronic noncontagious suppurative infection	Immunofluorescent antibody stains of drainage or necrotic debris *Actinomyces israelii* or anaerobic culture	Hard, circumscribed, inflammatory masses (chronic); multiple fistulas (chronic)	I & D; large long-term doses of penicillin
Histoplasmosis (*Histoplasma capsulatum*)	Septic fever; pulmonary involvement; enlargement of spleen, liver, lymph nodes; contaminated soil in semi-Tropics	Histoplasmin skin test; serological tests Cultures	Ulcerations, nodular lesions	
Blastomycosis (*Blastomyces dermatidis*)	Skin papules; sometimes fatal pulmonary involvement; contaminated soil		Ulcerative papules	0.02% amphotericin-B ointment for oral lesions

Tuberculosis (*Mycobacterium tuberculosis*)	Droplet spread; fatigue, decrease in weight, fevers	Chest radiograph; Ziehl-Neelsen stain; Mantoux skin test; Caseous avascular necrotic nodule surrounded by multinucleated giant cells	Oral lesions rare; painless nodule ulcerates; osteomyelitis with tubercle bacilli on histology	Dental rehabilitation after sputum becomes negative; Ethambutol, isoniazid, streptomycin, aminosalicylic acid
Syphilis (*Treponema pallidum*)	Spread by sexual intercourse and through oral cavity	Physical examination, dark-field examination of chancre, serological examination of blood; dark field examinations of oral lesions difficult due to presence of other acquired spirochetes	Congenital (linear scars at angles of lips, hypoplasia of permanent incisors and molars, deafness [CN VIII], interstitial keratitis, increased corneal opacity); Acquired (indurated nodule ulcerates, often painful; mucous patch, painful raised gray lesion with erythematous base, ulcerates; gumma, indurated, ulcerated, enlarging lesion; loss of taste, paresthesias, neurological involvement)	Penicillin, follow-up with physical and serological examinations

CONNECTIVE TISSUE DISEASES

Collagen diseases	Clinical features and diagnostics	Oral manifestations	Treatment

Lupus erythematosus Chronic (discoid)	Reddish macular skin lesions with yellow scales; "butterfly pattern" in malar area
	Histological
	  Hyperparakeratosis
	  Perivascular lymphocytes
	  Hyaline degeneration of connective tissue
	LE prep
		Mucocutaneous disease; 25% have oral lesions; erythematous keratinized lesions on buccal mucosa and lower lip	Antimalarials suppress but do not cure

Systemic	Especially affects heart and kidneys; altered immune reactivity; hemolytic anemia; fever, weakness, decreased weight, anorexia LE prep	Similar to those of discoid lupus, particularly in acute form; hyperemia, edema, and extension of lesions more pronounced	Antimalarials, steroids, therapies of specific organ involvement failure

Dermatomyositis	Degenerative disease of connective tissue, skin, skeletal muscles; 25% associated with malignancy	Muscles of tongue and deglutition degenerate, may undergo necrosis and hyaline degeneration; mucosal lesions similar to lupus; painful tongue involvement with swelling, degeneration, atrophy, diffuse mucosal erosion	Systemic steroids suppress but do not cure; may end spontaneously or progress to fatality
Scleroderma	Disease of collagenous connective tissue; results in hardening of skin and subcutaneous tissues, atrophy, and pigmentation; indurated lesions of neck, trunk, extremities following distribution of peripheral nerves; osteoporosis, soft tissue calcifications, especially at joints; collagen fibers atrophy and compress into compact masses histologically; decreased elastic tissue; disappearance of most skin appendages (e.g., hair) in affected areas	Indurations of mucosa and submucosa, atrophy, pigmentation, false ankylosis of TMJ, painful induration of tongue and gingiva, thickening of periodontal ligament at radiography	Physiotherapy; systemic steroids may repress but not cure

ANEMIAS

Type	Causes and diagnostic	Oral manifestations	Treatment
Microcytic hypochromic (iron deficiency)	Blood loss resulting in iron deficiency (GI bleeding); rarely from dietary deficiency of iron; decreased HCT; decreased Hgb; small faint RBCs on smear	Plummer-Vinson syndrome (glossitis with dry indurated tongue and dysphagia, atrophy of mucous membrane of mouth and pharynx)	Oral ferrous salts, identify and correct any acute or chronic blood loss
Megaloblastic (pernicious)	Decreased vitamin B_{12} because of decreased absorption due to lack of gastric intrinsic factor; arrest of erythrocyte maturation; megaloblasts and macrocytes on smear	Smooth tongue, painful, atrophy of papillae, pale oral mucosa, petechiae	Vitamin B_{12} injections
Aplastic	Aplasia of bone marrow shown at needle biopsy; leukopenia occurs first because of shorter life-span of leukocytes; caused by extrinsic chemicals, antibiotics, radiation	Pallor, petechiae, opportunistic infections	Control infections (because of leukopenia)

Normocytic	Toxins inhibit RBC formation and decrease life-span of RBCs; may be secondary to chronic inflammatory disease or renal failure	Pallor, mucositis	Remove etiological factors; hygiene; improved diet
Polycythemia vera	Absolute increase in number of circulating RBCs; etiology unknown; splenomegaly most constant feature	Gingiva deep purplish red, often swollen; tongue may also be involved as well as all mucosa; cyanosis due to presence of reduced hemoglobin in excess of 5 g/100 ml	Symptoms relieved by phlebotomy
Thalassemia	Hereditary, especially in people of Mediterranean descent; thalassemia major (impaired hemoglobin synthesis, hemolipids), thalassemia minor (mild chronic anemia)	Pallor; few if any oral symptoms	Patients with thalassemia major may need frequent transfusion
Sickle cell	Hereditary hemolytic type; misshapen RBCs can cause embolism and thrombosis; happens when hemoglobin reduces during decreased oxygen tension	Pallor and icterus, petechiae, osteoporotic changes on jaw radiographs and periapical films	Avoid hypoxia; in acute crisis, administer oxygen by nasal cannula and IV fluids

HEMATOLOGICAL LESIONS

Type	Oral manifestations
Infectious mononucleosis (Epstein-Barr virus)	Palatal petechiae, lymphadenopathy
Agranulocytosis (arrested maturation of granulocytes in marrow)	Gangrenous stomatitis, sore throat
Hodgkin's disease (lymphoma)	Cervical (and other) adenopathy
Hemophilia	Spontaneous bleeding, excessive continuous bleeding after minor mucosal trauma
Thrombocytopenic purpura	Spontaneous bleeding, mucosa bleeds easily and excessively from minimum trauma, petechiae
Acute leukemia	Ulcerative stomatitis, progressively worsening, gangrenous necrosis of gingiva; swollen, edematous, painful gingiva; frequent, chronic herpetic lesions; bleeding, petechiae; lymphadenopathy
Chronic lymphocytic leukemia	As above, marked tonsillar enlargement with hard cervical lymphadenopathy
Chronic myelogenous leukemia	Gingival bleeding and enlargment, toothache, ulcerative lesions, petechiae

RETICULOENDOTHELIOSES (HISTIOCYTOSIS X)

	Oral manifestations	Other considerations
Eosinophilic granuloma	Oval or round, irregular, sharply demarcated radiolucencies of maxilla and mandible; extrabony lesions may occur as tender swelling	Usually solitary granuloma (usually) of bone consisting of histiocytes and eosinophils
Hand-Schüller-Christian	Swelling of gingiva, early necrosis, maxillary and mandibular osseous xanthomatosis, tooth extrusion	Reticuloendothelial cell proliferation inflitates and replaces bone and soft tissue; exophthalmos, diabetes insipidus, defects of membranous bones; histiocytes are lipid laden
Letterer-Siwe	Hemorrhage and ulceration of gingiva; lytic destruction of alveolar bone	Progessive, acute, disseminated proliferation of histiocytes

COMMON ENDOCRINE AND STORAGE DISEASES

Type	Oral manifestations	Other considerations
Diabetes mellitus	In uncontrolled or poorly controlled patient, exaggerated periodontal response to common irritants (plaque), producing fulminant suppurative periodontitis and acetone breath; xerostomia results in mucositis	Maintain dentition to avoid infections
	In controlled diabetic, no special oral manifestations, periodontium reacts to irritants same as in nondiabetic	
Amyloidosis	Nodules of gingiva (50%), tongue (50%), pharynx, respiratory and GI tracts; tongue purpura	Diagnosis by biopsy
Lipidoses (Gaucher's disease)	Osteoporosis of mandible with large radiolucencies, yellowish patches on mucosa (histiocytes engorged with cerebroside lesions)	Cerebroside accumulation in spleen, liver, bone marrow, lymph nodes causing portal cirrhosis
Niemann-Pick disease	Jaws infiltrated with lipid-containing cells; large radiolucencies	Sphingomyelin accumulates in RE system
Mucopolysaccharidoses (Hurler syndrome, Hunter syndrome, etc.)	Broad mandible; localized areas of destruction in jaws may be seen	Primarily genetically determined disburbance of mucopolysaccharide metabolism; a range of diseases

Laboratory Values

HEMATOLOGY

Hematocrit (HCT)
    42–53%, males
    37–48%, females
Hemoglobin (Hgb)
    13–18 g/100 ml, males
    12–16 g/100 ml, females

Methemoglobin	0.4–1.5% of total hemoglobin
Erythrocyte (RBC) count	4.2–5.9 million/mm³
Mean corpuscular hemoglobin (MCH)	28–30 $\mu\mu$g
Mean corpuscular hemoglobin concentration (MCHC)	32–36%
Mean corpuscular volume (MCV)	86–98 mμ^3
Serum hemoglobin	2–3 mg/100 ml

White blood count (WBC), normal differential screen

Granulocytes	52–79%
Lymphocytes	11–39%
Monocytes	4–15%

    Differential leukocyte count (adults)

PMNs	40–75%
Bands	0–4%
Lymphocytes	20–45%
Monocytes	2–10%
Eosinophils	1–6%
Basophils	<1%
Eosinophil count	70–440/mm³
Reticulocyte count	0.5–2.5%

Erythrocyte sedimentation rate (ESR)
    1–13 mm/hr, males
    1–20 mm/hr, females

Special hematology studies

Vitamin B_{12}	205–876 pg/ml
Folic acid (serum)	>3.3 ng/ml
Serum ferritin	0–12 ng/ml (iron deficiency)
	13–20 ng/ml (borderline iron deficiency
	21–50 ng/ml (normal range; however, could be consistent with iron deficiency if liver disease or inflammation is present)
	>400 ng/ml (iron excess)
Iron	50–150 μg/100 ml (higher in males)
Iron-binding capacity	250–410 μg/100 ml

Coagulation studies

Prothrombin time (PT)	±2 sec of control value (normal 11 sec)
Partial thromboplastin time (PTT)	25–40 sec
Platelet count	150,000–350,000/mm³
Thrombin time	±5 sec of control value
Bleeding time test	2–9.5 min
Fibrin split products (FSP)	1:4 or less
Protamine sulfate	1:20 or less
Circulating platelet aggregates (CPA)	0.8 or greater
Ristocetin cofactor	>40%

Hepatitis-related studies

Antibody to hepatitis-A virus (anti-HAv)

IgG detectable	Infection with hepatitis-A in remote past
IgM detectable	Infection with hepatitis-A currently or recently

Antibody to hepatitis-B core antigen (anti-HBc)

Detectable	Current or past hepatitis-B infection

Hepatitis-Be

Antigen (HBe Ag)	Detectable: High infectivity
Antibody to HBe	Detectable: Low infectivity

Blood plasma and serum chemistries

Electrolytes

Calcium	8.5-10.5 mg/100 ml (children slightly higher)
Chloride	100-106 mEq/L
Lithium	0.5-1.5 mEq/L
Magnesium	1.5-2.0 mEq/L
Potassium	3.5-5.0 mEq/L
Sodium	135-145 mEq/L
Phosphorus	3.0-4.5 mg/100 ml (infants up to 6 mg/100 ml)

Carbon dioxide content	24-30 mEq/L infants 20-26 mEq/L)
Osmolality	280-296 mOsm/kg H_2O

Protein

Total	6.0-8.4 g/100 ml
Albumin	3.5-5.0 g/100 ml
Globulin	2.3-3.5 g/100 ml
Electrophoresis	Percent of total protein
Albumin	52-68

Globulins

Alpha-1	4.2-7.2
Alpha-2	6.8-12
Beta	9.3-15
Gamma	13-23

Bilirubin	Direct up to 0.4 mg/100 ml
	Total up to 1.0 mg/100 ml
Glucose	70-110 mg/100 ml (fasting)
Triglycerides	40-150 mg/100 ml
Cholesterol	120-220 mg/100 ml
Lipoproteins (as cholesterol)	
HDL	30-65 mg/100 ml, males
	35-80 mg/100 ml, females
LDL	70-190 mg/100 ml

Cardiac enzymes

CPK (creatine phosphokinase)	17-148 U/L, males
	10-79 U/L, females
CPK isoenzymes	5% MB band or less
LDH (lactic dehydrogenase)	45-90 U/L
SGOT (aspartate aminotransferase)	7-27 U/L
SGPT (alanine aminotransferase	1-21 U/L

Renal-related studies

Urea nitrogen (BUN)	8-25 mg/100 ml
Creatinine	0.6-1.5 mg/100 ml
Uric acid	3.0-7.0 mg/100 ml
Acid phosphatase	0-0.5 Fishman-Lerner unit/100 ml
Alkaline phosphatase	13-39 U/L (infants and adolescents up to 104 U/L)
Carbon monoxide	Less than 5% total hemoglobin (symptoms with over 20% saturation)
Copper	70-150 μg/100 ml
Lead	Up to 50 μg/100 ml
Ammonia	12-55 μmol/L

Medications and drugs

Carbamazepine (Tegretol)	2.0-8.0 μg/ml
Chloramphenicol	10-20 μg/ml
Ethosuximide (Zarontin)	40-100 μg/ml
Phenobarbital	15-50 μg/ml
Phenytoin (Dilantin)	5-20 μg/ml
Procainamide (Pronestyl)	4.0-10.0 μg/ml
Propranolol	100-300 μg/ml
Quinidine	1.2-4.0 μg/ml
Salicylate	Therapeutic 20-25 mg/100 ml (25-30 mg/100 ml to age 10 yr)
	Toxic over 30 mg/100 ml (over 20 mg/100 ml after age 60 yr)
Serum digoxin	1.2-1.7 ng/ml
Serum digitalis	17 ± 6 ng/ml
Sulfonamide	5-15 mg/100 ml
Valproic acid	50-100 μg/ml
Vitamin A	0.15-0.6 μg/ml

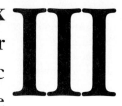
Endocarditis prophylaxis recommended:
    Prosthetic cardiac valves (including biosynthetic valves)*
    Most congenital cardiac malformations
    Surgically constructed systemic-pulmonary shunts*
    Rheumatic and other acquired valvular dysfunction
    Hypertrophic cardiomyopathy
    Previous history of bacterial endocarditis*
    Mitral valve prolapse with insufficiency†
Endocarditis prophylaxis not recommended:
    Isolated secundum atrial septal defect
    Secundum atrial septal defect repaired without a patch 6 or
       more months earlier
    Patent ductus arterosus ligated and divided 6 or more
       months earlier
    Postoperative coronary artery bypass graft (CABG)

    This list gives just the common conditions. It is not meant to be all-inclusive.

•These patients are at high risk for developing bacterial endocarditis.

†Definitive data is limited. Individuals with mitral valve prolapse associated with thickening and/or redundancy of the valve leaflets may be at increased risk, particularly men over the age of 45.

SUMMARY OF RECOMMENDED ANTIBIOTIC REGIMENS FOR DENTAL OR RESPIRATORY TRACT PROCEDURES

Standard regimen

For dental procedures that cause gingival bleeding, and oral-respiratory tract surgery

Amoxicillin 3.0 g orally 1 hr before procedure, then 1.5 g 6 hrs after initial dose

Special regimens

Parenteral regimen for use when maximum protection desired (e.g., for patients with prosthetic valves)

Ampicillin 2.0 g IV or IM plus gentamicin 1.5 mg/kg IV or IM (not to exceed 80 mg) one-half hr before procedure, followed by 1.5 g oral amoxicillin 6 hrs after initial dose. Alternatively the parenteral regimen may be repeated 8 hrs after the initial dose

Oral regimen for penicillin-allergic patients

Erythromycin 1.0 g orally 1 hr before, then 500 mg 6 hr after initial dose

Erythromycin ethylsuccinate 800 mg or erythromycin stearate 1.0 g orally 2 hrs before procedure, then one-half the dose 6 hrs after initial dose. Or: clindamycin 300 mg orally 1 hr before procedure, then 150 mg 6 hrs after initial dose

Parenteral regimen for penicillin-allergic patients

Vancomycin 1.0 g IV administered over 1 hr, starting 1 hr before the procedure. No repeat dose is necessary

Parenteral regimen for patients unable to take oral medication

Ampicillin 2.0 g IV or IM 30 minutes before procedure, then 1.0 g ampicillin IV or IM (or 1.5 g amoxicillin orally) 6 hrs after initial dose

If penicillin allergic: clindamycin 300 mg IV 30 minutes before a procedure and 150 mg IV (or orally) 6 hrs after initial dose

Pediatric doses: Ampicillin 50 mg/kg per dose; erythromycin 20 mg/kg for first dose; then 10 mg/kg; gentamicin 2.0 mg/kg per dose; penicillin-V full adult dose if greater than 60 lb (27 kg), one-half adult dose if less than 60 lb (27 kg); aqueous penicillin-G 50,000 units/kg (25,000 units/kg for follow-up); vancomycin 20 mg/kg per dose. The intervals between doses are the same as for adults. Total doses should not exceed adult doses.

Emergency Care of the Oral and Maxillofacial Surgery Patient

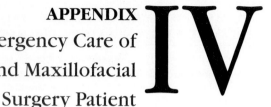

The oral and maxillofacial surgeon like all health care providers is caring for a greater percentage of patients with chronic diseases who are older and taking more medications. For these reasons the practitioner must not only be more familiar with medical illness in general, but must have the ability to manage a variety of medical emergencies. The material in this appendix deals with these emergencies. The reader is referred to other sources for the current protocols for basic and advanced cardiac life support.

LOSS OF CONSCIOUSNESS
I. Etiology. Diverse causes include syncope, hypotension, drug reaction, seizure, insulin reaction, cerebrovascular accident, hyperventilation, and acute adrenal insufficiency. Mechanisms involved are psychic, diminished cerebral perfusion, metabolic alterations, and drug reactions.
II. Physical findings. Lack of response to auditory and physical stimuli, loss of protective reflexes, lack of ability to maintain an airway.
III. Management
    A. Activate office or local emergency system
    B. Place patient in supine position
    C. Begin cardiopulmonary resuscitation (CPR)
    D. Assess response to treatment and treat for specific etiology as soon as it is recognized, e.g., hypoglycemia
IV. Prevention
    A. Rigorous medical evaluation to recognize all important medical conditions
    B. Reduction of physical and psychological stress of procedure, e.g., pain control
    C. Make patient comfortable by position and environment, e.g., supine position

SYNCOPE (FAINTING, VASOVAGAL REACTION)
I. Etiology. Transient cerebral ischemia leading to loss of consciousness, often related to peripheral pooling of blood.
II. Physical Findings
    A. Presyncopal signs are characteristic and include:
        1. Transient, sudden loss of consciousness

    2. Loss of color, pallor

    3. Diaphoresis

    4. Nausea

    5. Yawning and hyperpnea

    6. Tachycardia followed by hypotension and bradycardia

  B. Syncopal signs include:

    1. Irregular and decreased ventilation

    2. Convulsive movements

    3. Hypotension and bradycardia

III. Management

  A. Place patient in supine position

  B. Establish a patent airway by lifting chin and tilting head

  C. Loosen restrictive clothing

  D. Monitor vital signs

  E. Administer supplemental oxygen

  F. Administer reflex stimulants such as ammonia inhalants and cold compresses

  G. Assess recovery. (If recovery does not occur within a few minutes, continue basic life support and consider other causes of unconsciousness.)

IV. Prevention

  A. Minimize patient's anxiety and stress; use sedation and pain control methods appropriately

  B. Advise appropriate food intake before a procedure

  C. Put patient in supine or semisupine position whenever possible

HYPERVENTILATION SYNDROME

  I. Etiology. Rapid breathing characterized by an increased depth and/or frequency of ventilation. Usually anxiety-related but may occur with metabolic acidosis, hypercarbia, drug reaction, central nervous system disturbances, or pain.

 II. Physical findings

  A. Chest tightness

  B. Dyspnea

  C. Apprehension

  D. Palpitation

  E. Chest or abdominal discomfort

  F. Hyperventilation (25–30 breaths/min)

  G. Paresthesia of mouth, hands, or feet

  H. Carpopedal spasm

  I. Loss of consciousness

III. Management

  A. Place patient in comfortable position, sitting up is usually better than supine

  B. Reassure patient

  C. Guide patient in slow breathing, may include intermittent breath-holding

    D. Let patient rebreathe his or her own exhaled air by using paper bag or full-face mask on anesthesia machine without oxygen turned on to let patient correct respiratory alkalosis

    E. If no improvement, consider sedation to reduce anxiety

IV. Prevention

    A. Assessment of previous medical history

    B. Appropriate pain control and sedation techniques to reduce anxiety

ASTHMATIC REACTION

  I. Etiology. A paroxysmal state of hyperactivity of the tracheobronchial tree. *Extrinsic asthma* is bronchospasm as a result of an extrinsic allergin that is antibody-mediated and usually occurs in children. *Intrinsic asthma* is bronchoconstriction caused by non-allergic factors such as infections, irritating fumes, and emotional stress. It is more likely to be seen in adults.

 II. Physical findings

    A. Chest tightness

    B. Sudden or slow onset

    C. Coughing

    D. Wheezing, usually greater with expiration

    E. Dyspnea

    F. Anxiety

    G. Tachycardia*

    H. Cyanosis*

    I. Use of accessory muscles of respiration*

    J. Nasal flaring*

    K. Supraclavicular retraction*

    L. Agitation*

    M. Hypoxia*

    N. Status asthmaticus—prolonged asthma attack

    O. Fatigue

    P. Hypoxia

    Q. Shock

    R. Airway obstruction

III. Management

    A. Place patient in most comfortable position.

    B. Administer inhalant therapy with aerosol bronchodilator; use patient's own medication if available; if not, use emergency kit medicine (epinephrine, isoproterenol, metaproternol).

    C. Administer supplemental oxygen.

    D. Administer epinephrine 0.2–0.4 mg subcutaneously if attack continues.

    E. Start aminophylline 5–7 mg/kg and give slowly if attack continues after epinephrine has been given.

---

* In severe cases

IV. Prevention
   A. Minimize anxiety with appropriate pain control and sedation techniques
   B. Ensure patient has been taking medications for asthma
   C. Have patient's own medication available for use
   D. Avoid large doses of barbiturates or narcotics if sedation is being used
   E. Attempt to remove or eliminate possible allergens in environment

ACUTE HYPOGLYCEMIA (INSULIN REACTION)

   I. Etiology. Rapid decrease in serum blood sugar usually seen in diabetics. Related to overdose of insulin or lack of normal dietary intake following normal insulin dosage. Commonly called insulin "shock."
  II. Physical findings
   A. Sudden decreased cerebral function characterized by mental confusion, lethargy, diminished cerebral function, or slurred speech
   B. Hunger
   C. Nausea and increased gastric motility
   D. Diaphoresis with cold, clammy extremities
   E. Tachycardia
   F. Belligerent non-cooperative behavior
   G. Eventual unconsciousness
   H. Seizures
   I. Hypotension, shock, and eventual death
 III. Management
   A. Early recognition by history and physical examination.
   B. In conscious patient, administer oral carbohydrate such as orange juice or sugar-containing soft drink; give slowly.
   C. In unconscious patient, start IV infusion and administer 50mL of 50% dextrose over 2 min; recovery should be rapid.
   D. In situations without IV access, glucagon 1 mg IM may be given continual observation of the patient.
  IV. Prevention
   A. Careful history of diabetes, insulin dosages, and schedule and dietary habits.
   B. Provide specific insulin and dietary guidelines for the perioperative period, e.g., patients who are NPO may be given half their normal insulin dose and an infusion with D_5W begun at the time of surgery.
   C. Monitor blood or urine glucose levels in pre-, peri-, and postoperative periods.

ACUTE HYPERGLYCEMIA (DIABETIC COMA)

   I. Etiology. Elevated blood glucose usually a manifestation of diabetes mellitus. Other specific precipitating factors include pregnancy, exercise, hyperthyroidism, overdose of thyroid replacement drugs, epinephrine, steroid therapy, or infections.

II. Physical Findings. Signs of hyperglycemia, in contradistinction to those of hypoglycemia, are usually slow to develop, often taking days. The final emergency phase is usually ketoacidosis and coma.

History or signs and symptoms of diabetes, including polydypsia, polyphagia, polyuria, and weight loss. Additional symptoms include:

A. Fatigue
B. Headache
C. Abdominal pain, nausea, vomiting
D. Dyspnea (pulmonary compensation for metabolic acidosis)
E. Warm, dry skin
F. Acetone smell on breath (sweet or fruity)
G. Weak, thready pulse
H. Loss of mental acuity
I. Coma and death

III. Management. Abnormal or bizarre behavior or unconsciousness in a patient with a history of diabetes warrants treatment for hypoglycemia until proven otherwise. It will have little effect on the treatment of hyperglycemia if that is the problem.

If hyperglycemia is established:

A. Assess airway, respiration, circulation, and manage appropriately.
B. Begin an IV infusion with normal saline to facilitate definitive treatment in office setting; patient should immediately be transported to an emergency facility for management with constant serum glucose measurements.
C. In hospital setting, patient can be treated with regular insulin with the dosage dependent on the level of hyperglycemia.

IV. Prevention

A. Obtain detailed history of diabetic patients
B. Avoid stress through appropriate pain control and sedation techniques
C. Treat infections aggressively
D. Avoid use of steroids in diabetic patients

SEIZURES

I. Etiology. Paroxysmal neuronal discharge in the brain characterized by altered consciousness, uncoordinated muscle activity, or abnormal sensory phenomena, behavior, or perception. May be focal or generalized. Seizures may be idiopathic or caused by fever, cerebrovascular accidents, central nervous system infection, head injury, toxic and metabolic disorders, or drug overdose. Epileptic seizures must be differentiated from syncope, cerebrovascular accident, or hypoglycemia.

II. Physical findings. Several types of seizures must be recognized.

A. Grand mal seizures (tonic-clonic) may be divided into three phases:

1. Prodromal phase
    a. May occur several minutes to several hours before motor activity
    b. May see minor or overt changes in personality, with anxiety or depression
    c. Patient may have an aura immediately before motor activity; this may be visual, auditory or olfactory
2. Ictal (convulsive) phase
    a. Loss of consciousness
    b. Extensor rigidity of extremities
    c. May see stertorous breathing
    d. May see cyanosis
    e. Generalized clonic movements
    f. Frothing of the mouth
    g. Usually lasts 2–5 min
    h. Urinary or fecal incontinence
3. Postictal phase
    a. Gradual return of consciousness
    b. Generalized relaxation and deep sleep
    c. Disorientation and confusion
    d. Amnesia

B. Petit mal seizures
    1. Primarily in children
    2. Patient appears distracted or confuse
    3. May see intermittent blinking
    4. May see blank stare
    5. No prodromal or postictal phase

C. Status epilepticus
    1. Recurrence of seizures without any recovery period
    2. Seizure activity is the same as in generalized seizure
    3. May last hr to da
    4. Most commonly seen with metabolic disturbances of drug or alcohol withdrawal
    5. Hyperthermia, tachycardia, and hypertension
    6. May lead to death from cardiac arrest or brain damage from cerebral hypoxia or decreased cerebral blood flow

III. Management
    A. Grand mal seizures—management based upon protecting patient from injury
    B. Place patient supine on floor with head turned to side
    C. Place soft object under head
    D. Consider placing a soft object between teeth to prevent tongue biting, avoid hard objects or placement in such a way as to cause airway obstruction
    E. Remove nearby objects that may cause harm
    F. Gently aspirate secretions in the buccal sulcus
    G. Consider supplemental oxygen if condition warrants it (e.g., cyanosis)
    H. Check airway, breathing, and circulation, and support as needed

    I. Monitor vital signs during recovery
    J. Petit mal seizures—no emergency treatment needed
    K. Status epilepticus—consider terminating any seizure activity lasting >5 min
    L. Treat initially as for grand mal seizure
    M. Begin IV infusion and administer diazepam 2 mg/min until seizures terminate or a dose of 10–15 mg is reached (divide dose in half for child)
    N. If diazepam not available, consider a short-acting barbiturate (pentobarbital 25 mg/min or methohexital 10–20 mg/min); not first choice for these drugs are more prone to increase postictal cerebral and respiratory depression

IV. Prevention
    A. Good medical history and knowledge of medication compliance
    B. Avoid toxic doses of local anesthetics because this is the most likely cause of a seizure in the office setting
    C. Avoid factors that may cause physical or psychologic stress or fatigue
    D. Avoid hypoglycemia with good dietary advice

ANGINA PECTORIS

    I. Etiology. Acute onset of chest pain associated with insufficient coronary blood flow secondary to ischemic coronary artery disease. Associated factors include emotional or physical stress, smoking, fever, and hypoxia.
    II. Physical findings
        A. Chest pain, usually a crushing substernal pain
        B. Radiation to left shoulder, arm, neck, jaw, and face
        C. Episodes usually characteristic and consistent for each patient; variation may indicate an impending infarction
        D. Tachycardia
        E. Hypertension
        F. Diaphoresis
        G. Occasional dyspnea
        H. May see dysrhythmia
    III. Management
        A. Aimed at increasing coronary blood flow and decreasing myocardial oxygen demand
        B. Position patient in most comfortable position, usually sitting upright
        C. Administer supplemental oxygen
        D. Administer a coronary vasodilator: nitroglycerin is the initial drug of choice. Patient should take one of his or her own tablets sublingual, if available, since nitroglycerin comes in three dosages. If the patient does not have nitroglycerin, 1/150 gr tablets should be used from the emergency cart
        E. A second and third tablet may be given at 5-min intervals if relief is not obtained

    F. Failure to respond to three doses of nitroglycerin or amyl nitrate in a 10-min period suggests myocardial infarction and the patient should be transported to an acute care facility for treatment and monitoring

IV. Prevention
    A. Knowledge of previous history of angina or myocardial infarction
    B. Eliminate stress and anxiety with appropriate pain and sedation techniques
    C. Consider administering prophylactic nitroglycerin before stressful procedure

MYOCARDIAL INFARCTION

I. Etiology. Infarction and necrosis of heart muscle caused by coronary artery insufficiency and inadequate myocardial oxygen supply.

II. Physical findings
    A. Chest pain of a crushing, tightening, pressing, or aching but ominous nature
    B. Variation of the chest pain from patient's typical angina
    C. Tachycardia or bradycardia
    D. Hypertension or hypotension
    E. Diaphoresis
    F. Dyspnea
    G. Dysrhythmia
    H. May lead to cardiac arrest

III. Management
    A. Initial treatment the same as for angina pectoris
    B. After failure of third dose of nitroglycerin, infarction must be assumed
    C. Continue oxygen supplementation
    D. Monitor ECG for specific dysrhythmia and treat as per ACLS protocols
    E. Consider morphine, 2–8 mg, to relieve pain and anxiety
    F. Transport to an acute care facility for monitoring and definitive treatment

IV. Prevention. Same as for angina pectoris.

ALLERGY/ANAPHYLAXIS

I. Etiology. Hypersensitivity state caused by exposure or reexposure to a particular antigen. Possible causative agents include antibiotics, analgesics, barbiturates, local anesthetics, acrylics, and preservatives. Reaction may be immediate or delayed.

II. Physical findings
    A. Allergy
        1. Itching
        2. Rash
        3. Redness
        4. Angioedema

      5. Dyspnea

      6. Wheezing

      7. Tachycardia

   B. Anaphylaxis

      1. Skin

         a. Pruritus, intense

         b. Conjunctivitis

         c. Rhinitis

         d. Piloerection

      2. Gastrointestinal and genitourinary

         a. Diarrhea

         b. Nausea and vomiting

         c. Incontinence

      3. Respiratory

         a. Dyspnea

         b. Cyanosis

         c. Wheezing

         d. Substernal tightness

      4. Cardiac

         a. Palpitation

         b. Tachycardia

         c. Hypotension

         d. Dysrhythmia

         e. Cardiac arrest

III. Management

   A. Allergy

      1. Assess airway, breathing, circulation

      2. Administer diphenhydramine (Benadryl) 50 mg IM

      3. Continue diphenhydramine 50 mg orally every 4 hr for 2 da

   B. Anaphylaxis/immediate allergic reaction

      1. Assess ABCs; provide basic life support as indicated

      2. Administer epinephrine 0.3 mg (0.3 mL of 1:1000 solution) subcutaneously or intramuscularly; may repeat this in 3–5 min if needed

      3. Administer 100% oxygen; intubate if necessary

      4. Consider diphenhydramine 25–50 mg IV or IM and hydrocortisone 100 mg IV or IM to help prevent a recurrence of symptoms

      5. In case of cardiac arrest, define specific rhythm and treat using appropriate ACLS protocol

      6. Transport patient to appropriate acute care facility

IV. Prevention

   A. Obtain medical history and family history of allergy

   B. Consider skin testing before using suspicious drugs

NARCOTIC OVERDOSE

  I. Etiology. Level of a narcotic resulting in an absolute or relative blood level producing adverse clinical reactions. Dosage varies depending on many factors, including body weight, age, sex, route of administration. The main effect is based on direct depressant effect of narcotics on the medullary respiratory center.

II. Physical findings
   A. Oversedation or unconsciousness
   B. Bradypnea
   C. Decreased tidal volume
   D. Hypercarbia
   E. Hypoxia
   F. Hypotension
   G. Respiratory arrest
   H. Cardiac arrest

III. Management
   A. Position patient in supine position
   B. Assess ABCs; administer assisted ventilation, controlled ventilation, or CPR as indicated
   C. Maintain patent airway, intubate if needed
   D. Administer supplemental oxygen
   E. Administer naloxone (Narcan) 0.2–0.4 mg IV; if IV route not possible, IM is acceptable although slower
   F. If naloxone is given IV, consider an additional slower acting 0.4 mg IM dose to prevent renarcotization, especially with longer acting narcotics like morphine
   G. Monitor vital signs and observe for renarcotization

IV. Prevention
   A. Obtain past history of adverse reaction drug intolerance or addiction
   B. Titrate narcotics slowly
   C. Carefully monitor respiratory parameters when using narcotics

ACUTE ADRENAL INSUFFICIENCY

I. Etiology. Originally associated with primary adrenal disease (Addison's disease) with depressed serum level of adrenocortical steroids. Uncommon now other than as a secondary problem related to suppression of adrenal gland by exogenous steroid administration. Stressful situations may increase the relative need and cause an acute insufficiency syndrome. Stress may be physiological or psychological. Magnitude of stress is important.

II. Physical findings
   A. Progressive confusion
   B. Fatigue
   C. Muscle weakness
   D. Nausea and vomiting
   E. Extracellular fluid depletion
   F. Hyperkalemia
   G. Syncope
   H. Hypotension and tachycardia
   I. Coma and death

III. Management
   A. Assess ABCs and administer basic life support as needed

B. Position patient in supine position
C. Administer supplemental oxygen
D. Begin an IV infusion of D_5W and replace extracellular volume aggressively
E. Administer hydrocortisone (Solu-Cortef) 100 mg IV (or IM if IV route not possible)
F. Administer additional steroids as needed
G. Examine electrolytes and correct appropriately
H. Administer a vasopressor as needed (e.g., dopamine 1–4 µg/kg/min)

IV. Prevention
A. Careful medical history essential, especially looking for exogenous steroid use.
B. If a patient has been on 20 mg of cortisone (or its equivalent) for a continuous period of 2 wk or greater within the last 2 yr, a supplemental dose of steroid should be administered. Hydrocortisone 100 mg IV or IM may be given preoperative, intraoperatively and postoperatively. Patients having general anesthesia are primarily candidates for this regimen. A patient currently on oral therapy may take an additional oral dose the night before and the day of surgery. Most office procedures in oral and maxillofacial surgery fall in this latter category.
C. Appropriate sedation and pain control methods should be used to decrease stress.

CEREBROVASCULAR ACCIDENT (CVA)

I. Etiology. A neurologic disease state caused by infarction and necrosis of brain tissue. Causes included thrombosis, embolism, vascular spasm, or vascular insufficiency, atherosclerosis, or intracranial hemorrhage. Transient ischemic attacks (TIAs) are short episodes of CVA symptoms without necrosis of brain tissue.

II. Physical findings. Usually related to the specific area of the brain involved. Can have gradual or acute onset. Findings include:
A. Headache
B. Nausea and vomiting
C. Dizziness
D. Sweating
E. Chills
F. Focal neurologic signs like hemiparesis or paralysis, difficulty with speech, incontinence, and facial weakness
G. Hypertension
H. Loss of consciousness

III. Management. Treatment is symptomatic
A. Assess ABCs and implement basic life support if warranted
B. Position patient supine
C. Administer supplemental oxygen if unconsciousness or respiratory distress if present
D. Guard against high oxygen concentration, which may cause cerebral vasoconstriction

E. If symptoms persist, transfer patient to an acute care facility

IV. Prevention

    A. Obtain history of any previous cerebral ischemia

    B. Avoid central nervous system depressants, which may cause hypoxia in high-risk patients

    C. Avoid hypotension or hypertension

    D. Use pain control and sedation techniques appropriate to diminish stress of procedure

Index